The Professional Nurse

Issues and Actions

Ann Boyle Grant, RN, PhD
Dean of Instruction, Health, Science and Nursing
Cuesta College
San Luis Obispo, California

Faculty Member
Statewide Nursing Program
California State University, Dominguez Hills

Springhouse Corporation
Springhouse, Pennsylvania

STAFF

EXECUTIVE DIRECTOR, EDITORIAL

Stanley Loeb

SENIOR PUBLISHER, TRADE AND TEXTBOOKS

Minnie B. Rose, RN, BSN, MEd

ART DIRECTOR

John Hubbard

CLINICAL CONSULTANT

Cindy Tryniszewski, RN, MSN

EDITORS

David Moreau, Kathy Goldberg, Rick Stull

COPY EDITORS

Diane M. Armento, Barbara Hodgson, Pamela Wingrod

DESIGNERS

Stephanie Peters (associate art director), Mary Stangl, Lesley Weissman-Cook

COVER ILLUSTRATION

Cindy Marczuk

MANUFACTURING

Deborah Meiris (director), Anna Brindisi, Kate Davis, T.A. Landis

EDITORIAL ASSISTANTS

Caroline Lemoine, Louise Quinn, Betsy K. Snyder

Library of Congress Cataloging-in-Publication Data

Grant, Ann Boyle.
The professional nurse: issues and actions / Ann Boyle Grant
  p. cm.
Includes bibliographical references and index.
I. Title [DNLM: 1. Nursing. 2. Nursing Care. 3. Nursing Process. WY 100 G761p 1994]
RT82.G73 1994
610.73'069--dc20
DNLM/DLC   93-26276
0-87434-504-9   CIP

CONTENTS

Acknowledgment iv

Foreword v

Preface viii

1. Communication and Interpersonal Relations 1

2. A Conceptual Base for Nursing Practice 42

3. How Organizations Are Structured 74

4. Health Care Delivery 114

5. Cultural Implications for Nursing Practice 148

6. Legal Implications for Nursing Practice 187

7. Ethical Implications for Nursing Practice 225

8. The Nurse as Teacher 260

9. The Nature of Leadership 290

10. Decision Making in Nursing 322

11. The Nurse as Change Agent 348

12. Using Power 382

13. Using Research Findings 411

14. Nursing as a Developing Profession 443

Index 466

ACKNOWLEDGMENT

To Don: for his patience, his humor, his encouragement, and his love

FOREWORD

Transitions can be exhilarating and enhancing. At the same time, they can be rife with anxiety and sometimes downright scary. Thousands of nurses today willingly place themselves in transition as they enter the profession or reenter the educational setting to further their professional goals. Such programs include that offered by the Statewide Nursing Program of California State University, Dominguez Hills, which currently has 3,200 RNs studying for their BSN degree, many while working full-time. This popular program has been operating for 10 years, graduating about 150 students per year, proving that successful transitions are possible.

The Professional Nurse: Issues and Actions contains the content identified as necessary for socialization into professional nursing. It also contains the most recent concepts identified as essential to understanding the world of health care and of professional nursing. Dr. Grant has organized the content logically and in palatable increments to appeal to the adult learner. Objectives are clearly stated to guide self-paced learning. An application exercise and review questions at the end of each chapter allow the reader to check for content mastery.

In the 1970s, much discussion centered around identifying a common core of nursing knowledge and skills required to deliver direct client care. This common core was perhaps more concentrated on the technical aspects of nursing practice. Today, we are seeking to understand the core knowledge for a vastly more complex and constantly changing health care arena. Our colleagues in Nursing Service Administration are demanding a more professionally informed practitioner. Nurses themselves realize the need for greater preparation to become and remain marketable practitioners in an increasingly competitive environment. Dr. Grant's readers will be well served by *The Professional Nurse: Issues and Actions*. It contains that core knowledge so necessary for professional practice in today's environment. I would recommend that it become a well-used part of the student's personal library.

Colleen Ehrenberg, RN, EdD
Associate Professor and Curricula Coordinator
Statewide Nursing Program
California State University
Dominquez Hills

Dr. Ann Grant's professional pathway exemplifies the new-era nurse. Prepared by a combination of traditional and innovative educational modes and with years of experience preparing nurses through "non-traditional" means, Dr. Grant shares her knowledge of nursing's essential conceptual ground.

Nurses continue to achieve baccalaureate preparation by various routes. Such educational flexibility is important, especially in a society as varied as ours will be in the next decade. Providing a basis and opportunities for professional advancement at all nursing levels guarantees not only individual access but also a cadre of well-prepared nurses ready to serve society.

Our educational system is challenged to produce graduates with the skills needed to succeed in today's and tomorrow's world. Like other demanding professions, health care requires well-prepared practitioners with an understanding of both quality and economy. This book offers the practical and conceptual knowledge to equip students and practitioners with an integrated approach for successfully meeting the needs of today's fast-paced and complex health care environments.

This text is especially useful for those students making the transition from registered to baccalaureate nurse. However, any nurse exploring the socialization process as well as the expectations and responsibilities of professional practice will find it an invaluable and enlightening source.

The first chapter, for example, concentrates on the importance of inculcating caring values: personal responsibility, the valuing of all individuals, and professional self-care. These concepts are critical core ingredients of any personal, professional, and departmental philosophy. The book goes on to cover other far-reaching topics, such as ethics, teaching, culture, change, power, and research, in a manner succinct yet sufficient to offer even the busy nurse executive guidance through the complicated and sometimes turbulent transformations in current health care.

Thought-provoking objectives focus the reading of each chapter so that salient themes are not missed. The author also includes review questions to spark the reader's curiosity and interest, both of which can be easily satisfied through the recommended readings listed at the end of each chapter in an extensive, current bibliography. Application exercises are also included to provide immediate use of the theoretical knowledge covered in the chapter.

Learning from an expert's experiences is always a pleasure. Equally satisfying is seeing such a combination of solid theory, an array of practical nursing understanding, and opportunities for immediate application. This book makes great sense and is right on target for our times.

Malcolm R. MacDonald, RN, EdD
Vice President, Patient Care Services
Grey Bruce Regional Health Centre
Owen Sound, Ontario, Canada

PREFACE

Health care is experiencing its most dramatic changes since the 1930s. Hospitals and other health care agencies are evolving in new and unforeseen ways: technology continues to outstrip society's ability to decide when and how it should be used; new social legislation is altering the way in which health care is achieved and who receives such care.

To respond to these significant developments, nursing must also change. Drawing upon its roots, its extraordinary capacity for adaptation and persistence, and its guiding principle of advocacy for those needing care, nursing must develop new models, new ways of relating to employers, clients, and colleagues, and an awareness of the change process and the opportunities it affords.

This book presents a foundation for professional nursing that looks to the next century. It begins with the most fundamental nursing skills, communication and interpersonal relations, exploring the ways in which nurses, clients, employers, and colleagues can more effectively communicate and work together in the highly competitive and stressful climate of the future. The book concludes by asking the prospective nurse to approach the future with a changed paradigm, or vision, of how nursing and health care should be accomplished.

The intervening 12 chapters discuss nursing theory, organizational structure, and the health care delivery system. They also cover current cultural, legal, and ethical implications for nursing; the nurse's role as teacher, leader, decision-maker, and change agent; and finally, the uses of power and research as two important ways for adapting to and promoting constructive change.

The book can be used by students in a four-year institution or a diploma or associate-degree institution as well as by registered nurses beginning their baccalaureate studies in a second-step or completion program. All nurses need to know the principles, theories, and applications of nursing if the profession is to grow and prosper.

Each chapter begins with a series of learning objectives to guide reading. Interspersed throughout each chapter are sidebars that direct the reader to important topic-related concepts. Each chapter also includes an application exercise by which the reader makes practical use of the information learned. This exercise is followed by review questions that cover important concepts and by a list of references and readings recommended for further study. To enable readers to become more familiar with different cultural groups, an additional reference list of important works by ethnic writers is included at the end of Chapter 5, "Cultural Implications for Nursing Practice."

True learning occurs only when knowledge is made personally relevant. Toward this end, the application exercises enable the reader to apply the concepts covered in the chapter. In Chapter 5, "Cultural Implications for Nursing Practice," for example, students perform a beginning cultural assessment in cooperation with a client who self-defines his cultural group. Together, the student and client examine the client's definitions of health and illness and identify how cultural elements influence these definitions. The application exercise for Chapter 13, "Using Research Findings," has readers examine published research from the standpoint of its application to their own practice. Some chapters provide alternate application exercises, so that complexity can be varied according to the desires of the student or instructor.

This book was undertaken with the hope that it would help to make the concepts essential to professional nursing practice available to all students. Presenting the underpinnings of nursing practice at all levels may make students' move from one educational level to another easier.

The author notes with special appreciation the work of the nursing directors, deans, and faculty who served on the Articulation Committee of the California Joint ADN/BSN

Deans and Directors Association. They prepared the way for the cooperation development by the nearly 100 baccalaureate and associate degree nursing schools of a coherent, compassionate, and highly professional career mobility model for the state's nursing students.

Ann Boyle Grant

COMMUNICATION AND INTERPERSONAL RELATIONS

OBJECTIVES

After studying this chapter, the reader should be able to:

1. Define communication, including verbal and nonverbal components.

2. Analyze a specific communication, using the sender-receiver model, Maslow's hierarchy of needs model, or the transactional analysis model.

3. Describe the components of nonverbal communication.

4. Explain the importance of simplicity, clarity, timing, relevance, adaptation, and credibility in enhancing communication.

5. Identify specific techniques to help clients communicate their conditions and problems.

6. List barriers that inhibit clients from disclosing information about themselves.

7. Describe written communication trends in health care settings.

8. Describe the therapeutic relationship and the importance of communication to this relationship.

9. Analyze a situation involving confrontation, and plan a communication to address the problem assertively.

INTRODUCTION

Communication and relating to other people are closely linked behaviors. Effective communication enhances interpersonal relations; conversely, good interpersonal relations promote effective communication. By the same token, poor communication can impair a relationship between two people, and a difficult relationship may make communication nearly impossible.

In a professional setting, poor communication can be particularly harmful. Consider, for instance, a nurse who has a strained relationship with a particular physician. Disliking the physician, the nurse does not communicate changes in client status to the physician in a timely, effective manner. This problem damages the relationship further, ultimately endangering client care.

This chapter begins by examining several models of communication. After discussing various types and aspects of verbal and nonverbal communication, it explores nonverbal communication, including such aspects as kinesics, proxemics, and touch. Next, it explains how to establish therapeutic relationships. The chapter concludes by describing how to cope with difficult communications, such as telephoning physicians, confronting, saying no, making requests, and stating opinions.

COMMUNICATION DEFINED

Communication is the verbal or nonverbal transmission of information—the process by which people exchange information. It may involve behaviors, symbols, or signs held in common by the communicating parties. Communication can range from a simple declaration (such as a client telling the nurse, "I need a drink of water") to a complex, multistage communication regarding the budget for an intensive care unit. In the latter case, communication may involve such electronic media as facsimile machines and interactive video in addition to traditional verbal and nonverbal communication methods.

Verbal communication can be spoken (oral) or written. Examples of verbal communication include care plans, nurses' notes, and written policies and procedures. *Nonverbal communication* includes physical, spatial, and other unspoken but expressive behaviors that communicate meaning and feeling. For example, to communicate the message "No, you may not enter" nonverbally, a person may hold up one hand in the universal "no" gesture, block the entrance, or make a facial expression conveying the negative.

MODELS OF COMMUNICATION

Communication can be described in various ways to help evaluate its effectiveness and identify communication problems. Three of the most useful models with which to examine communication are the sender-receiver model, the human needs model, and the transactional analysis model.

SENDER-RECEIVER MODEL

In 1949, Shannon and Weaver described communication based on messages, or signals, passing between the sender and the receiver. Based on the same concepts, Gerrard, Boniface, and Love (1980) described a similar five-step sequence of exchanges making up a single communication.

The initial step, *message formation*, occurs when the message develops in the mind of the sender. The second step, *message encoding*, takes place when the sender decides how to communicate the message using verbal and nonverbal elements. The third step, *message transmission*, occurs when the spoken, written, or nonverbal communication is expressed. In the fourth step, *message reception*, the receiver hears the spoken element, sees the nonverbal element, or reads the written element. In the final step, *message decoding*, the receiver interprets the message that was sent. To be effective, the message formed must be identical to the message that is sent and subsequently received.

Problems can occur at any step in this process. Miscommunication (sometimes called communication error) can occur if elements included during message encoding are misinterpreted later. For example, suppose a nurse wants to find out if a male postoperative client is comfortable, and asks, "You're comfortable, right?" Because the question is phrased in a way that suggests the nurse expects the client to be comfortable, the client may decode the message to mean that he should not be uncomfortable. Therefore, the client may not acknowledge discomfort.

The client would have been less likely to misinterpret the inquiry if the nurse had worded it more objectively, such as by asking, "Are you comfortable?" This question does not suggest that the client is expected to be comfortable.

Similarly, miscommunication may occur if nonverbal elements seem at odds—are not *congruent*—with verbal elements. In the above example, if the nurse appears rushed and harried when asking the client if he is comfortable, the client might assume the nurse has no time for his problems. Thus, he will be less likely to communicate his degree of comfort or discomfort.

A *congruent* message is one in which verbal and nonverbal elements communicate the same message. An *incongruent* message occurs when one element conveys an impression or feeling contrary to the other. Incongruence is a major cause of miscommunication.

HIERARCHY OF NEEDS MODEL

A second communication model is based on the hierarchy of needs described by Abraham Maslow (1954). Maslow described human needs as pyramidal (see *Maslow's hierarchy of needs*). The most *basic needs*—those relating to such physiologic requirements as eating, sleeping, and breathing— are at the bottom of the pyramid. Just above basic needs, at the second level, are *safety needs,* which include the need to be safe from fear of physical harm. Next, above safety needs, are *belonging needs,* including the need for love and association. At the fourth level of the pyramid are *esteem needs,* such as the need for achievement and independence. At the final level (top) of the pyramid are *self-actualization needs,* or the

Maslow's Hierarchy of Needs

This diagram shows the various levels of needs according to Abraham Maslow's hierarchy of needs model. Basic physiologic needs (food, water, sleep, and freedom from pain) are at the bottom of the pyramid. Above basic needs are safety needs (involving the need to be free of fear or harm). Belonging needs (the needs for affiliation and love) are at the next highest level at the hierarchy. Esteem needs (the needs to achieve independence and respect) are at the second highest level. At the top of the pyramid are self-actualization needs—the needs to achieve personal potential and accomplishment. According to Maslow, needs at the bottom of the hierarchy must be met before those at higher levels can be addressed.

The nurse can use Maslow's hierarchy as a guideline for tailoring communication to a client's level of need. For instance, basic needs, such as pain relief, must be met before a client can understand a communication that addresses higher-level needs, such as discharge teaching.

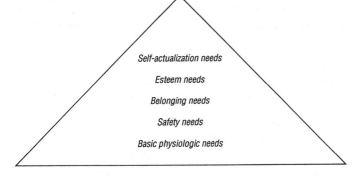

needs to achieve a sense of personal fulfillment and accomplishment. According to Maslow, needs at lower levels of the pyramid must be fulfilled before those at higher levels can be addressed.

When used to analyze communications, Maslow's hierarchy of needs helps us understand and interpret the needs or frame of reference of parties involved in a communication or interaction. Suppose, for example, that a female client is scheduled for surgery in 3 hours. She may be functioning at the level of safety needs, focusing on the amount of postoperative pain she expects to experience or the extent of surgery that will be performed. Therefore, the nurse should not expect her to focus on a communication that addresses independence needs, such as how to care for her dressings after discharge, because independence is a fourth-level need. To address the client's second-level needs, the nurse might provide appropriate preoperative teaching that will help alleviate the client's anxiety. The appropriate time to address independence needs is after the client's basic and safety needs have been met.

Maslow's hierarchy of needs can be used to tailor a particular communication—for example, one between a nurse and a client. First, the nurse identifies the level of need from which the client might be expected to operate. To do this, the nurse must determine which needs are most important by asking the client, "What concerns you most right now?"

Then the nurse identifies the level of need that was addressed in the unsuccessful communication. For instance, client teaching commonly focuses on independence and achievement, a fourth-level need. Yet a client at a more basic need level (such as the need to breathe without exhaustion or finish a meal unaided) may not value or even understand a communication that addresses a higher-level need.

Finally, the nurse matches communication with the client's need level. This may mean deferring a communication regarding independence skills until the client's basic, safety, or belonging needs have been met.

By recognizing the level of need at which a client is operating, health care professionals can develop more appropriate messages when caring for clients and can time messages to coincide with periods of greatest client receptivity.

TRANSACTIONAL ANALYSIS MODEL

A third communication model is based on transactional analysis theory, developed by Eric Berne in 1964. Berne proposed that personality is composed of three elements, or *ego states,* that are consistent patterns of feeling, thinking, and behaving.

PARENT EGO STATE

The first ego state, the *parent ego state,* includes thoughts, feelings, and emotions communicated during childhood by parents, teachers, and other authority figures. It includes both censoring and nurturing elements; Berne described these two elements as substates, which he called the *nurturing parent ego state* and the *critical parent ego state.* A person functioning in the critical parent ego state may voice expressions reminiscent of the censorious statements made by authority figures during childhood. Examples include "You never do anything right" and "Haven't you learned anything?" Uttered uncritically, they reflect childhood experiences. Typically, people make such statements without examining whether they are appropriate to the present situation, and they may be surprised to hear themselves say these things. ("Now, why did I say that? I always said I'd never say that to my kids.")

The nurturing parent ego state intercedes, comforts, rescues, and protects. At first glance, this state might seem appropriate for a nurse or other caregiver. However, like the critical parent ego state, it is unthinking and reflects childhood experiences. A person in a nurturing parent ego state may make such statements as "Don't worry, everything will be all right" or "I'll take care of you."

ADULT EGO STATE

A person in the *adult ego state* responds in a rational and considered way. The adult ego state is objective and emotionless, engaging in problem solving and decision making on a factual basis. Frequently, it is compared to the processes carried out by a computer. When confronted with a communication reflecting a critical parent ego state, someone in the adult ego state might ask, "What exactly did you find wrong with my performance?"

For example, suppose nurse Claire Morris has conflicting demands on her time. In the adult ego state, she objectively and unemotionally requests help: "I've been asked to admit a new client from the emergency room, and I also need to change Mr. Jenkins's dressing before he's discharged in a half hour. I see that you did his dressing change yesterday. If I help you ambulate Mrs. Entridge at 11 o'clock, will you return the favor by doing Mr. Jenkins's dressing change now while I admit the new client?" By communicating in this way, Claire is likely to get a positive response.

In contrast, if Claire had been communicating from the critical parent role, she might have said something like, "They shouldn't assign new admissions to us before they check to see how we're doing with the clients we've already got! I think you should take this new client."

CHILD EGO STATE

The *child ego state*—the third ego state Berne described—has several substates. The *natural child ego state* reflects unmodified feelings and expressions. Communications arising from this substate are spontaneous and unreserved ("Gee, that's a cute car the new pharmacist has!"). An example of someone in this state is the new father who dances around the delivery room with his arms in the air, shouting, "We did it! Hooray, we did it!"

Communications from the natural child state typically are exuberant and may be hard for nurses to contain. A communication that redirects the person's activity rather than censures the expression may be most effective; an appeal to the adult ego state often suffices. In the above example, the nurse might say to the new father, "Congratulations! Would you like to use this washcloth to wipe your wife's forehead?"

The *adapted child ego substate*, in contrast, reflects change resulting from experience with parents and the environment. One part of the adapted child wants to please and thus exhibits "good" behavior designed to win approval. A second part of the adapted child state is the *rebellious child ego state*, which exhibits feelings and behaviors typical of those of a rebellious, resistive child.

Many clients are dependent when admitted to health care facilities; thus, they commonly exhibit behaviors that characterize child ego states. The "good" client, like the adapted child, attempts to win the nurse's concern and caring by acquiescing to schedules and requirements, always trying to please. The "difficult" client, like a rebellious or spoiled child, is emotional, demanding, and hard to deal with. (In contrast, a client functioning in an adult ego state would work with health care personnel in developing schedules and making plans for care.) Both the "good" and "bad" clients reflect the adapted child ego state.

Miscommunication may occur when persons communicate from different ego states. However, the following example shows how one party in the communication may adjust the response to meet the communication level of the other. (This example also shows the abrupt change in communication style that such an adjustment may cause.)

Nurse Barbara Sulzberger, concerned about a change in her client's condition, calls Dr. Breyer, the attending physician, at 2:00 A.M.

> *Barbara:* "Dr. Breyer, I'm calling to report a change in Mrs. Medford's status. Her temperature is still going up despite the antipyretics you prescribed, and she's getting quite agitated." (This communication reflects the adult ego state.)
>
> *Dr. Breyer:* "I don't know why you had to wait until 2:00 A.M. to call me about this. You nurses never seem to know how to do timely assessments." (This communication reflects the critical parent ego state.)
>
> *Barbara:* "Doctor, I realize it's unpleasant to be awakened in the middle of the night, but Mrs. Medford's condition was stable until an hour ago. With this rapid rise in her temperature, I knew you'd want to be informed." (This communication reflects an adult ego state.)
>
> *Dr. Breyer:* "Yes. Thank you, Ms. Sulzberger. I'm awake now and will be in to see Mrs. Medford shortly." (In response to the nurse's adult ego state, the physician shifts abruptly from a critical parent ego state to an adult ego state.)

By recognizing that the physician was responding from a parent ego state—and by *not* responding in kind—the nurse elicited a rational, considered response from the physician's adult ego state. Had she responded from an adapted child ego state ("I'm so sorry, Doctor, I shouldn't have bothered you") or a rebellious child ego state ("What do you expect me to do, let the client suffer so you can get your sleep?"), the physician's response might have been inappropriate.

VERBAL COMMUNICATION

Verbal communication can be spoken or written. In both cases, certain qualities may enhance communication and others may inhibit it.

QUALITIES THAT ENHANCE COMMUNICATION

- *Simplicity*
- *Clarity*
- *Timing*
- *Relevance*
- *Adaptation to circumstance*
- *Credibility*

QUALITIES THAT ENHANCE COMMUNICATION

The chance for successful communication is enhanced by simplicity, clarity, appropriate timing, relevance, adaptation to circumstance, and credibility (Kozier, Erb, and Olivieri, 1991).

SIMPLICITY

Communication should be direct, jargon-free, and understandable. The health care setting poses a challenge in this area. For example, suppose a client is admitted to the hospital for surgery, and the nurse says, "Mr. Rivers, I understand you're here for a TURP; I need to get a UA and then I'll get you ready for the OR."

Unless Mr. Rivers has a medical background, he has little chance of understanding this jargon-filled message. The communication would have been much more effective if the nurse had said, "Mr. Rivers, I understand you're here for surgery on your prostate gland." The nurse then might say, "To get you ready for surgery, we need to take a sample of your urine." After making sure he understood the process of obtaining the sample, the nurse might add, "I'll be back to help you with your urine sample and answer any questions you might have, then help get you ready for your operation."

By indicating that the nurse expects the client to have questions, she makes it easier for him to ask such questions.

Even the jargon-free message presented in the last paragraph might be ineffective, however, if Mr. Rivers does not understand the terms *prostate gland* or *urine sample*. In this case, the nurse must use more basic terms. By avoiding jargon and speaking simply, the nurse can help ensure that the client understands the communication.

CLARITY

Ambiguity, obscurity, and indirectness compromise clarity. Effective communication requires a clear, unambiguous, direct approach.

In an ambiguous communication, the intended meaning is obscured by the possibility of multiple interpretations. Ambiguity can result from poor word choice or lack of congruence between verbal and nonverbal elements of communication. For example, in a change-of-shift report, a nurse might state that a client "had a quiet night." This communication is ambiguous. To one listener, it might mean that the client was comfortable and slept well; to another, it might mean merely that the client did not express discomfort or sleeplessness.

Indirectness also reduces clarity. During a difficult communication, a person may take an indirect approach out of discomfort with the information that needs to be conveyed, believing such approach will make the information more acceptable to the listener. However, indirectness usually just increases the apprehensiveness of the other party, who senses that something is wrong but cannot figure out exactly what it is.

For example, suppose Karen Jantzen, a nurse supervisor, wants to talk to John Briggs, a staff nurse, about his incorrect pediatric assessments. Taking an indirect approach, she might ask, "John, have you had much experience with pediatric clients? Do you have any children yourself?" Believing that this is a casual conversation, John replies, "No, I'm not ready to tie myself down. I like kids, but most of the time, they're a mystery to me." Karen might respond, "I'd like to talk to you about this sometime. I think I may be able to help you with a problem."

Instead of clarifying the problem, Karen's communication makes John wonder exactly what the problem is and why Karen is concerned about his personal interest in children. He may have the impression that Karen believes that high-quality care for pediatric clients can be provided only by nurses who are parents. Karen's message can only serve to confuse John and cause problems when she ultimately broaches the topic of John's incorrect pediatric assessments.

If Karen instead uses a direct approach, she can avoid this problem. Choosing an appropriate time and setting, she might say: "John, your assessments of pediatric clients are not as thorough as those of your adult clients. What experience have you had with pediatric clients? Would you be interested in spending some time next week working with Sharon Pettit in the pediatric unit and observing her do some assessments?"

Intelligibility also is crucial to the clarity of a communication. Speech must be slow and loud enough to be understood. Written text must be legible.

TIMING AND RELEVANCE

Clients may be more receptive to a particular communication at a certain time, based on their needs. For instance, before impending surgery, a preoperative client may not be receptive to teaching about dressing changes after discharge. A wise nurse would delay such teaching until after surgery, then make it timely and relevant by showing its immediate importance, usefulness, and relevance. For instance, the nurse could teach the client how to reduce postoperative discomfort by splinting with a pillow and how to perform self-care immediately after surgery by turning, coughing, and deep breathing.

To do this, the nurse must assess timing and client receptivity to communication, then delay the communication if timing or receptivity seem poor. In some cases, the nurse may be able to alter the situation to increase client receptivity—for instance, by showing the client that the communication is relevant.

ADAPTATION TO CIRCUMSTANCE

To be effective, communication must be adapted to the situation at hand. An obvious example involves the hearing-impaired client; if speech is not an effective way to communicate with this client, the nurse should attempt written communication. Another example is the client who speaks only a foreign language that the nurse does not know; in this case, the nurse must find an interpreter. With a client who is fearful, the nurse should communicate slowly and succinctly, combining an authoritative manner with sensitivity.

CREDIBILITY

Both the communicator and the information being communicated must be perceived as believable. The credibility of the communicator sometimes is overlooked by researchers who focus mainly on the message rather than on the person who is doing the communicating.

Clients consider many factors when judging health care providers, including how professional they look and seem, knowledgeable information sharing, and apparent competence. Suppose, for example, staff nurse Myra Crane is teaching Julia Muller, a diabetic client, how to prepare an insulin injection. During the teaching session, Myra must interrupt the session to obtain a missing supply, then appears clumsy when handling the equipment. This causes Ms. Muller to question Myra's credibility and professional competence and consequently to resist the teaching, sensing that Myra does not fully understand the information she is communicating.

AVOIDING MISCOMMUNICATION

Grensing (1990) summarized ways to avoid miscommunication when dealing with clients. She identified the main obstacles to effective communication as lack of congruence between verbal and nonverbal elements, inadequate time to make the communication clear, neglect of important elements in the communication, and the effect of personality on communication. Grensing proposed a three-stage approach to communicating thoroughly and accurately:

Verify. Make sure that the received message has been interpreted accurately by asking the client to repeat the message.

Clarify. Ask questions, and encourage the client to ask questions.

Follow up. Determine what should happen next and what expectations resulted from the communication.

Grensing's model focuses on the nurse as a receiver of communication. However, it can also apply when the nurse is the sender. In this case, in the second step (clarify), the nurse should ask questions to confirm that the client understood the nurse's message correctly.

VERBAL HELPING TECHNIQUES

Certain techniques can encourage clients to engage in conversation by promoting self-disclosure and allowing them to express themselves freely. Each technique guides and encourages the client to provide information while promoting the client's confidence in the communication process. The techniques include:

- recognizing—formally acknowledging a person, typically by name
- observing—describing what one sees or perceives
- using a general lead—providing an opening that lets the other person enter the conversation from a comfortable starting point
- using a broad opening—providing an opening with minimal suggestion of where to begin
- restating—repeating what the other party has communicated to encourage the person to elaborate or proceed
- focusing—concentrating on a specific point, narrowing the scope of inquiry
- exploring—enlarging a discussion around a particular point

- validating—affirming that the receiver has interpreted the other person's message accurately
- refocusing—returning to a main point when the conversation has strayed
- clarifying—correcting perceptions by expanding, refining, or revising
- reflecting—mirroring the words and feelings of the other party
- summarizing—reviewing a communication, impression, or observation.

The following example shows how a nurse might use these verbal techniques when communicating with a client to determine the cause of a problem.

> Mrs. Ellison arrives at the emergency department accompanied by her family. The nurse who escorts her into the examination room finds her noncommunicative and unwilling to respond to questions about why she is here. Mrs. Ellison sits with hands clasped in front of her, with her head lowered. A frequent visitor to the hospital, she is being treated for an anxiety disorder.
>
> *Nurse:* "Good morning, Mrs. Ellison." (*Recognizing*)
>
> "You seem very sad." (*Observing*)
>
> "Can you describe what the problem is?" (*Using a general lead*)
>
> "Please begin with what happened this morning." (*Using a broad opening*)
>
> "You say you're feeling anxious and afraid." (*Restating*)
>
> "Try to describe what is making you feel afraid." (*Focusing*)
>
> "Can you tell me more about feeling anxious? Is this something that happens to you a lot?" (*Exploring*)
>
> "I think I understand what you're saying: You woke up feeling that something bad had happened, and this made you anxious. Is that right?" (*Validating*)
>
> "Can we talk some more about the kinds of things that make you anxious? You say that staying alone by yourself makes you feel that something bad might happen?" (*Refocusing*)
>
> "You say you weren't angry when you learned your family would be away for the weekend and that Mrs. Jones, the nursing attendant, would be staying with you for 2 days. But you say that this made you afraid. Is that right?" (*Clarifying and reflecting*)

"If I understand you correctly, you began to feel anxious when your family made plans to be away for the weekend and you learned that Mrs. Jones would be staying with you. You didn't want your family to feel badly about going, so you didn't say anything to them. Then this morning, you woke up feeling that something bad was going to happen. Your family brought you here because they didn't know what was wrong, and you couldn't tell them. Is that correct?" (*Summarizing*)

FACTORS THAT HINDER COMMUNICATION

Just as some qualities promote and enhance communication, others hinder it. Hindering factors typically distract the person who is communicating, interject unhelpful advice, or negate the other party or the importance of the communication.

Specific behaviors that hinder communication include offering inappropriate reassurance, rejecting, agreeing, probing, responding defensively, offering inappropriate advice, stereotyping, using cliches, belittling, and showing egocentrism. These behaviors are most harmful when they cut off communication prematurely or remove the other party's decision-making power.

Offering inappropriate reassurance. This occurs when a listener inhibits or discourages a person who is describing a problem or concern by suggesting that the problem or concern is not serious or does not exist. Typically, the listener is well-meaning ("Everything is going to be all right"). However, the inappropriate reassurance suggests that the other party has no real basis for concern or reason for action. In a health care setting, inappropriate reassurance commonly is offered because a caregiver feels uncomfortable with what the client is saying or feels helpless to solve the client's problem.

Instead of offering inappropriate reassurance, the listener should allow the person to complete the self-disclosure, then use other techniques, such as reflecting or clarifying, to help the person express feelings.

Rejecting. Although caregivers rarely reject a client's communication intentionally, they may do this for the same reasons that they sometimes offer inappropriate reassurance: discomfort with what the client is saying. For example, if a child says, "I hate her" when her mother is admitted while intoxicated, the nurse who says "You shouldn't feel that about your mother" negates the child's feelings. Transactional analysis might view a rejecting response as an unexamined response coming from the parent ego state. It suggests that what the person feels is wrong; it also inhibits the person from expressing feelings and interferes with progress toward dealing with such feelings.

Agreeing uncritically. This behavior cuts off discussion prematurely and focuses attention on the listener rather than on the person who is communicating. For example, a nurse who has just listened to a client say that she has run away from her husband might say, "You did the right thing. I'd have done exactly what you did." Another example would be a nurse who responds to a postmastectomy client who says she feels mutilated, "Everybody feels that way after breast surgery." In both examples, the nurse's response suggests that the client's concern or problem does not warrant examination or exploration. In fact, by exploring the concern or problem, the nurse might have helped the client find a more positive course of action or perception. At certain points in a therapeutic relationship, validating a client's perceptions and feelings can be helpful. Validating differs from offering uncritical agreement in intent and timing. Validating occurs after thorough examination of the problem has confirmed the person's worth; it acknowledges feelings and actions. Uncritical agreement, in contrast, occurs before the problem or concern has been explored; typically it occurs because the listener is uncomfortable with the communicated problem or concern.

Probing. This occurs when the listener seeks additional information that distracts from the communicator's main focus of concern. For instance, the listener may respond in a way that focuses on minutiae or conveys suspicion of what the person is communicating. Examples of probing include asking such questions as "Are you sure you didn't have more calories than you've recorded on your diet log?" and "When exactly did you begin to feel suicidal?"

Although the nurse should strive to obtain accurate and detailed information about a client's status and problems, focusing mainly on details rather than substance or questioning the client's veracity can inhibit communication.

Responding defensively. Defensive responses typically come from the child ego state described by transactional analysts. For instance, a client suggests that the caregivers seem insensitive; the nurse responds defensively, "If you don't like this hospital, you can go somewhere else" or "The nurses on this unit are among the most qualified I've ever known." These responses prevent examination of the client's communication and perceptions. Instead of responding defensively, the nurse should try to find out why the client feels that way—determining, for instance, which actions suggest a caring attitude to the client and how caregivers might alter the client's perceptions of the staff and environment.

Offering inappropriate advice. Offering advice before the other person's problems have been explored or options are considered inhibits communication and problem solving. Suppose a nurse learns during an admission interview that a client's husband has just lost $10,000 gambling. Examples of inappropriate responses by the nurse would include, "Tell him you'll leave him if he can't stop gambling" and "I wouldn't put up with him for one moment longer if I were you." These responses, like other forms of inappropriate advice, make no attempt to help the client solve the problem independently.

Stereotyping. Like offering inappropriate reassurance or uncritical agreement, stereotyping dismisses a client's feelings and perceptions. Suppose a postmastectomy client tells the nurse that her husband is having trouble coping with her surgery. The nurse replies, "All men are like that." Instead of promoting an exploration of the client's problem, this response implies that the situation cannot be changed and thus dismisses the client's feelings and perceptions.

Offering cliches. Although cliches usually are well-intended, they seem false, trite, and uncaring when offered in response to communication of feelings or concerns. Examples of cliches include "Where there's life, there's hope" and "Every cloud has a silver lining." Caregivers typically offer cliches when at a loss for what to say. However, in such situations, silence may be the best response.

Belittling. Typically arising from the unexamined parent ego state, belittling statements mimic those of a critical parent: "Think of people who have *real* problems" or "It doesn't help to cry about it." Belittling responses suggest that the communicator's feelings or actions are inappropriate and do not warrant examination or discussion.

Showing egocentrism. An egocentric response is one in which the listener changes the focus of the communication from the sender to the listener (self). Although self-disclosure and sharing by a caregiver can be useful when offered appropriately, it is egocentric when offered in a way that makes the other party feel "one-upped" or inhibits self-disclosure. For example, an anxious client wants to talk about her perceptions of surgery with a nurse. However, instead of encouraging the client to explore her feelings, the nurse says, "My surgery was much more extensive than yours" and proceeds to tell the client about her own experience, thus preventing the client from discussing her experience.

Clients commonly ask caregivers personal questions in an attempt to establish a relationship—and also to try to balance the disclosures that they typically are asked to make by caregivers. For instance, a client asks if the nurse is married or has children or how long the nurse has worked at the hospital. However, if the focus of the conversation shifts from the client's condition to that of the nurse, egocentrism has displaced the client as the appropriate center of discussion.

WRITTEN COMMUNICATION

Much verbal communication occurs through written means; frequently, it is the main source of communication among caregivers and forms the legal documentation of client care. Nonetheless, written communication has been examined less thoroughly than spoken, or oral, communication. As technology brings dramatic changes to written communication, nurses must make sure they know how to avoid pitfalls.

Examples of written communication in health care settings include entries in clients' charts, such as physicians' orders and progress notes; nurses' notes; medication, laboratory, and other service records; formal descriptions of policies and procedures; job descriptions; and informal communications (such as communication logs and suggestion notebooks).

The same considerations described for oral communication apply to written communication, and the factors that enhance or inhibit oral communication can enhance or inhibit written communication as well. Just as speech must be understandable to the listener, written communication must be legible to the reader to be effective. Like oral communication, written communication must be timely, clear, and credible.

Most health care facilities have specific policies and guidelines regarding written communication. The nurse must learn how to record entries in official documents and follow the required forms. Guidelines regarding use of abbreviations, for example, may vary among health care facilities, and misinterpretation may occur if the established policy is not followed. For example, in some facilities, the abbreviation *w.c.* means *without complaints*; in others, it means *wheel chair*. To someone from Britain, *w.c.* may mean *water closet*, a term for bathroom or toilet.

Written communication is evolving rapidly; many health care facilities now use computerized charting. Although the use of computers simplifies such matters as format, it also requires nurses to become familiar and comfortable with the technology so that they can use it appropriately and skillfully.

Citing changes in the expectations of the Joint Commission on Accreditation of Healthcare Organizations (JCAHO), Iyer (1991) predicts that nurses will spend less time preparing individually written care plans. She also predicts increased use of standardized care plans addressing common illnesses and injuries and foresees wider use of critical path plans to expedite treatment and discharge. Critical path plans aid in outlining the expected course of client treatment, indicating which elements must be accomplished during a specific timeline. Thus, these plans promote early identification of problem areas and use of appropriate measures to address them. For example, a critical path plan for a postoperative cholecystectomy client might specify that the client should be able to get out of bed and into a chair 1 day postoperatively and should be able to walk down the hall 2 days postoperatively. (For more information on critical path methodologies, see Chapter 10, Decision making in nursing.)

Iyer also predicts that nurses will work more efficiently, focusing on outcome and documentation of teaching, evaluation of client response to treatments, and preventive care. She foresees a decrease in duplicative charting and less use of "handmaiden" charting, such as documentation of physician visits. She predicts that nurses increasingly will use flow sheets to document diagnostic tests and visits by other health care professionals.

Nursing diagnoses are predicted to be used more widely, and there will be a continued shift from narrative and problem-oriented charting to focus charting and charting by exception. These last two methods streamline communication by using a shorthand method for documenting normal findings and focusing on significant findings or exceptions to established norms.

Finally, the use of facsimile (FAX) machines and computers also will increase. FAX machines can transmit written orders rapidly and accurately; thus, telephone relay of orders will become less common. Computers increasingly will be used at the client's bedside, standardizing data entry and making the information more legible and timely.

NONVERBAL COMMUNICATION

Nonverbal communication can reinforce, negate, or exist independently of verbal communication. Although it contributes significantly to communication, its value sometimes goes unrecognized.

Nonverbal communication includes all aspects of behavior "that contribute to the meaning of messages, including such things as body movement, gesture, proxemics, facial expression, eye contact, posture, and certain paralinguistic cues associated with vocal quality and intonation" (Mortensen, 1972).

Northouse and Northouse (1985) describe five components of nonverbal communication—kinesics, proxemics, paralinguistics, touch, and physical and environmental factors.

KINESICS

Kinesics is the study of body motions—such as gestures, posture, facial expressions, and eye movements—as part of communication. The nurse who raises her eyebrow when asked to accept an additional client assignment is using kinesics to communicate her feelings about the assignment. The client who looks at the floor when asked about his job status may be communicating discomfort with the question.

Body motions can be used to communicate in various ways. *Emblems* are motions with generally accepted meanings; for instance, nodding the head indicates "yes." *Illustrators* are motions that convey through gestures what is being expressed in words. For example, a physician describing the dilation of the cervix may use hand motions to illustrate' the concept. *Affect displays,* such as wringing the hands, are motions that suggest the nature of the emotion involved in the communication. *Regulators* are motions that punctuate the conversation; for example, rising to shake hands signals that a conversation is over. *Adaptors* are motions that are used to adapt to stress or discomfort associated with a communication; an example is drumming the fingers on a table (Ekman and Friesen, 1969).

The following example shows each of the kinesic elements described above:

> Nurse Winona Pullman is performing an admission assessment on Suzanne Clarke, a preoperative client. She begins the interview by sitting down and leaning forward (affect display: welcoming). Ms. Clarke shifts her weight from one foot to another (affect display: nervousness) and asks if she can have a glass of water. Nurse Pullman shakes her head (emblem: no) and explains that Ms. Clarke cannot have any water until after her surgery. Nurse Pullman then begins preoperative teaching. Stating that an I.V. line will be placed in Ms. Clarke's vein, she indicates its likely placement on her own forearm (illustrator). After completing the assessment and preoperative teaching, Nurse Pullman stands (regulator), signalling that the interview is nearing completion. Because she noted that Ms. Clarke tapped her foot (adaptor) and bit her lip (adaptor) during the interview, Nurse Pullman decides to return to her room shortly to see if Ms. Clarke has any more questions or concerns and to reinforce teaching.

FACIAL EXPRESSIONS

Facial expressions can confirm or negate the verbal element of a communication. If, for example, Nurse Pullman had smiled broadly at Ms. Clarke at the start of the admission interview, this would have reinforced her attempt to convey welcome. If she had frowned during the interview, Ms. Clarke might have felt that Nurse Pullman was reluctant to help her prepare for surgery. Using congruent verbal and nonverbal elements helps ensure accurate communication of the intended message.

Interpretation of facial expressions is influenced by culture. In one culture, a given expression may convey seriousness; in another culture, it may convey worry. An expression that conveys indifference in a culture where feelings are expressed openly may be perceived as calm and untroubled in a culture that frowns on open display of feelings. When in doubt about the meaning of a nonverbal element of communication, the receiver should validate the message by requesting verbal clarification.

GAZE

Gaze—a fixed, intent look—also can be used to communicate a particular meaning or emotion. In some cultures, a person may be uncomfortable meeting the gaze of an unfamiliar person or authority figure. In mainstream American culture, a person is expected to look another directly in the eye; failure to meet another's gaze may be interpreted as a sign of indirection, dishonesty, or withholding of information. However, in other cultures, gaze aversion is a sign of respect. Thus, misunderstanding may occur when people from cultures with opposing expectations about gaze communicate.

However, even Americans do not expect gaze to be continuous. For example, in most normal conversations, direct eye contact occurs only 50% to 60% of the time. The listener looks at the speaker 75% of the time; the speaker looks at the listener 40% of the time (Argyle and Ingham, 1972).

PROXEMICS

Proxemics is the study of the effects of spatial separation (distance) that people maintain when interacting and of their orientation toward each other. The distance between individuals in conversation is influenced by many factors, including culture, age, status, and comfort level. In mainstream American culture, distance typically depends on the type of conversation. According to Hall (1966), participants stand roughly $1\frac{1}{2}'$ apart during an intimate conversation, $1\frac{1}{2}'$ to $2\frac{1}{2}'$ during a personal conversation, 4' to 12' apart during a social conversation, and 12' to 25' apart during conversation at a large, public gathering. If one party breaches the conventionally accepted distance, the other may become uncomfortable and feel that personal space is being invaded. On the other hand, someone who maintains excessive distance may be perceived by the other party as disinterested. Thus, when conversing, each party should watch the other closely for signs of discomfort related to proxemics.

ENVIRONMENT

The environment in which a communication occurs can affect the participants' comfort level. A tidy hospital room with comfortably arranged furniture conveys concern for the client; a cluttered room with furniture arranged haphazardly in one corner suggests a disorderliness and may engender apprehension in the client.

Noise level also affects communication and comfort. If a nurse attempts to teach a client in a noisy environment, the client will have trouble hearing the information and may feel that the nurse regards understanding as secondary to finishing the teaching session.

Other components of environment include privacy, ambient temperature, formality, familiarity, and the degree to which the parties are free to leave. Disclosing personal information is much easier for the client when privacy is ensured; questioning a client about bodily functions when another client is lying in the next bed just a few feet away may cause discomfort and inhibit disclosure.

The importance of ambient temperature often is overlooked. A client who is asked to disrobe in a cold room may feel uncomfortable and inhibited from communicating fully, as may the client who must endure an intake interview in an overheated room. To an active, fully-clothed nurse, the ambient temperature may feel comfortably warm—yet a client seated in a chair wearing only a hospital gown may be quite chilly.

The degree of formality of the environment also influences communication. Many childbirth centers strive for a familiar homelike environment to help couples to relax during labor and delivery and to enhance communication (between the partners as well as between the couple and staff members). By the same token, a client may feel uneasy discussing a medical problem in an examination room, which can seem impersonal compared to the client's own hospital room or a physician's consulting office.

A client who is not free to leave the environment, such as one who has been committed for treatment involuntarily, may feel inhibited when communicating. However, in some cases—such as when the client is concerned about harming the self or others—constraint can promote communication by making the client feel safe. Thus, when gathering data on a client who is present by constraint, the nurse should assess its effects on the client and on communication.

PARALINGUISTICS

Paralinguistics refers to the study of optional vocal effects that are used as adjuncts to language but are not part of formal verbal construction. Such vocal effects accompany speech and may convey meaning; they include "ah," "um," and "uh"—sounds used almost unconsciously (just as people vary the quality and intensity of spoken communications without conscious thought). Although audible, such effects are considered nonverbal components of communication because they do not convey precise information in the same way as does ordinary written or verbal communication (Northouse and Northouse, 1985).

Paralinguistic elements include vocal qualities, vocal characterizers, vocal segregates, and vocal qualifiers (Trager, 1958). Vocal qualities include the rhythm and tempo of speech. Vocal characterizers include individual ways of groaning, sighing, laughing, or crying. Vocal segregates are interjections, such as "er" and "eh," used to punctuate and regulate speech. Vocal qualifiers include the volume (loudness or intensity) of speech, the pitch ("highness" or "lowness," or relative vibration frequency), and the length of vocalization (may range from a long Southern drawl to a clipped New England accent).

Paralinguistic elements communicate information in the same way as do other nonverbal components of communication; they may be congruent or incongruent with the formal verbal message. In the following example, the verbal message is incongruent with the paralinguistic elements:

A nurse asks a colleague to help turn a heavy client in bed. The second nurse, although busy, feels it would be unacceptable to decline the request. The second nurse groans, then replies with an elevated pitch and rapid tempo, "Okay, I'll be there in just a minute."

The verbal part of the nurse's response is positive: "Okay, I'll be there in just a minute." The paralinguistic elements (prefatory groan and altered pitch and tempo) are negative, communicating the message that the nurse does not want to help move the client.

TOUCHING

Touching is a crucial form of nonverbal communication. However, because it involves physical contact between people, it also is the most problematic. Like other elements of communication, touching can be perceived differently depending on the recipient's cultural background and other factors. Although touching can convey caring, it also can alienate or offend if used injudiciously. To determine how a particular client might perceive touching, the nurse should consider the client's cultural norms related to touching and show sensitivity to the client's feelings.

Other elements that might influence how touching is perceived include gender, age, intent, and relationship with the recipient. A female client who is touched by a female caregiver may react differently than would a male client. However, the nurse should not assume that touching a client is acceptable simply because the client is of the same gender.

Similarly, the nurse should not assume that a pediatric client will respond positively to being touched. Not all young clients appreciate being touched or held; in each case, the nurse should evaluate relevant factors to anticipate how the client might respond. Similarly, a nurse may believe that touching an elderly client is acceptable; however, some elderly clients may perceive touching as an invasion of privacy or a sign of lack of respect.

Intent, or the reason for touching, also influences the recipient's perception. Touching a client during a physical examination, such as when the nurse palpates the pulse or assesses the strength of a uterine contraction, has a specific purpose. By explaining why touching is necessary in this case, the nurse can decrease the client's resistance.

The relationship between participants also influences the recipient's response to touching. People with greater power or authority generally touch those with less authority or power more frequently than the reverse (Henley, 1973). However, this does not mean that such touching is acceptable. For instance, a male physician may pat a female nurse on the shoulder to convey appreciation for assistance; the nurse may perceive this as a condescending, harassing, or sexist gesture.

Touching can substitute for or augment a verbal message. It can be a powerful, eloquent communication tool when words are inadequate to convey the sender's message. Consider the following example:

> A Spanish-speaking couple come to the emergency department with their infant, age 6 months. The infant is pronounced dead on arrival; the official diagnosis is sudden infant death syndrome (SIDS). When an articulate Spanish-speaking physician offers a clinical explanation for the child's death, the couple show little response. Then the nurse, who speaks only English, places a sympathetic hand on the shoulder of the dead infant's mother. The mother turns to the nurse and begins to cry because her touch conveyed the caring that the physician could not express in words.

When deciding whether or not to touch a client, the nurse should consider:

- the client's culturally influenced attitudes toward touching
- the client's response to previous verbal and nonverbal elements of communication
- the client's need for distance
- the client's apparent degree of receptivity to the nurse.

Careful evaluation of these factors and sensitivity to the client's responses are the best predictors of how the client might perceive touching. It also will help the nurse choose the specific type of touch to use.

THERAPEUTIC RELATIONSHIPS

Communication is a vital element in the therapeutic relationship. Also called the helping relationship (Brammer, 1985), the therapeutic relationship is characterized by trust, respect, empathy, and autonomy. Besides providing a supporting, self-validating setting, it helps the client to explore and deal with all types of concerns and problems and to decide on an appropriate course of action.

According to Brammer, the caregiver in a therapeutic relationship has an awareness of self, values, and cultural experiences, can analyze personal feelings, serves as a role model, is altruistic, and has a strong sense of ethics and responsibility. Brammer suggests that a caregiver's ability to enter into a therapeutic relationship depends on the level of self-knowledge, dedication to helping, and understanding of the caregiver's role and responsibility in the therapeutic relationship.

REQUIREMENTS FOR A THERAPEUTIC RELATIONSHIP

According to Carl Rogers (1957), a therapeutic relationship requires congruence, unconditional positive regard, empathic understanding, and communication of this understanding. Warmth and caring also are essential to the relationship.

CONGRUENCE

As discussed earlier, congruence refers to the state or quality of being in agreement; congruence of verbal and nonverbal elements enhances communication. Similarly, Rogers defines congruence in a relationship as the degree of consistency and genuineness. Thus, the caregiver who strives for congruence demonstrates a consistent, honest approach to the client.

Congruence helps establish trust; if the client perceives the caregiver as consistent and dependable, the relationship is more likely to involve honest communication and will help the client make appropriate choices. If, on the other hand, the client perceives the caregiver as untrustworthy (such as by

REQUIREMENTS FOR A THERAPEUTIC RELATIONSHIP

- *Congruence: consistency and genuineness*
- *Unconditional positive regard: valuing of the individual*
- *Empathic understanding: perceiving things as others see them*
- *Warmth and caring*

failing to provide medications or care measures when expected) or inconsistent (such as by sometimes seeming preoccupied or dismissing client concerns), the client may not trust the caregiver as a source of dependable help.

UNCONDITIONAL POSITIVE REGARD

Unconditional positive refers to valuing an individual regardless of all other factors. The nurse demonstrates this principle by upholding the client's right to appropriate, compassionate care in all cases—even when disapproving of the client's actions. Unconditional positive regard is especially crucial when a nurse provides care for a client whose behavior is unethical or illegal, such as a client who was injured while attempting to rob a bank or an alcoholic client who has been readmitted to the hospital for detoxification.

Brammer suggests that unconditional positive regard may be inappropriate for some clients—such as those who refuse to comply with attempts to change behavior—because the caregiver's approval of the client might impede the client from changing the behavior. Generally, however, the nurse can best establish and maintain a therapeutic relationship by acknowledging the individual worth of all clients and by providing compassionate, skillful care regardless of other factors.

Some nurses may be reluctant to care for clients whose values and actions conflict with their own. Dealing with such clients is one of the greatest challenges in health care. To help cope with these situations, the nurse can use ethical problem-solving strategies (see Chapter 7, Ethical implications for nursing practice).

EMPATHIC UNDERSTANDING AND ITS COMMUNICATION

Empathic understanding refers to the ability to understand or be aware of the feelings, thoughts, or behavior of another person. Brammer (1985) describes two stages of empathic understanding. In the first stage, a person must "feel into" (experience empathically) another's emotions and perceptions. In the second stage, a person gains cognitive awareness or understanding of the other person's frame of reference. To move from the first to the second stage, one must consider the reflected emotions within the other person's context of understanding.

For instance, during the first stage of empathic understanding, a nurse may experience feelings of sadness, hurt, or anger similar to the client's feelings. During the second stage, the nurse reflects back to information based on the client's frame of reference, enhancing self-understanding. Communicating this empathic understanding, the nurse might state, "From your point of view, that must have seemed like a very hurtful thing for your wife to say" or, "Considering what happened earlier in the day, that must have felt like the last straw."

WARMTH AND CARING

Warmth and caring are crucial to a therapeutic relationship. Without them, care-giving may seem mechanical and impersonal—and therefore less effective. Suppose, for example, a nurse is caring for a client who has an altered self-concept after radical neck surgery. For such a client, warmth and caring from the nurse may be as important as clinical care measures. If the nurse provides care that is competent technically but lacks warmth and caring, the client may believe that he lacks value as a person and thus may fail to achieve the treatment goal of resuming a maximally functional life.

In Rogers's view, the therapeutic relationship fosters individual growth by providing warmth and caring. The client perceives a constant and genuine concern (congruence) on the part of the caregiver, who understands (through empathic understanding) the clients' feelings and frame of reference and who has unconditional positive regard for the client simply because the client is a human being.

DIFFICULT COMMUNICATIONS

Certain types of communication are more difficult than others. Working collegially with other health care providers is a long-established goal; however, the different levels of authority and role expectations sometimes make this goal hard to achieve.

Unpleasant communications frequently are avoided; as a result, problems are dealt with indirectly. Rather than deal directly with an abusive physician, for instance, a nurse may complain to colleagues about the physician and take pains to avoid working with the physician. However, this approach does not address the problem constructively. As described below, experts recommend specific techniques for coping with difficult communications.

TELEPHONE CALLS TO PHYSICIANS

Murphy (1990) suggests that one type of difficult communication—telephone contact between nurse and physician—can be more effective if the nurse uses the following approach:

- Identify yourself to the physician at the start of the call.
- Do not apologize for calling; keep in mind that you have a specific purpose—a purpose that also should be important to the physician.
- State the reason for your call succinctly but completely. Make sure you have all necessary information available.
- Ask the physician for specific orders when appropriate. When making a request, be specific; do not hint or insinuate, hoping that the physician will know what you are suggesting. If you believe the physician should examine the client, state this specifically.
- If the physician is coming to the health care facility to see the client, ask the anticipated time of arrival so that you can alert other staff and family members as appropriate.
- Document the telephone call. (If you were unable to reach the physician, document the attempts.)

If the physician is rude or abusive, Murphy suggests that the nurse should express that perception to the physician, then report the telephone call to the appropriate supervisor. If the physician cuts off the conversation, the nurse should call again, remaining calm and polite. If the nurse fails to reach a physician or if the physician refuses to offer the assistance the nurse seeks, Murphy suggests that the nurse contact the appropriate supervisor.

ASSERTIVE COMMUNICATIONS

Assertive communication skills are crucial to health care professionals. Such skills include confrontation, saying no, making requests, and expressing opinions. Gerrard, Boniface, and Love (1980) suggest specific techniques to make such communications more effective and direct.

CONFRONTATION

Gerrard, Boniface, and Love (1980) describe two types of confrontation.

DESC confrontation. DESC stands for *D*escribe, *E*xpress, *S*pecify, outline *C*onsequences. A DESC confrontation occurs when the confronting parties are of equal authority or have mutual regard for one another. In such a confrontation, one party seeks a specific change in the behavior of the other party. In a DESC confrontation, the first party:

- describes the behavior in question
- expresses the feeling aroused by the behavior
- specifies the behavior that is expected
- outlines the anticipated consequences (both positive and negative) of the desired behavior change as well as the anticipated consequences if the other party fails to make the desired behavior change

The following example shows what occurs in a DESC confrontation:

> Janet Strong, a new nurse in the medical-surgical unit, notices that Dr. William Donaghy always excludes her from discussions regarding her client. Instead, he communicates orders and assessment findings to Margery Ballost, a former charge nurse on the unit. Janet finds this disconcerting because the hospital recently decentralized authority and responsibility, making staff nurses responsible for communicating with physicians. Ms. Ballost no longer has supervisory responsibilities; staff nurses are expected to interact directly with physicians, as needed.

Janet decides to use the DESC confrontation method to clarify her responsibilities with Ms. Ballost and to ask her assistance in talking with the physician.

Describe: "Ms. Ballost, I've noticed that when Dr. Donaghy has finished rounds, he gives his orders to you, even though some of the clients are assigned to me."

Express: "This is difficult for me because I then have to ask you for information or wait until Dr. Donaghy has written a progress note and orders. Also, it means I don't get a chance to share my own observations with him or ask him questions. This makes me feel that I can't be responsible for my clients directly in the way I'm expected to be."

Specify: "The next time Dr. Donaghy talks to you about one of my clients, would you please introduce him to me and help clarify that I am the one who is caring for his client? He may not understand our decentralized system, so he may not know that he should work directly with me."

Outline consequences: "Doing this will save you time and effort because you won't have to find me to repeat what Dr. Donaghy has told you. It will help me develop a better working relationship with him and provide care to his clients in a more timely fashion.

"If we don't clarify the situation, I'll continue to have trouble establishing an appropriate relationship him; also, it will hinder the relationship between you and me."

DISC confrontation. DISC stands for *D*escribe, *I*ndicate, *S*pecify, outline *C*onsequences. A DISC confrontation occurs when the parties lack equal authority or mutual regard for each other—for instance, when one party is not concerned about the other's feelings. In such a confrontation, the confronting party *indicates* the problem rather than expressing feelings.

The following example shows what occurs in a DISC confrontation:

Dr. Lila Gerhart repeatedly complains that Melanie Tanner, a staff nurse, is late in entering daily weights in her clients' charts. She tells other staff members that Melanie is ignoring her requests to have data recorded in a timely fashion. When Melanie hears about this, she becomes upset. She understands Dr. Gerhart's need to have weights recorded as ordered, and feels that she is judging her performance unfairly. Melanie decides to confront Dr. Gerhart with her concerns directly to explain the circumstances and communicate her intention to ensure that clients weights are recorded properly.

Describe: "Dr. Gerhart, I understand from other staff members that you believe I've been ignoring your orders to record daily weights on your clients by 7:30 each morning."

Indicate: "When you don't come directly to me with a concern about my performance, it's hard for me to address it. I may not hear about it until much later, and your concerns may not be communicated properly."

Specify: "I'd prefer that you let me know when you feel a change needs to be made or when something should be brought to my attention. In this case, I'd like to explain why it wasn't possible to record weights as you wanted. I want to work with you to ensure that your clients receive the care they need. I've asked the other staff members to alert me if you have questions about clients assigned to me so that I can work with you directly."

Outline consequences: "If you come to me when you feel I'm not doing something properly, I'll be happy to talk to you about the situation. This will help me learn your established preferences for care. I also can inform you of any problem, such as with getting all daily weights done by 7:30, and we can come up with a solution.

"If you *don't* bring your concerns to me, we'll have trouble working together. This will impose a burden on the other nurses you might approach because they're not responsible for your clients and will have to communicate your instructions to me."

SAYING NO, MAKING REQUESTS, AND EXPRESSING OPINIONS

Despite the current emphasis on client autonomy and the need for nurses to assume responsibility for their own practice, nursing sometimes overlooks the skills required to exercise such basic options as saying no, making requests, and expressing opinions. Many nurses have as much trouble saying no appropriately, making requests, and expressing opinions as they do in handling assertive confrontation.

Like confrontation, these actions involve assertive rather than aggressive or submissive responses. From a transactional analysis viewpoint, an assertive response originates from the adult ego state, whereas an aggressive response might stem from the rebellious child or critical parent ego state and a submissive response from an adapted child ego state. An aggressive response goes beyond assertive, rational communication; frequently, it is a personal attack. A submissive response, on the other hand, fails to assert needs and concerns, pacifying the immediate situation rather than addressing the problem.

Saying "no". When saying "no," a person can be aggressive, submissive, or assertive. Consider the differences in effect as shown in the following example:

> Barry Albright, a night nurse on a busy medical unit, is preparing to give his report at the end of a long shift. He is looking forward to going home, taking a shower, having a special breakfast with his family, and going to bed. Today his daughter Laura turns 5, and his wife is going to serve Laura's favorite foods, including a cake that Barry plans to pick up on his way home from work. As Barry completes his charting, his supervisor approaches him:
>
> "Barry, we're going to be short-staffed on the day shift, so I'd like you to stay on for a few hours until we can call in more nurses."
>
> Barry's response might range from aggressive to submissive to assertive.
>
> *Aggressive responses:* "What do you mean I have to stay on? My family is waiting for me to get home and I'm not going to stay here and work a minute longer than my shift requires."
>
> "You should have thought of the staffing problem hours ago. I don't know why you can't organize things properly and avoid these last-minute emergencies. I can't be expected to make up for your inadequacies as a supervisor."
>
> *Submissive response:* "Do I really have to? I need to get home on time this morning. Isn't there any way you can let me go?"
>
> *Assertive response:* "I won't be able to stay late today because of important plans I've made with my family. Have you checked with Cindy Kolb on the surgical unit? She mentioned earlier that she was looking for some overtime. If she's not available, I know that the staffing agency is open 24 hours a day. I'll help you make sure we have staff available before I leave."

The assertive response avoids a personal attack on the supervisor, states a decision clearly and dispassionately, and suggests alternative ways in which the other party might handle the problem. Such a response is more likely to evoke a similarly objective response from the supervisor, who will realize that Barry has said no to her request to stay on and that other options are available. (However, in an emergency situation where client safety is at risk, saying no might be inappropriate.)

Making requests. Making requests also requires objectivity and directness. Many nurses have trouble requesting help from others because their socialization has led to the belief that doing so would show a lack of self-sufficiency. However, the nurse who develops a collegial working relationship with peers typically is more comfortable asking for or offering help; these behaviors are appropriate in an environment in which colleagues routinely assist each other.

Consider the situation of staff nurse Carol, whose obese client must be repositioned often. Carol would like assistance from Sara Hunt, her colleague, in repositioning the client. However, she hesitates to ask because she knows Sara has a heavy case load. Using an indirect, nonassertive approach, Carol might complain to Sara about her client's weight, stating, "Mr. Dickinson is a real problem. He's so heavy that it's almost impossible to move him in bed. I'm worried about hurting him—or more likely myself."

Sara might react to Carol's comments by perceiving her to be a complainer; worse, she probably will remain unaware that Carol is requesting help. If Carol instead used a direct approach, Sara would know that she was asking for help. For instance, Carol might say, "Sara, Mr. Dickinson is too heavy for me to reposition by myself. I know you're very busy, but could you help me reposition him? In return, I'll do Mrs. Baird's preoperative teaching for you."

Expressing opinions. Expressing opinions about work-related situations is hard for many nurses to do because they fear that they will be perceived as criticizing others for lack of competence or self-sufficiency. Also, in the past, nurses who expressed their opinions sometimes have been labeled troublemakers.

A direct, objective style is best for expressing opinions. An assertive opinion is clear and unambiguous and avoids attacking or complaining about others. For example, suppose that Barry, the night nurse in the example above, wants to express his opinion about the need to examine the way his supervisor calculates staffing requirements. Barry might arrange a meeting with his supervisor and tell her, "I've noticed lately that we've had a shortage of staff members scheduled to take over from the night shift on our unit. I'm wondering if there's been any change in the way admissions are being scheduled and if there's a way we can better predict what our census is going to be. Could we schedule time at our staff meeting to discuss these problems and ask for help in reexamining how decisions are made on staffing levels?"

Barry's comments suggest that a problem exists in calculating staffing needs and that this problem can be dealt with through positive action. He has avoided making the supervisor the scapegoat and has enlisted her support for the proposed analysis. Because Barry has not criticized her directly, the supervisor may be more willing to examine and possibly adopt Barry's opinion and suggestions.

SUMMARY

Communication is one of the most important skills that nurses use. Cultivating the characteristics that promote effective communication and avoiding those that inhibit it or cause miscommunication can help the nurse become a more effective communicator.

Communication is a part of the therapeutic relationship, which involves congruence, positive regard, empathy, and communication of understanding. The successful communicator avoids aggressive and submissive styles and uses an objective, direct approach. This approach can help a person handle confrontations, say no, make requests, and offer opinions and suggestions effectively.

APPLICATION EXERCISE

After reading the following description, develop a plan for using the DISC confrontation format to deal with the situation.

You are a staff nurse on the surgical unit. Yesterday, Dr. Browning became annoyed when a triple-lumen catheter set was not immediately available for him to use on a client. He embarrassed you in front of the staff by calling you inept for not having the kit at hand. You had not been aware that he had intended to insert the catheter that morning, and a set was not available in the department. You feel that Dr. Browning should have voiced his feelings in a more professional manner, and you want to ensure that this does not happen again.

Describe: Objectively describe the behavior you dislike, taking care not to attack the other party personally.

Indicate: Indicate the nature of the problem the person's behavior has caused, both for you individually and for the nursing unit as a whole.

Specify: Specify the behavior change you desire, again taking care not to cast blame or be defensive. Also specify the actions you might take to help alleviate the problem.

Outline consequences: Describe the positive consequences that will result if the person changes the behavior as requested and the negative consequences that will result if the person continues the offensive behavior. Also identify how you and the other party can work together to address the problem.

REVIEW QUESTIONS

1. Which factors distinguish effective communication from ineffective communication?

2. How does the sender-receiver model of communication differ from that based on Maslow's hierarchy of needs?

3. What are the elements of nonverbal communication, and how do they contribute to the communication process?

4. How do body motions affect communication?

5. What problems might occur regarding the use of touch in a health care setting?

6. How can nurses ensure that touching is acceptable to clients?

7. Which factors enhance communication with clients?

8. Which factors impede communication with clients?

9. What types of written communication occur in health care settings?

10. What assertive communication techniques can the nurse use to communicate requests and opinions and to say "no" when appropriate?

REFERENCES

Argyle, M., and Ingham, R. (1972). "Gaze, mutual gaze, and proximity." *Semiotica,* (6), 32-49.

Berne, E. (1964). *Games people play.* New York: Grove.

Brammer, L. (1985). *The helping relationship.* Englewood Cliffs, N.J.: Prentice Hall, Inc.

Ekman, P., and Friesen, W. (1969). "The repertoire of nonverbal behavior: Categories, origins, usage, and coding." *Semiotica,* 1, 49-98.

Gerrard, B., Boniface, W., and Love, B. (1980). *Interpersonal skills for health professionals.* Reston, VA: Reston Publishing Co.

Grensing, L. (1990). "A formula to avoid miscommunicating." *Nursing,* 20(9), 122-127.

Hall, E.T. (1966). *The hidden dimension.* Garden City, N.Y.: Doubleday.

Henley, N. "The Politics of Touch." In *Radical Psychology,* edited by P. Brown. New York: Harper & Row, 1973.

Iyer, P. (1991). "New trends in charting." *Nursing,* 21(1).

Maslow, A. (1954). *Motivation and personality.* New York: Harper and Row.

Mortensen, C. (1972). *Communication: The study of human interaction.* New York: McGraw-Hill.

Murphy, T. (1990). "Improving nurse/doctor communications." *Nursing,* 20(8), 114-118.

Northouse, P., and Northouse, L. (1985). *Health communication in nursing.* Englewood Cliffs, New Jersey: Prentice-Hall.

Rogers, C. (1957). "The necessary and sufficient conditions of therapeutic personality change." *Journal of Consulting Psychology,* 21: 95-103.

Trager, G.L. (1958). "Paralanguage: A first approximation." *Studies in Linguistics,* (13), 1-12.

RECOMMENDATIONS FOR FURTHER STUDY

Greve, P. "Documentation: Every Word Counts." *RN,* 55(7):55-60, July 1992.

Jones, K. "Confrontation: Methods and Skills." *Nursing Management,* 24(5):40-44 May 1993

Town, J. "Changing to Computerized Documentation—PLUS!." *Nursing Management,* 24(7):44-48, July 1993.

Trofino, J. "Voice-Activated Nursing Documentation: On the Cutting Edge." *Nursing Management,* 24(7):40-42, July 1993.

A CONCEPTUAL BASE FOR NURSING PRACTICE

OBJECTIVES

After studying this chapter, the reader should be able to:

1. Identify four philosophical systems that have influenced nursing.

2. Describe nursing theories based on client needs, using as an example the theory developed by Hildegard Peplau.

3. Discuss nursing theories based on nurse-client interactions, using as an example the theory of Orlando or King.

4. Identify and describe nursing theories based on nursing outcomes, using as an example the theory of Johnson or Levine.

5. Describe the four major concepts used by nursing theorists to develop conceptual frameworks, models, and theories.

6. Apply a nursing theory to interpreting a client-care situation.

INTRODUCTION

Nursing is a complex process based on the application of scientific knowledge. It calls for an integration of technical skills, complex understandings, intuition, values, and perceptions. To organize these elements into a congruent whole, nurses rely on a basic conceptual framework, or theory, of nursing. A theory is a "logically interconnected set of propositions used to describe, explain, and predict a part of the empirical world" (Riehl and Roy, 1980).

A person who practices nursing or conducts nursing research without the basic organizing principles of nursing theory will achieve less predictable and possibly less effective results than someone who relies on nursing theory. A staff nurse who sees the nurse's role simply as carrying out a physician's orders may let many client needs go unidentified and unmet. In contrast, the nurse who relies on a comprehensive nursing theory as a framework for action will assess all potential client needs, not merely those reflected in the physician's orders.

Similarly, a nurse researcher who merely wants to determine which of two procedures is quicker or more efficient may fail to ask more basic questions related to the purpose of the procedure and whether the procedure is appropriate in the given situation. The nurse who bases research on theory, however, will be led by the theory to examine all aspects of the situation—not just those that are connected superficially to efficiency. The outcome will be a more comprehensive understanding of the problem. To begin to understand nursing theory, it is important to understand the similarities and differences between theory and the nursing process, and between theory and philosophy.

NURSING THEORY AND THE NURSING PROCESS

The nursing process is a framework for problem solving that helps to structure everyday nursing practice. It has specific steps—assessment, diagnosis, planning, implementation, and evaluation—that provide guidelines for dealing with specific client problems.

The nursing process differs from nursing theory in several ways. The nursing process provides guidelines for approaching a particular client-care situation. It identifies the series of actions through which the nurse can make decisions. Nursing theory, while providing a way to understand a particular client-care problem, also provides a comprehensive view of nursing as an entity in itself. While the nursing process provides the steps in problem solving, nursing theory provides a way of viewing the major phenomena of nursing and provides answers to various questions: What is health? What is illness? What is the nature of human beings? How do people affect the environment? How does the environment affected human beings? What is nursing?

PHILOSOPHY AND NURSING

To function most effectively, nurses must have a basic understanding of what nursing is and how it is practiced. This knowledge, in turn, hinges on an understanding, or philosophy, of the nature of the world. Such philosophical grounding provides the basis for developing concepts, or ideas, about nursing, mankind, health, and the environment.

A philosophy is a system of thought that reflects beliefs, values, and knowledge, which form the basis for understanding specific phenomena or concepts. Such understanding varies with the particular philosophy adopted. For example, a framework for nursing based on the humanistic and existentialist philosophies would stress the importance of self-determination and individual worth, both important trends in these philosophical systems. Conversely, a culture whose dominant philosophy does not recognize individuals as intrinsically worthy of care or does not value life highly will not place much importance on self-determination and individual worth. Consequently, beliefs about the duty to provide care and the nature of nursing responsibilities would differ from those in a humanistic or existentially based culture.

CONCEPTS, CONCEPTUAL MODELS, AND THEORIES

Before theories can exist, concepts must exist. Concepts are abstract ideas generalized from specific instances. Propositions describe relationships between concepts; in turn, propositions can be elaborated to form models and theories that describe, explain, predict, or control phenomena. A model generally is less elaborate than a theory and can be thought of as the skeleton, or basic structure, of the theory.

CONCEPTS

In nursing, four concepts are crucial:
- caring/nursing
- client (clients, person, patient)
- health (or the health-illness continuum)
- environment.

Fawcett (1989) calls this grouping of the four important concepts the "metaparadigm of nursing," a superstructure under which all of nursing can be described.

CARING/NURSING

The concept of caring incorporates the right of clients to make decisions about their health and illness and the obligation to provide care to all clients regardless of their individual state—a concept that reflects the humanistic and existentialist philosophies. Caring requires nursing action based on moral value, not just empathy or intellectual understanding. A nurse who upholds the concept of caring takes action to address client needs.

Ismeurt, Arnold, and Carson (1990) define nursing as the science of caring and view caring as an overarching umbrella that includes everything the nurse does in the process of nursing. Leininger (1981) suggests that caring is the core and unifying concept for both the body of nursing knowledge and the practice of nursing, proposing that it is "at the heart of all health care services." She defines caring as "those assistive, supportive, or facilitative acts toward or for another individual or group with evident or anticipated needs to ameliorate or improve a human condition or lifeway" (1991).

According to Leininger, although human caring is a universal phenomenon, its expression varies among cultures; what is experienced as caring in one setting may be perceived as uncaring in another. To provide therapeutic care and serve as an effective client advocate, the nurse must be familiar with the clients' values and beliefs.

Caring, then, refers to providing assistance to individuals, families, or communities to help prevent illness and to maintain or restore health in its fullest meaning.

Other important aspects of caring include the understanding that the nurse assists clients within the framework of a helping relationship and that the nurse must care for himself or herself. Caring for one's self also is part of the caring process. Nursing involves not merely doing something to or for a client; but the interaction and relationship between two people, both of whom are valued and whose individual beliefs, needs, and rights are respected. A nurse who does not practice self-care may experience job "burnout," becoming so exhausted that he or she cannot continue to practice nursing. Nursing can be stressful as well as rewarding; by providing for one's own needs, the nurse can continue to give effective care to others throughout the career.

According to Veatch and Fry (1987), caring has the force of a moral value and serves as an ethical standard for nursing. Caring-based philosophy identifies and values nursing behaviors and actions that are supportive, empathic, and compassionate. To practice nursing that is caring, the nurse must go beyond delivering expert technical care, developing a relationship with the client that assists the client to optimal health in ways that recognize individual worth and responsibilities.

CONCEPTS CENTRAL TO NURSING THEORY

- *Caring/nursing*
- *Client*
- *Health*
- *Environment*

CLIENT

The client—the second concept crucial to nursing—may be a person, a person in the context of the family, an entire family, or even an entire community or society. This definition makes the task of providing nursing care much more complex. Nurses are responsible for a range of client-care situations both in structured settings (such as the medical floor of a general acute-care hospital) and unstructured settings (such as the homes that a visiting nurse may encounter). They provide care to clients with both routine and unusual problems. Nurses who care for clients with complex problems in unstructured settings have responsibilities that range from routine and structured to complex and unstructured. Thus, they require more knowledge and preparation to practice more independently as the situation demands. Generally, they gain such advanced knowledge in baccalaureate or higher programs, in such courses as pathophysiology, physical assessment, leadership, and management.

HEALTH

The American Nurses Association (1980) defines health as "a dynamic state of being in which the developmental and behavioral potential of an individual is realized to the fullest extent possible." Thus, health is more than just the absence of disease; it also includes the drive toward optimal functioning and achievement. Health and illness are points along a continuum and not distinctly different; during the course of a life, a person may move from one end of the continuum to the other.

The concept of health, like that of caring, is culturally mediated: What is considered healthy in one culture may not be what is considered healthy in another. In a culture that views pain as a symptom of ill health, people who experience pain typically define themselves as ill. In a culture that views pain as a fact of life that one should cope with unless it interferes with functioning, people do not consider themselves ill simply because they are in pain.

ENVIRONMENT

Environment refers to the setting in which a person functions. One might consider the environment to be separate and distinct from the people who live in it. However, a more comprehensive perspective recognizes that individuals interact with the environment constantly in what is called an *open system*. Hall and Fagan (1968) define a system as a set of parts or components and the relationships between the parts and the properties of the parts. In an open system, the system and the surrounding environment exchange energy. Living beings are open systems, taking in energy and returning it to the environment. (For more information on open systems, see Chapter 3, How organizations are structured.)

Including the environment as a concept in nursing theory allows a more comprehensive approach to problem solving. Suppose a client has a pulmonary disease. Although some nurses might carry out ordered treatments without considering environment, optimally they would consider various environmental factors—a spouse who smokes, a drafty home, an unhealthy diet, or a family income insufficient to permit preventive medical care—when developing the plan of care for this client.

Environment can include all the factors that affect the client, including physical surroundings and social relationships. Florence Nightingale was the first author to describe the importance of the environment on individual health, stressing clean air and surroundings in the recovery of wounded soldiers (1869).

CONCEPTUAL MODELS

Once concepts are identified, propositions (statements of relationship) can be developed (Jacox, 1974). Suppose, for example, that a nurse-theorist develops a concept of self-worth, then links this concept to another concept—successful maternal-infant bonding. The relationship between the two concepts may be described by the proposition that an adult's perception of self-worth may be influenced directly by the success or failure of early maternal-infant bonding.

A proposition can be developed further to show specifically in what way success or failure of early bonding may influence self-esteem. The description of the interrelationships between concepts is called a conceptual model or framework. In the example above, the nurse-theorist might develop a conceptual model that attempts to encompass all the concepts, propositions, and interrelationships involved in analyzing the attainment of self-worth. From conceptual frameworks, it is then possible to develop more elaborate descriptions about phenomena which take on the characteristics of theory. A theory has the power to describe, explain, predict, or control, depending on its level of development.

THEORIES

Theories of nursing, like those of other disciplines, start by describing the nature of nursing, including the major concepts and the relationships between them. This provides a way to explain phenomena that nurses confront and, as theories are refined and tested, increases the ability to predict and control client outcomes.

Experts continue to debate the question of whether one universally espoused theory of nursing is better than many different theories. Because no one theory satisfactorily explains all the phenomena of nursing, most nursing theorists recognize the value in having numerous theories.

TYPES OF THEORIES

Depending on its level of complexity, a theory can be descriptive, explanatory, predictive, or controlling. A *descriptive theory* identifies and describes phenomena. When little is known about a given phenomenon, a theory addressing the phenomenon is likely to be descriptive. A descriptive theory can be used to develop an explanatory theory. An *explanatory theory* describes relationships among phenomena. When a theory is put into practice and tested in real situations, uncovering more information about the given phenomenon, the theory is refined—eventually, to the point where it predicts the phenomenon (*predictive theory*) and, finally, allows for control of the phenomenon (*controlling theory*).

Using the example of maternal-infant bonding, once a conceptual framework is developed to show the concepts and their relationships, a descriptive theory can be developed to identify the elements of maternal-infant bonding. Then, an explanatory theory could be developed to explain how maternal-infant bonding is accomplished. Predictive theory could be used to predict who might have problems with self-image in later life as a result of deficient maternal-infant bonding. Finally, a theory could be formulated to provide a basis for intervening in a problematic bonding between mother and infant; this would provide an opportunity to affect—and potentially control—successful bonding and later development of a positive self-image.

LEVELS OF THEORY

Nursing theories exist at several levels. At the highest level are highly abstract theories that define broad philosophical and methodologic issues; at the lowest level are practical theories that describe specific nursing interventions to produce predictable nursing outcomes (Walker and Avant, 1983).

Metatheory, the most abstract level of theory, addresses the nature of theory itself and the types of theory that nursing needs. *Grand theory*, slightly less abstract, describes the practice of nursing in global terms, using the concepts of client, nursing, health, and environment. *Middle-range theory* focuses on nursing practice, attempting to provide more specific information for nursing actions and research. *Practice theory*, the most concrete level of theory, addresses nursing actions necessary to achieve specific outcomes and how the theory can be tested in nursing practice (Dickoff and James, 1968).

Again using the example of maternal-infant bonding, a metatheory might address the nature of and need for a theory that addresses bonding. A grand theory would address the concepts of bonding and self-image, offering propositions that describe the relationships between these concepts, and the resulting structure of the developing theory. A middle-range theory might describe how to evaluate and foster bonding, and a practice theory might describe specific nursing strategies to enhance maternal-infant bonding.

Having multiple levels of theory helps address nursing concerns at different levels of complexity. Also, advancements and changes in theory resulting from implementation at the practice level might reveal the need to reexamine a theory at other levels. For example, suppose a middle-range theory suggests that early physical contact between mother and infant is an element required for successful maternal-infant bonding. However, applying the practice theory derived from this middle-range theory might show that physical contact is less important to bonding than is positive verbal support of the anxious new mother by family members and nursing staff. This finding might lead nursing theorists to reexamine and make changes in both practice theory and middle-range theory.

EVOLUTION OF NURSING THEORY

Nursing theory has its roots in the work of Florence Nightingale in the late 19th century. However, in the subsequent period, when romanticism and pragmatism held sway, nurses paid little attention to the theoretical bases of nursing actions. After the second World War, nursing research—a prime source for nursing theory—focused mainly on the education of students rather than the practice of nursing itself.

As nursing education programs developed and expanded, more nurse-scholars were educated in doctoral programs, typically in the social or biological sciences. These nurse-scholars were exposed to—and borrowed from—theories from these disciplines to help explain phenomena of concern to nursing. Many theories from other disciplines—including education, sociology, psychology, and developmental theory—still are useful to nursing.

Nursing theory continues to evolve, largely as a result of the establishment of nursing doctoral programs and the work of nurse-researchers and nursing theorists. Conceptual models continue to be expanded and elaborated on. Nursing theories—whether borrowed from other disciplines or unique to nursing—are being tested in practice.

Florence Nightingale. Florence Nightingale developed the first formal pre-theoretical formulations regarding nursing based on environmental concepts. Although she did not develop a formal theory, she described the interchange between people and the environment and stressed the importance of clean, warm, quiet, light surroundings. Her book *Notes on Nursing* (1869) inspired later writers and researchers by focusing on the client rather than disease and by recognizing that the practice of nursing requires a conceptual framework, not just technical skill.

Hildegard Peplau. After Nightingale, nursing theory remained stagnant for nearly a century. In 1952, Hildegard Peplau described nursing in terms of the relationship between nurse and client in her book *Interpersonal Relations in Nursing*. Peplau used concepts from developmental and psychological theory to help explain how such a relationship develops, allowing further examination and description of the nurse's role.

Peplau described the development of interpersonal relationships in four phases. During the *orientation phase*, the client experiences a need and asks for assistance. During the *identification phase*, the client identifies and responds to persons who can provide assistance. During the *exploitation phase*, the nurse-client relationship is exploited to its fullest extent to create changes that will benefit the client. During the *resolution phase*, the client reestablishes independence.

Peplau's theory foreshadowed the articulation of the nursing process, with its steps of assessment, diagnosis, planning, implementation, and evaluation. In Peplau's schema, the client identifies a problem, identifies the individuals who can assist in addressing the problem, uses the relationship with that person to effect change, then resumes independence. In the nursing process, the nurses assesses the client for problems, diagnoses each problem from a nursing standpoint, engages in planning, addresses the problem through appropriate interventions, then evaluates the effectiveness of the nursing action.

During roughly the time of Peplau's writing, the journal *Nursing Research* began publication. This was an important milestone because the journal provided a venue for the exchange of information about nursing research and theory. In the middle to late 1950s, the U.S. Public Health Service began offering predoctoral research fellowships, and many nurses took advantage of nurse-scientist training programs for doctoral education.

During the 1960s and 1970s, nursing theoretical work advanced. Meleis (1985) classifies the theories developed during this period as:

- theories based on human needs
- theories based on interaction
- theories that seek to describe the outcome of nursing.

THEORIES BASED ON NEEDS

The earliest nursing theorists used an approach to nursing based on client needs. For instance, Faye Abdellah (1961) developed a problem-solving approach for addressing 21 nursing problems through nursing actions that included sustenal, remedial, restorative, and preventative activities. Sustenal care involves psychosocial needs; remedial care, the provision of such substances as oxygen, fluid, nutrition; restorative care, assistance in coping with illness and life adjustment; and preventative care, such factors as safety, hygiene, activity, and rest. According to Abdellah, the goal of nursing is to help the individual meet health needs and adjust to health problems using a problem-solving approach.

Virginia Henderson described nursing in similar terms. In her book *The Nature of Nursing* (1966), she states, "The unique function of the nurse is to assist the individual, sick or well, in the performance of those activities contributing to health or its recovery (or peaceful death) that he could perform unaided if he had the necessary strength, will or knowledge, and to do this in such a way as to help him gain independence as rapidly as possible" (1966). These activities are:

- breathing normally
- eating and drinking adequately
- eliminating body wastes
- moving and maintaining desirable postures
- sleeping and resting
- selecting suitable clothing, dressing and undressing
- maintaining body temperature within normal range by adjusting clothing and modifying the environment

- keeping the body clean and well-groomed and protecting the integument
- avoiding dangers in the environment and avoiding injury to others
- communicating with others to express emotions, needs, fears, and opinions
- worshiping according to one's faith
- working in a way that brings a sense of accomplishment
- playing or participating in various forms of recreation
- learning, discovering, or satisfying the curiosity that leads to normal development and health and use of available health facilities (Henderson, 1966).

THEORIES BASED ON INTERACTION

Other nursing theories focus on the nurse-client interaction. Although interaction theorists also address client needs, they stress the importance of the nurse-client relationship. They propose that nursing involves more than just providing technical help in meeting a client's needs; it also includes providing care that recognizes the autonomy of the client, who contributes to decisions about care. Nurses must be knowledgeable about their own values and needs to enter into the therapeutic relationship. According to interaction theorists, the goals of nursing include helping clients find meaning in their experience.

Peplau, an early interaction theorist, addressed healthcare problems in terms of the therapeutic relationship between the nurse and client. Ida Jean Orlando, author of *The Dynamic Nurse-Client Relationship* (1961), described nursing as a dynamic interaction in which the nurse uses a deliberate approach to help clients who have needs they cannot meet on their own. The client's perceptions and feelings are important in the nurse-client interaction; nursing action is structured and based on the nursing process. Nursing involves the nurse's perception of the client's thoughts, feelings, and actions and the nurse's actions to address the client's needs.

Another theorist who emphasized the nurse-client interaction was Imogene King, who wrote two influential books—

Toward a Theory for Nursing: General Concepts of Human Behavior (1971) and *Theory of Nursing: Systems, Concepts, Process* (1981). King based her theory on systems theory, which defines the client as either an individual (called a personal system) or a group (called an interpersonal system). The client interacts with the environment in such a way that health problems develop; the personal and interpersonal systems cannot cope with these problems effectively. Health is the ability to perform the usual roles; the nurse and client set mutual goals. Nursing involves the interaction between client and nurse, in which mutual goal setting occurs. The focus of nursing is on human beings in interaction with the environment; this interaction leads to a state of health, which she defined as the ability to function in social roles (King, 1981).

THEORIES BASED ON NURSING OUTCOMES

According to Meleis (1985), theories based on needs attempt to describe the "what" of nursing, whereas theories based on interaction attempt to describe the "how" of nursing. In contrast, the third group of theories—those based on nursing outcomes—describe the "why" of nursing.

Dorothy Johnson, for instance, drew on theories from the biological and social sciences to develop a model of nursing based on behavioral systems. A behavioral system is "the person, composed of interactions among and between seven subsystems" (Leddy and Pepper, 1989). Johnson sees illness as an imbalance within the larger system and its seven subsystems. These subsystems include:

- the ingestive subsystem, involving nutrition
- the eliminative subsystem, involving excretion
- the sexual subsystem, involving procreation and sexual behaviors
- the aggressive subsystem, involving safety and self-preservation
- the achievement subsystem, involving success and accomplishment
- the dependency subsystem, involving physical and emotional nurturing and assistance

- the affiliative subsystem, involving social relationships.

Johnson views nursing as an external force that acts to maintain equilibrium and integration when health is threatened. The goal of nursing is to preserve the balance within the system and it seven subsystems (Johnson, 1967, 1974).

Myra Levine, whose book *Introduction to Clinical Nursing* was published in 1973, also focused on nursing outcomes. Like Johnson, Levine applied theories from the social and biological sciences to develop four principles of conservation, or preservation. These principles hold that nursing intervention is based on conserving the client's energy, structural integrity, personal integrity, and social integrity (1967).

Levine describes nursing as client advocacy in conserving energy and integrity. The client must be respected as an individual; "client-centered nursing care means individualized nursing care" (1973). Levine stressed the need for nurses to individualize nursing care and to perform nursing care with compassion and commitment.

CONTEMPORARY NURSING THEORIES

Besides Johnson and King, other contemporary nursing theorists have had a major influence on nursing education, research, and practice. These theorists include Dorothea Orem, Martha Rogers, Sister Callista Roy, and Jean Watson. The following discussion of the theoretical models developed by each of these theorists includes interpretations of a clinical situation based on each model.

DOROTHEA OREM'S SELF-CARE MODEL

Dorothea Orem wrote *Guides for Developing Curriculae for the Education of Practical Nurses* (1959) and *Nursing: Concepts of Practice* (1980) to define content for the nursing curriculum. Based mainly on the concept of client needs, Orem's theory may be the most widely used nursing theory in the practice arena. Incorporating concepts from the medical model of practice, it mainly addresses the client during illness.

Orem sees nursing as actions that are deliberately selected and performed to help clients who have self-care needs that they cannot meet on their own because of illness. Orem introduced the term *self-care* defining it as the activities that a person performs to promote health. The client, or patient, is an individual who cannot meet self-care needs to sustain life and health, to recover from disease or injury, or to cope with the effects of disease or injury.

The *therapeutic self-care demand* refers to actions required to meet the requirements to sustain life and health. *Self-care agency* refers to the person—either the client or the nurse—who provides the needed actions. If the client cannot meet the needs of the therapeutic self-care demand, the nurse or other care-giver must meet do this. *Self-care deficit* is the difference between the client's needs and the ability to meet them. Health is the ability to meet self-care needs for structural integrity, functioning, and development.

Orem views self-care actions as "activities that individuals initiate and perform on their own behalf in maintaining life, health, and well-being" (1980). These activities fall into three categories—universal self-care requisites, developmental self-care requisites, and health-deviation self-care requisites.

Universal self-care requisites include:
- maintaining sufficient intake of air, water, and food
- providing care associated with elimination processes and excrements
- maintaining a balance between activity and rest and solitude and social interaction
- preventing hazards to life, functioning, and well-being
- promoting functioning and development within social groups in accord with human potential, known limitations, and the desire to be normal (1980).

Developmental self-care requisites include:
- bringing about and maintaining living conditions that support life processes and promote development; that is, progress toward higher levels of the organization of human structures and toward maturation. These requisites include

CONCEPTS CENTRAL TO OREM'S SELF-CARE MODEL

- *Universal self-care requisites*
- *Developmental self-care requisites*
- *Health-deviation self-care requisites*
- *Wholly compensatory nursing actions*
- *Partially compensatory nursing actions*
- *Supportive educative nursing actions*

such needs as a safe social and physical environment in which a person can develop in an optimal manner.
- providing care either to prevent deleterious effects or conditions that can affect human development or to mitigate or overcome the effects from various conditions (1980).

Health-deviation self-care requisites include:
- seeking and securing appropriate medical assistance in the event of exposure to specific physical or biological agents or environmental conditions associated with pathologic events and states, or when evidence exists of genetic, physiologic, or psychological conditions linked with pathology
- being aware of and attending to the effects and results of pathologic conditions and states
- effectively carrying out medically prescribed diagnostic, therapeutic, and rehabilitative measures directed to preventing specific types of pathology, to the pathology itself, resolution of human integrated functioning, correction of deformities or abnormalities, or compensation for disabilities
- being aware of and attending to or regulating the discomforting or adverse effects of measures performed or prescribed by the physician
- modifying the self-concept in accepting oneself as being in a particular state of health and in need of specific forms of health care
- learning to live with the effects of pathologic conditions and the effects of medical diagnostic and treatment measures in a life-style that promotes continued personal development (1980).

Although Orem's concept of environment is not well-developed or defined specifically, she generally views the environment as the setting in which a person has unmet needs for self-care. However, she also describes it in a therapeutic light, stating that it can manipulated to provide for developmental self-care requisites.

According to Orem, nurses who intervene to assist clients can be considered self-care agents (Meleis, 1985). Thus, nursing is therapeutic self-care that supplements the client's self-care requisites when the client cannot provide for these.

In Orem's model, nursing actions exist on three levels. *Wholly compensatory nursing actions* are self-care actions performed by the nurse when a client is wholly incapable of performing self-care. Nursing actions are wholly compensatory when the client cannot perform self-care without continuous guidance.

Partially compensatory nursing actions are self-care actions that assist those of the client. For example, a client may be able to perform activities of daily living but may need partly compensatory nursing actions to help with other activities, such as bathing, ambulating, or self-administering an insulin injection.

Supportive educative nursing actions address client needs for assistance with decision making, behavioral control, knowledge, or skill development. For example, a client can be taught to develop skill in independently measuring blood pressure.

Orem's model can be used to analyze the following client-care situation:

> Joan, age 22, has just had a miscarriage. She and her husband Rob had been looking forward to their first child with great excitement. Now, each has trouble coping with individual feelings of loss while at the same time trying to support the other. Joan begins to withdraw and refuses to eat. Early one evening, Rob decides to takes her to the hospital, after consulting with her physician, because she has refused to eat or talk since noon.

Interpreting Joan's situation using Orem's self-care theory, we can see that Joan is experiencing a self-care deficit that she and her husband cannot meet independently. By taking Joan to the hospital, Rob recognizes that self-care must be provided by other care-givers. The nurse's role is to diagnose Joan's self-care deficits, which include the following:

- current reduced food intake (universal self-care requisite: maintenance of a sufficient intake of food)
- interrupted developmental task of becoming a mother (developmental self-care requisite: provision of care so as

to mitigate the effects from conditions having deleterious effects on human development)

- health-deviation self-care requisites, which include not only Joan's current physiologic problems but the potential need to modify her self-concept and to accept herself as being in a particular state of health and in need of specific forms of health care.

The nurse may assist Joan using wholly compensatory, partially compensatory, or supportive-educative actions. Such actions would address Joan's physiologic needs for sustenance and help her deal with her grief and altered self-image. The nurse also could use these actions to assist Rob to support Joan more effectively at a time when she cannot meet her needs for self-care independently.

Contributions and Limitations. Perhaps the greatest contribution of Orem's theory is its focus on clients' responsibility for their own health care. A descriptive theory, it provides information about nursing concepts and has been of particular use to nurses in practice. It has led to development of measures that assess the ability of clients to meet their own self-care needs (Kuriansky, Gurland, Fleiss, and Cowan, 1976).

However, Orem's theory fails to consider the effects of culture. Perceptions of self-care during illness vary; in some cultures, the family assists with self-care of an ill family member rather than expecting the ill person to provide self-care. Also, the theory is illness-focused and does not address issues of health and illness prevention. Although it may be possible to identify self-care needs to prevent illness using Orem's theory, this has not been the focus of the theory's development or application.

MARTHA ROGERS'S UNITARY MAN MODEL

Another nurse-theorist whose work has had considerable influence is Martha Rogers, who wrote *An Introduction to the Theoretical Basis of Nursing* (1980). Whereas Orem describes nursing from the standpoint of education and curriculum, Rogers identifies the unique body of knowledge encompassed by nursing. She views nursing not merely as a synthesis of other sciences but as a separate body of knowledge. Influenced by systems theory, Rogers holds that man is greater than the sum of his parts (a concept also central to humanism) and is in constant interaction with the environment. Rogers's writing is highly theoretical and sometimes is difficult to apply in practice. Also, definitions of key concepts continue to evolve and change.

Rogers describes nursing as the art and science of promoting the symphonic, or harmonious, interaction between human beings and the environment. The client is unitary man—an irreducible whole. Man is an energy field with four dimensions, in constant interaction with the environment. Health results from harmonious interaction between a person and the environment. When this interaction is disrupted, interventions are needed. Such interventions may necessitate dealing with external factors in an action Rogers terms repatterning of the human environmental fields or with internal factors which Rogers terms mobilizing inner resources.

Rogers holds that health and illness are points on a continuum and expressions of the life processes. The environment, like mankind, is a unitary energy field; irreducible, it includes everything that exists outside a given human energy field.

The concepts of integrality, helicy, and resonancy are central to Rogers's model. *Integrality* refers to the constant interaction between the human and environmental energy fields, which constantly influence and are influenced by each other. *Helicy* is the continuous and innovative nature of change. As a person ages and behavior becomes more complex, behavior may recur, but the conditions in which it does so will have changed. *Resonancy* suggests that changes in pattern and organization of both the human field and the environmental field can be described as waves. These waves start out as low-frequency, long-wave patterns but change to short-wave, high-frequency patterns as complexity increases. The concept of resonancy suggests that as individuals develop, change becomes more frequent and more profound.

CONCEPTS CENTRAL TO ROGERS'S UNITARY MAN MODEL

- *Integrality*
- *Helicy*
- *Resonancy*

Interpreting the situation of Joan and Rob using Rogers's theory, we might describe Joan's situation as one in which the interface between client and environment lacks integrality. A disjuncture in the expected development has occurred. The nurse's function is to help restore the balance between Joan and her environment. To do this, the nurse must strengthen "the coherence and integrity of the human field" and "direct and redirect patterning of the human and environmental fields" (1970). Nursing interventions should focus on supporting Joan and changing the client-environment interchange.

Although Rogers's theory does not lend itself to an explicit blueprint for specific nursing action, it does emphasize the importance of focusing on the client-environment interchange. This could lead the nurse to evaluate the role of the environment in producing Joan's miscarriage or to examine the contribution of the environment to Joan's problem in coping with her experience. By emphasizing the interchange between the client and the environment, Rogers's theory potentially broadens the scope of nursing practice and nursing research.

Contributions and Limitations. Perhaps the greatest contribution of Rogers's theory is its emphasis on interchange between human beings and the environment. Also, its view of man and the environment as energy fields suggests another way of viewing both entities.

The drawback of Rogers's work is the highly abstract language, which makes understanding and applying her theory more difficult for researchers and practicing nurses.

ROY'S ADAPTATION MODEL

Sister Callista Roy sees nursing as the process of promoting adaptation, or beneficial change, in response to stimuli. Her article "Adaptation: A Basis for Nursing Practice," published in *Nursing Outlook* (1971), was followed by her book *Introduction to Nursing: An Adaptation Model* (1976).

Roy proposes that the client can be an individual, families, groups, or communities who demonstrate ineffective coping.

Individuals, she proposed, are beings with biological, psychological, and social elements who are in constant interaction with a changing environment. Health is a state of adaptation in which energy is free to deal with stimuli—the state and process of integration. When the individual is not adapting and shows ineffective coping responses, nursing intervenes to help restore health.

Roy views the environment as everything that influences the client and describes it in terms of stimuli (either internal or external). Roy classifies stimuli as:

- focal stimuli, or stimuli confronting a person immediately; for example, an injection
- contextual stimuli, or stimuli in the background; in the case of a client receiving an injection, contextual stimuli include sounds, heat, and cold
- residual stimuli, or stimuli involving attitudes and previous experiences; for example, memories of an earlier painful injection.

Roy holds that the individual uses two subsystems to adapt. The first subsystem, called the regulator subsystem, functions mainly through the autonomic nervous system. It receives stimuli from the internal or external environment and responds to allow the person to adapt physiologically.

The second subsystem, called the cognator subsystem, allows a person to adapt through perceptual/information processing, learning, exercising judgment, and manifesting emotion. As with the regulator subsystem, the cognator subsystem responds to both internal and external stimuli.

In the above example of the client receiving an injection, both subsystems would come into play. The stimulus would evoke a physiologic response, which might involve an increased heart rate, sweating, and nervousness. A perceptual/information processing response also would result, which might cause the person to realize that this injection is not nearly as difficult or painful as the remembered one.

Thus, the client receives both external and internal stimuli and uses both regulator and cognator subsystems to respond. According to Roy, this is accomplished through four modes. The *physiologic mode* addresses the need for appropriate

**CONCEPTS
CENTRAL TO
ROY'S
ADAPTATION
MODEL**

- *Focal stimuli*
- *Contextual stimuli*
- *Residual stimuli*
- *Regulator mechanisms*
- *Cognator subsystem*
- *Effector modes*

activity and rest, nutrition, and elimination. The *self-concept mode* addresses such concerns as self-esteem and the self-ideal. The *role function mode* involves primary and secondary roles or responsibilities, role performance, role mastery, and social integrity. The *interdependence mode* involves nurturing, support systems, and significant others.

Interpreting Joan and Rob's situation from the perspective of Roy's adaptation model, the nurse would identify that they are not coping effectively. Joan is receiving both internal and external stimuli relating to her miscarriage. Such stimuli may be focal, related to the immediate experience of losing her baby; contextual, related to returning home to an environment that emphasizes her loss; or residual, based on existing attitudes and early experiences. Both her regulator and cognator systems are engaged in attempting to respond to the changes that have occurred; her body is responding with physiologic changes, and she is attempting to solve problems, express emotion, and learn.

The nurse's role is to assist Joan and her husband to adapt to the stimuli appropriately. This could be done by assisting the cognator and regulator systems through any of the four modes. For example, the nurse could attempt to address changes in Joan's self-concept and role that were affected by the miscarriage. The goal is to help Joan make the most positive long-term adaptation possible to her changed situation.

Contributions and Limitations. Roy's theory focuses on the outcome of adaptation and on the individual's ability to respond to external and internal stimuli in constructive ways. Thus, her theory broadens the focus of nursing, in terms of both problems and potential interventions. By identifying modes, including self-concept and interdependence, it allows examination of the various ways in which individuals can be assisted to adapt.

JEAN WATSON'S HUMAN CARING MODEL

As described in Watson's book *Nursing: the Philosophy and Science of Caring* (1979), Watson sees nursing as a transpersonal process whose aim is to help the client gain self-knowledge and control, to promote self-healing through inner harmony, and to help the client find meaning. According to Watson, the practice of caring "integrates biophysical knowledge with knowledge of human behavior to generate or promote health and to provide ministrations to those who are ill." The client is the person who enters into the transpersonal process with the nurse. Watson views individuals as inherently good and capable of growth and development. Health refers to unity of mind, body, and soul and involves congruence between the perceived self and experienced self.

Watson does not focus specifically on the environment but implies that environment is the setting in which nurse and client interact. She identifies the caring environment as "one that offers the development of potential while allowing the person to choose the best action for himself or herself at a given point in time."

Watson's theory represents a shift toward an existential-phenomenologic perspective (Deloughery, 1991). This perspective emphasizes experience as it is perceived by the individual and stresses human experiences that transcend the physical body and rational mind. Watson proposes that the client's unique subjective and objective experiences are of interest and must be examined from a holistic standpoint. She focuses on the individual as a whole (including mind, body, and soul) rather than on the disease.

Watson holds that the following assumptions underlie the science of caring in nursing (1979, 1985):

- Caring can be demonstrated and practiced effectively only in terms of the interpersonal relationship.
- Carative factors (factors that are caring in nature) result in satisfaction of human needs, which promotes health and growth.
- Caring responses recognize not only what the individual is in the present but what the individual may become. That is, they recognize the human potential for growth and change.
- Caring is more health-centered ("healthogenic") than curing.

- The caring environment allows for personal development and individual choice.
- The practice of caring is central to nursing.

Watson proposes that 10 primary carative factors underlie nursing as the science of caring:

- formation of a humanistic-altruistic value system that recognizes the importance of the individual and has regard for others' interests
- instillation of faith and/or hope, which are important to individual motivation
- cultivation of sensitivity to one's self and others, because an awareness of one's own and others' needs and values is crucial to the ability to act as client advocate
- development of a helping-trusting relationship
- promotion and acceptance of the expression of positive and negative factors
- freedom and encouragement to discuss both positive and negative elements within a given situation
- systematic use of the scientific problem-solving method for decision making; as exemplified in the nursing process and the research process, scientific problem-solving provides important information for making decisions
- promotion of interpersonal teaching and learning; nurses and clients learn from each other in the interpersonal process, promoting both teaching and learning
- provision of a supportive, protective, and/or corrective mental, physical, sociocultural, and spiritual environment
- assistance with gratification of human needs
- allowance for existential-phenomonologic-spiritual forces (1979).

Analyzing Joan and Rob from the perspective of Watson's caring model, we see that the nurse must focus on Joan's experience as it has meaning for her. To assist Joan, the nurse must create an environment that provides for growth and gives Joan choice. By establishing a relationship with Joan in which Joan is valued for what she can become as well as for what she now is, the nurse can help her address not only the biological needs created by her physical experience but the emotional, cultural, and spiritual needs of her own individual experience.

Contributions and Limitations. Watson's major contribution is her emphasis on the importance of viewing experience from the standpoint of the individual who is perceiving and experiencing it. She focuses mainly on what the experience means to the individual, not just on external assessments or judgments. She views the goal of transpersonal caring as nursing that promotes the preservation of humanity, dignity, and freedom of self (Watson, 1985). This goal is much broader than simply dealing with disease or promoting health. For example, the nurse can provide transpersonal caring to a terminally ill client for whom no curative interventions exist. Transpersonal caring allows for nursing that is respectful, honors the client's wishes, and treats the client as an individual worthy of regard even in the act of dying.

Another important contribution of Watson's work is its emphasis on "meaning, relationships, context, and patterns" (Watson, 1985). By focusing on experience as perceived by the individual, Watson views events not in isolation but in terms of their meaning. Suppose, for example, that an elderly client has just died. This event can be viewed in isolation and in purely physiologic terms. However, its meaning to surviving family members may vary. Some family members might see the death as a comforting release while others might view it as cause for sorrow.

Watson's work is limited by its use of terminology that is unfamiliar to many readers. Also, because some of the concepts are hard to quantify and define concretely, its application and related research are problematic.

EVALUATING NURSING THEORIES

Huckabay (1991) suggests that nursing theories meet the following criteria:
- Concepts within the theory are interrelated in a way that provides a different view of a particular phenomenon.
- The theory is logical.

- The theory is relatively simple but also capable of providing generalizations (in other words, applicable to more than one setting).
- The theory provides hypotheses about reality that can be tested by research.
- The theory adds to the body of nursing knowledge through validation by research.
- The theory is useful to nurses in practice.
- The theory is consistent with other knowledge that has been tested and validated.

Huckaby's criteria underscore the importance of theories that are relevant to nursing practice. This introduces a new vision of nursing, one that is understandable yet comprehensive, logical and consistent with other knowledge.

Not all nursing theories may satisfy all of these criteria—especially during early development. However, as theories are applied, tested, confirmed, and integrated into the body of nursing knowledge, they will be evaluated in terms of their usefulness in advancing nursing knowledge, aiding nursing practice, and guiding nursing research.

LINKING THEORY, RESEARCH, AND NURSING PRACTICE

Theory, research, and nursing practice have reciprocal interrelationships; each affects and is affected by the other. For example, phenomena observed in nursing practice might give rise to concepts and understandings, which might, in turn, lead to formal hypotheses that can be tested by nursing research. Results of such research, in turn, might influence theory by confirming or failing to confirm the concepts and propositions of the theory.

Nursing theory influences nursing practice by providing a framework for action. Using a nursing model or theory "enables the nurse to see a unified view of the client" (Huckabay, 1991). The framework provides the structure within which assessments are made, as well as categorization and terminology for nursing diagnosis, intervention, and evaluation. Nursing theory provides a view of the world and a way of understanding the client, health, environment, and nursing itself (Huckabay, 1991).

Nursing theories also can be used as a framework for nursing research. Theory helps to identify important areas of study, to determine how such studies might proceed, and to determine how to interpret results of the studies. A nurse-researcher using Orem's theory might look for evidence of a previously unrecognized self-care deficit in adolescent mothers. The theory provides the basis for analyzing the situation and designing a study that would identify the various types of self-care deficits present; it then would provide the framework for presenting and interpreting data. An outcome might be identification of previously unrecognized and unmet needs—for example, the need for the adolescent to have time and a secure setting in which to be an adolescent and not necessarily a mother.

Nursing theories can prove helpful in education by providing information about the practice of nursing. They also can be used as conceptual frameworks for understanding the teaching and learning processes.

However, despite the advantages of using theory as a basis for nursing practice, education, and research, this happens less frequently than would be the case ideally. Causes for this include lack of familiarity with nursing theories and models by practicing nurses, lack of resources of health care facilities to undertake the training of all nursing staff in use of a particular model, and lack of agreement on which model to use in a particular setting. In addition, the degree of abstraction and lack of concreteness in some theories makes it difficult to apply them in practice or research.

SUMMARY

Nursing theories have guided nursing since the time of Florence Nightingale. Initially based on identifying client needs, they have progressed to focus on the nurse-client interaction and provide new ways of examining the four concepts central to nursing: caring, client, health, and environment.

Theories that focus on nursing outcomes are being applied in practice and research settings today and continue to provide the framework for nurses who function in many diverse roles.

APPLICATION EXERCISE

Based on one of the theories discussed in the chapter, describe a recent client-care situation, in which you were responsible for the client's overall care, in terms of the four basic concepts of nursing.

Client: Describe the client according to the theory you have selected.

Health: Discuss health issues according to the theory selected.

Environment: Discuss environmental issues according to the theory selected.

Caring/nursing: Summarize your role as the care-giver, according to the theory selected.

REVIEW QUESTIONS

1. How does nursing theory affect nurses in practice?

2. Using the concept of health, compare and contrast the theories of Orem and Roy.

3. Using the concept of caring (nursing), compare and contrast the theories of Rogers and Watson.

4. What problems might arise for the nurse who wishes to use nursing theory in practice?

5. How does nursing theory affect nursing practice and nursing research?

REFERENCES

American Nurses Association. (1980). *Nursing: A Social Policy Statement.* Kansas City, MO: Author

Abdellah, G., Beland, I., Martin, A., and Matheney, R. (1961). *Patient-centered Approaches to Nursing.* New York: Macmillan.

Bevis, E. (1982). *Curriculum Building in Nursing: A Process* (3rd ed.). St. Louis: Mosby.

Deloughery, G. (1991). *Issues and Trends in Nursing.* St. Louis: Mosby-Yearbook.

Dickoff, J., and James, P. (1968). "Theory of theories: A position paper." *Nursing Research,* 17(3): 197-203.

Fawcett, J. (1989). "Nursing conceptual frameworks." In J. Riehl-Sisca (Ed.), *Conceptual Models for Nursing Practice,* (3rd ed.). Norwalk: Appleton and Lange.

Fry, S. (1991). "The ethic of caring: Can it survive in nursing?" In R. Ismert, E. Arnold, and V. Carson, *Concepts Fundamental to Nursing.* Springhouse, PA: Springhouse Corp.

Hall, A., and Fagan, R. (1968). "Definition of a system." In W. Buckley (ed.), *Modern Systems Research for the Behavioral Scientist.* Chicago: Aldine Publishing Co.

Henderson, V. (1966). *The Nature of Nursing.* New York: Macmillan.

Ismert, R., Arnold, E., and Carson, V. (1991). *Concepts Fundamental to Nursing,* Springhouse, PA: Springhouse Corp.

Johnson, D. (1967). "Professional practice in nursing." In National League for Nursing, *The Shifting Scene: Directions for Practice.* NLN Publication #15-1252. New York: Author.

Johnson, D. (1974). "Development of theory: A requisite for nursing as a primary health profession." *Nursing Research,* 23(5), 372-377.

King, I. (1971). *Toward A Theory of Nursing: General Concepts of Human Behavior.* New York: John Wiley.

King, I. (1981). *A Theory for Nursing: Systems, Concepts, Processes.* New York: John Wiley.

Kuriansky, J., Gurland, B. Fleiss, J., and Cowan, D. (1976). "The assessment of self-care capacity in geriatric patients by objective and subjective methods." *Journal of Clinical Psychology,* 32, 95-102.

Leddy, S., and Pepper, J. (1989). *Conceptual Bases of Professional Nursing.* Philadelphia: Lippincott.

Leininger, M. (1978). *Transcultural Nursing Concepts, Theories, and Practices.* New York: John Wiley.

Leininger, M. (1990). "The phenomenon of caring: Importance, research questions and theoretical considerations." In R. Ismeurt, E. Arnold, and V. Carson, *Concepts Fundamental to Nursing.* Springhouse, PA: Springhouse Corp.

Levine, M. (1967). "The four conservation principles of nursing." *Nursing Forum,* 6:45-59.

Levine, M. (1973). *Introduction to Clinical Nursing* (2nd ed.). Philadelphia, F.A. Davis.

Meleis, A. (1985). *Theoretical Nursing: Development and Progress.* Philadelphia: Lippincott.

Nightingale, F. (1859). *Notes on Nursing: What it is, and what it is not.* London: Harrison and Sons. (1966 facsimile edition. Philadelphia: Lippincott.)

Orem, D. (1959). *Guides for Developing Curriculae for the Education of Practical Nurses.* Washington, D.C.: U.S. Department of Health, Education, and Welfare, Office of Education.

Orem, D. (1980). *Nursing: Concepts of Practice* (2nd ed.). New York: McGraw-Hill.

Orlando, I. (1961). *The Dynamic Nurse-Patient Relationship.* New York: G.P. Putnam's Sons.

Peplau, H. (1952). *Interpersonal Relations in Nursing.* New York: G.P. Putnam's Sons.

Riehl, J., and Roy, C. (1980). *Conceptual Models for Nursing Practice* (2nd ed.). New York: Appleton-Century-Crofts.

Rogers, M. (1970). *An Introduction to the Theoretical Basis of Nursing.* Philadelphia: F.A. Davis.

Rogers, M. (1980). "Nursing: A science of unitary man." In J. Riehl and C. Roy (eds.), *Conceptual Models for Nursing Practice* (2nd ed.). New York: Appleton-Century-Crofts.

Roy, C. (1971). "Adaptation: A conceptual framework for nursing." *Nursing Outlook,* 19(4), 254-257.

Roy, C. (1976). *Introduction to Nursing: An Adaptation Model.* Englewood Cliffs, N.J.: Prentice-Hall.

Stevens, B. (1984). *Nursing Theory: Analysis, application, evaluation.* Boston: Little, Brown.

Walker, L., and Avant, K. (1983). *Strategies for Theory Construction in Nursing.* Norwalk, CT: Appleton-Century-Crofts.

Watson, J. (1979). *Nursing: The Philosophy and Science of Caring.* Boston: Little, Brown.

Watson, J. (1985). *Nursing: Human Science and Human Care.* Norwalk, CT: Appleton-Century-Crofts.

Veatch, R., and Fry, S. (1987). *Case Studies in Nursing Ethics.* Philadelphia: Lippincott.

RECOMMENDATIONS FOR FURTHER STUDY

Fleury, J. "The Application of Motivational Theory to Cardiovascular Risk Reduction." *Image,* 24(3):229-239, Fall 1992.

Gilliss, C. (1991). "Family nursing research, theory and practice." *Image,* 22(4), 19-22, Spring.

Gortner, S. (1990). "Nursing values and science: Towards a science of philosophy." *Image,* 22(2) 101-105, Spring.

Morse, J., Solberg, S., Neander, W., Bottorff, J., and Johnson, J. (1990). "Concepts of caring and caring as a concept." *Advances in Nursing Science,* 13(1), 1-14.

Smith, M.C. "The Contribution of Nursing Theory to Nursing Administration Practice." *Image,* 25(1):63-67, Spring 1993.

Watson, J. (1990). "Caring knowledge and informed moral passion." *Advances in Nursing Science,* 13(3), 15-24.

How Organizations Are Structured

Objectives

After studying this chapter, the reader should be able to:

1. List the various approaches to the study of organizational structure.

2. Discuss the characteristics of a bureaucracy.

3. Compare and contrast the human relations, contingency, and systems approaches to analyzing organizational structure.

4. Discuss the various types and roles of groups in organizations, including primary and reference groups.

5. Analyze emerging organizational structures, such as nursing centers and magnet hospitals, in terms of their departure from typical bureaucratic models.

6. Discuss the implications of the American Nurses Association call for restructuring the health care delivery system (as it would affect clients and nurses).

Introduction

Successful organizations are those that can attract and keep highly skilled and motivated workers, produce a valued, sought-after product, and remain financially sound. Unsuccessful organizations, in contrast, are plagued with high staff turnover and discontent, have trouble attracting customers or clients, and are always teetering on the verge of financial calamity.

An important factor contributing to the success of an organization is its structure. Reitz (1987) defines structure as "a system that defines the division of labor and specialization and coordinates the relationships within an organization." Division of labor refers to the breakdown of a task into discrete subunits. In an acute-care hospital, for example, the task—providing client care—is broken down into such subunits as the business department, laboratory, maintenance department, and department of nursing services.

Once division of labor has been accomplished, worker specialization can occur. For instance, nurses receive special preparation for their responsibilities and employees in other subunits receive similar specialized preparation for their jobs. Thus, organizational structure specifies the way in which the various jobs within an organization are defined and identifies how those responsible for such jobs should interact.

The most concrete representation of an organization's structure is the organizational chart, which names the positions or individuals responsible for specific functions and identifies the relationships among them. In the broadest sense, structure also includes the rules, policies, and communication networks that govern these interactions.

This chapter examines various theories of organizational structure and traces the historical development of our understanding of organizational structure, beginning with classical organizational theory. Then it explores structure from the perspectives of the human relations school, the Carnegie approach, the Theory Y approach, the contingency approach, and the modern systems approach, and examines the role of groups as an important structural subset of organizations. The chapter concludes by discussing trends in the organizational structure of health care. The application exercise at the end of the chapter focuses on examining communication as one component of organizational structure from the viewpoint of classical bureaucratic or systems approaches.

COMPLEXITY, CENTRALIZATION, AND FORMALIZATION

The structure of an organization can be studied in terms of three basic characteristics: complexity, centralization, and formalization.

COMPLEXITY

Complexity refers to the degree of specialization and division of labor. A small nursing referral company with one manager and twelve registered nurses requires a much less complex organization than the typical acute-care hospital. One measure of complexity is *differentiation,* which can be horizontal or vertical. Horizontal differentiation refers to role differences based on levels of responsibility. The small nursing referral company may have two levels of vertical differentiation, manager and nurse. The large acute-care hospital, in contrast, may have many vertical levels of differentiation, ranging from head nurses to supervising nurses to director of nursing services and, finally, vice president for nursing and ancillary services.

Horizontal differentiation refers to role differences at the same level of responsibility. The large organization typically has greater horizontal differentiation than the small organization. In the latter, each employee has a similar responsibility and can substitute for one another as needed. The large organization has many employee classifications, which are divided into different departments and subunits. In the health care facility, these departments and subunits typically include the emergency department, medical department, pediatric department, and many other non-nursing departments.

CENTRALIZATION

Centralization refers to the degree to which authority is held by managers at the highest levels. In an organization that is highly centralized, most decision making occurs at the upper management level and decisions are communicated to employees at lower levels of the hierarchy. In a decentralized organization, decisions are made at the lowest level possible by those managers most closely involved with the issue at hand.

The benefit of centralized authority is greater control; decisions made by only a few managers are easier to monitor and evaluate. The drawbacks of centralization include the stress it places on high-level managers to make all decisions and the inflexibility that results when all decisions are made at the highest level. Also, centralized authority tends to diminish individual autonomy and may reduce employee morale if independence of action is seen as a desirable job characteristic.

Decentralization, on the other hand, allows a flexible response because each manager can make immediate decisions without going up the chain of command. It also leads to more equitable burden sharing in decision making.

Some experts believe decentralization puts less control in the hands of top management. In a centralized organization, decision-making powers are reserved for the highest levels of management. In a decentralized structure, decisions are made by those at lower levels of authority, potentially without the consultation of persons at higher levels.

FORMALIZATION

Formalization is the degree to which an organization regulates such things as schedules, manner of dress, and even employee interactions. A highly formalized organization may specify how employees at different levels are expected to dress; for instance, in a large health care facility, department heads may be expected to wear suits or dresses and all employees below that level may be expected to wear appropriate uniforms. Nurses may have to wear white uniforms, perhaps all of the same type and style; laboratory personnel may have to wear yellow; housekeeping personnel may have to wear blue.

In a less formalized organization, workers typically can choose their own style of dress as long as they meet basic requirements. For instance, nurses may be able to wear any type of uniform as long as it allows them to care competently for clients and projects a professional appearance.

In many highly formalized organizations, time cards are used to ensure that all employees arrive at work at the required time. In less formalized organizations, employees may be expected to work a specified number of hours but schedules are somewhat flexible. Obviously, health care facilities, which value continuity of care, have a greater need for formalized schedules than other types of organizations.

In highly formalized organizations, interactions between employees at different levels may be regimented. Commonly, titles or position names are used in communications between levels, and interactions tend to be formal. Typically, interactions between nurses and physicians in a large medical center typically are more formal than in a small rural clinic. For example, consider how the problem of inadequate pharmacy support during evening hours might be addressed; the nursing department might request that the pharmacy add staff members, while the pharmacy department suggests that nursing staff take on additional responsibilities. The large health care facility might address the problem in an interdisciplinary committee, selecting committee members through a formal process. During a committee meeting, participants might be addressed formally, such as "Dr. Michael Stevenson from the pharmacy" and "Ms. Jill Hunter, night supervisor for the medical unit." After an agenda is set and the issue discussed at the meeting, the committee might make a recommendation to the appropriate administrator. This person might decide to add a pharmacy aide from 4 to 7 P.M.; this decision then would be communicated through formal channels to all involved parties.

In contrast, in the small rural clinic, Michael Stevenson and Jill Hunter might discuss the issue privately over coffee in the staff meeting room. In other words, the individuals who discuss and solve the problem would be self-selected, and communication would be direct and informal. The two staff members might suggest to the administrator than an hourly aide be added on the busiest evenings; this administrator might communicate the decision to other staff members through regular channels.

Typically, large organizations have formalized expectations for behavior because authority is centralized and differentiation of horizontal and vertical authority and responsibility are formal.

In the large health care facility, staffing decisions typically are made at higher levels of authority because of the centralized approach to decision making and vertical differentiation of authority. Responsibilities of the nursing staff and pharmacy staff are differentiated horizontally. The smaller health care facility, in contrast, typically has a decentralized approach; the employees who are directly involved in an issue are responsible for addressing the problem themselves. Vertical and horizontal differentiation of authority are minimal.

HISTORICAL APPROACHES TO ORGANIZATIONAL STRUCTURE

The early Sumerians were the first to describe organizational structure and function. Luthans (1985) attributes much of the success of early Roman and Egyptian civilization to managers who developed effective organizational structure and processes. In modern times, the first important theory of organizational structure was the classical theory.

CLASSICAL THEORY

During the great industrial expansion of the nineteenth century, manufacturing and services became centralized in cities and towns. As the number of manufacturing workers grew, a class of employees evolved whose task mainly was to manage workers; this class consisted of managers. Organizations began to take on characteristics that maximized efficiency. To develop their structure, many borrowed from the military and the church. Industry adopted the structure of military troops, which divided into squads or platoons, then companies, battalions, regiments and divisions—each with a separate leader with specific responsibilities up and down the chain of command. In industry, subunits took on specific functions and were headed by a leader who had defined responsibilities to those up and down the corporate chain of command.

One of the first important analysts of this developing structure was Frederick Taylor, whose book *The Principles of Scientific Management* was published in 1911. Taylor began his career as a pattern-maker and machinist in a small shop. As a middle-level manager, he became interested in task design and efficiency when a dispute with workers erupted at the Midvale Steel Company in 1880 over what constituted a day's work. As a result of the dispute, Taylor began to analyze the components of work and identify the most efficient ways to perform a task.

Taylor's approach was to study the task to be performed, then design the organization accordingly to permit maximal efficiency. He proposed that every job could be analyzed scientifically to identify its components, and the work could be standardized by studying the motions required to produce it. In other words, he came up with a specific description of a job to be done or a product to be made and identified it as a standard; then he analyzed the job to identify the most efficient way to accomplish the task. Taylor then proposed that workers be selected and trained specifically for these highly structured tasks. He proposed that employers encourage workers by offering incentives and removing obstacles that impede their productivity.

Other pioneering scientific managers of the day, Frank Gilbreth and Henry Gantt, took Taylor's concept further, developing time and motion studies that broke down even the smallest tasks into individual physical motions, which then were analyzed to eliminate repetitive or inefficient patterns. This led to development of highly structured individual tasks within highly structured organizations.

Another person who influenced classical theory was Henri Fayol, whose book *Administration Industrielle et Generale* was published in 1916. A French engineer and geologist, Fayol did mining and geological research before becoming head of Comambault, a French firm on the verge of bankruptcy. With his management skills and understanding of the work environment, Fayol reversed the decline of the company, which subsequently contributed significantly to the French effort in World War I. After the war, he wrote and spoke extensively about his theories on organizational management.

Fayol proposed five guidelines for organizations:

- Plan for the future.
- Devise a structure that allows the organization to provide resources to implement its plan.
- Develop a command structure to implement the plan, selecting and leading the workers.
- Develop coordinating structures that permit actions and energies to promote attainment of the organizational goal.
- Develop control structures that allow verification of progress.

A command structure is a structure of authority and responsibility. A coordinating structure is a structure that promotes, supports, and encourages cooperation in reaching the organizational goal. Control structures are checkpoints and assessments that ensure that an organization is accomplishing its aims.

Fayol's guidelines—commonly summarized as *foresight, organization, command, coordination, and control*—resemble the steps of the nursing process. They start with development of a plan to meet specific goals, proceed to plans for implementation, and end with ongoing assessment (evaluation) to ensure that the plan is being followed successfully. Max Weber, the German sociologist, termed this developing organizational form *bureaucracy*. With some modifications, the bureaucratic structure remains the dominant form of organizational structure in health care facilities.

Robey (1986) suggests that 10 factors be considered when describing organizational structure. The following discussion of classical structure examines these factors in depth.

Division of labor. A bureaucracy fosters increased specialization, with workers having responsibility for specific parts of the overall task. At its best, division of labor allows workers to learn an individual task well and perform it with skill. However, task repetition, even when done skillfully, can contribute to decreasing attention and boredom and may cause job burnout.

In health care facilities, where increasing job specialization has been necessary, task repetition in isolation is blamed for staff turnover. In the operating room, for example, where task specialization and standardization are pronounced, nurses may feel disengaged from clients, whom they see for only a brief period; they may never learn the outcome of a client's surgery and may feel divorced from the larger picture of client care. On the other hand, specialization does allow development of highly trained specialists who can perform complex tasks with skill and precision—a crucial factor in operating-room nursing.

Standardization of tasks. A second characteristic of bureaucracies is a narrow division of labor in which job descriptions specify rather precisely how tasks are to be performed and who is authorized to perform them. In health care, this has led to fairly precise job descriptions; consider typical nursing procedure manuals, which delineates how a specific task is to be performed and which type of nurse (such as registered nurse, licensed vocational nurse, or certified nurse anesthetist) can perform it. A procedure manual may specify exactly how to care for I.V. sites, how often to change them, what solution to use to clean the skin, what type of bandage to use, and even how to affix tape to secure the dressing.

The advantage of task standardization is that it ensures that all employees perform tasks the same way, giving a high degree of predictability. The drawback is that it gives individual workers little discretion to adapt a task to different conditions.

Hierarchy of authority. Within a bureaucratic organization, decision making is highly regulated. The right to make decisions is a function of authority, which usually is centralized. As operations within an organization become more complex, levels of decision-making structure are added vertically; thus, over time, decision makers become increasingly removed from employee activity. For example, a small clinic may have three physicians, a nursing staff, and a general manager. If it expands, a nursing coordinator may be hired, adding a new level of decision maker. If the clinic evolves into a general hospital, it might hire a director of nursing services, further expanding the decision-making structure vertically.

In bureaucratic health care facilities, this distance from the client's bedside may contribute to unrealistic decisions that do not reflect the needs and constraints of practicing nurses. The advantage of hierarchical authority is that fewer decision-makers have greater control.

Equality of authority and responsibility. In bureaucracies, each employee who is responsible for a specific task has sufficient authority to accomplish it. Thus, an emergency department supervisor who is responsible for revising policies on staffing assignments typically has the authority to implement those assignment changes deemed necessary.

The benefit of equal authority and responsibility is that managers are not held responsible for outcomes they cannot control. Additionally, an employee given appropriate authority can he held accountable for accomplishing those tasks that fall within the purview of that responsibility.

Unity of command. This principle recognizes the importance of having each employee report to only one manager. Unity of command helps keep lines of authority clear and promotes orderly decision making. It results in the pyramidal structure typical of bureaucracies: the chief executive officer stands at the top, or apex, of the pyramid, middle-level managers at the middle, and remaining employees at the base.

In some organizations, notably acute-care facilities, unity of command is a matter of policy. An employee who has a concern must follow the chain of command, going to the immediate supervisor before broaching the matter with someone of higher authority. Take, for instance, an operating-room nurse who believes that a particular piece of equipment is unreliable. The nurse is responsible for bringing this matter to the attention of the nursing supervisor of the operating room; the nursing supervisor, in turn, may contact the maintenance department or the equipment company representative.

The advantage of unity of command is that employees know precisely to whom they are responsible. The disadvantage is that an unresponsive manager may be hard to circumvent. For example, the nurse needing a new part for a piece of equipment might find it easier to go directly to the department responsible for maintenance rather than through the O.R. manager, especially if the manager doesn't share the nurse's sense of urgency to have the equipment repaired.

Span of control. This refers to the number of employees over whom a supervisor has authority. To ensure close control and coordination, classical theorists recommend that this number not exceed seven (Robey, 1986). With more than seven employees, inefficiency may result because the manager cannot effectively oversee and evaluate the performance of all the employees. The importance of this principle is clear in health care environments today; as staff is reduced and nurse-managers assume responsibility for an increasing number of employees, efficiency and control may be compromised.

Line and staff differentiation. Employees with *line* authority are those with formal responsibility to make decisions. However, in some cases, information from sources outside the chain of command is necessary. These advisory sources, called *staff*, provide information and advice that assist line managers, who retain authority and responsibility. The nursing consultant, for instance, most commonly has staff responsibility, providing information about a particular client care situation—for example, wound care management—which then is used by the nurse-manager and staff nurses in making decisions about care.

Poor differentiation between line and staff responsibilities may cause confusion over who is in charge. Classical theory holds that formal assignment ensures clear differentiation between line and staff responsibilities. On many organizational charts, employees with staff responsibility are indicated by dotted lines, indicating that they have advisory—but not supervisory or decision-making—responsibility.

Decentralization. In a bureaucracy, each supervisor is responsible for the most important decisions—those necessary to retain control over crucial functions. Other decisions are delegated to managers closer to the operational level. This principle operates in tension with the principle of hierarchy of authority. In an effective organization, appropriate decentralization helps ensure that decisions are made by those with the most knowledge about the given situation; it also prevents supervisors at higher levels of the hierarchy from being overwhelmed with responsibility for a great number of decisions.

As described above, some organizations seek to maximize control by stipulating that decisions be made at the highest level and by minimizing decentralization. However, this can be inefficient if it results in decision making based on inadequate information about the specific circumstances involved. Although many researchers have criticized bureaucracies on these grounds, classical theory itself does identify appropriate decentralization as crucial to organizational effectiveness.

An ongoing concern for health care facilities is the degree to which control should be decentralized. Many newer organizational structures for health care facilities, described later in this chapter, emphasize a decentralized approach—both in terms of health care delivery and supervision of employees.

Departmentation. Large organizations, such as the typical health care facility, divide employees into subgroups to promote functioning. Departmentation may be made on the basis of process, purpose (or product), or clients served.

Where departmentation is by process, employees are organized by function. In the acute-care facility, larger differentiations usually are based on process; the facility is divided into smaller departments each with a specific function (such as the business, nursing and personnel departments).

In health care settings, departmentation by purpose and product resembles departmentation by process; the product, or purpose, is the provision of, for example, business services, nursing services, or personnel services. In organizations with more concrete products, departmentation according to product would produce departments responsible for each type of equipment, such as I.V. controllers, tubing, and solutions.

The third form of departmentation is by clients served. A health care facility reflects this type of departmentation through its division of nursing services into the medical unit, intensive care unit, emergency department, and other self-contained nursing units. Within each department and subdivision, the classical theory of organizational structure and function are applies.

Management processes. In addition to the structural characteristics discussed in the preceding nine points, some classical organizational theorists have described specific management activities necessary for effective operation. An example is Fayol's five rules of management, described earlier.

In an organization with classical structure, required tasks are identified, a structure in which tasks are carefully integrated is developed, and supervisors are given responsibility and authority to issue orders that are passed down the chain of command; each employee is held responsible for an individual part of the overall task (Luthans, 1985).

Although classical structure has many strengths, its weaknesses are many. Employees may feel like cogs in a machine; the focus on production and efficiency may make them feel that the company does not value their own interests and well-being. When employees are dissatisfied, managers in such an organization may have little recourse but to try to coerce them to conform with expectations through the use of hierarchical power.

Human Relations Approach

In the 1930s, recognizing the limits of classical organizational theory, the developing human relations school began to focus on the social and emotional aspects of organizations

(Robey, 1986). The human relations school got its name from its focus on the human dimensions of work rather than tasks to be performed. In the 1920s, Mary Parker Follett, an early advocate of this approach, proposed a version of participative management that allowed managers and workers to work according to mutual agreement (Sullivan and Decker, 1988). In her model, management and workers would agree mutually on what tasks workers should accomplish and how they would benefit. Follett proposed that this approach would increase productivity by giving employees a personal stake in achieving mutually developed goals.

An early study undertaken in the 1920s and 1930s showing the importance of the human element in organizational productivity involved the Chicago Hawthorne plant of Western Electric Company. Now known as the Hawthorne studies, they were performed with the intent of measuring the effect of lighting on productivity.

Under the assumptions of classical theory, an optimal level of illumination could be identified that would allow the greatest contribution to efficiency. However, instead of finding one optimal level, the researchers found wide fluctuations in productivity at different levels of illumination. Although they investigated other factors that could have contributed to such variation, they failed to find any that had a strong correlation to productivity. Finally, they determined that the study itself produced the variation; by focusing on and showing interest in the employees, the researchers had motivated them to perform at a higher level of productivity.

This effect now is called the Hawthorne effect—the effect of the experiment or study itself on the object under study. (Today, a similar result might occur if researchers investigated whether nurses appropriately discarded needles in "sharps" containers without recapping. The novelty of the study and interest in the phenomenon might increase the incidence of proper disposal.) Soon researchers demonstrated the effects of other factors on productivity, identifying them as psychological factors. Such factors might include employees' perception that they were valued by management and employee satisfaction in work.

Thus, the human relations school recognized that studying the mechanics of production is insufficient and that human factors also must be considered. This school suggested that organizational effectiveness is influenced not only by structural considerations but also by employees' personal needs, values, goals, and aspirations.

Studies conducted during the 1940s and 1950s compared the effects of democratic leadership on production. With democratic leadership, employees participate in decision making; with authoritarian leadership, managers are autocratic and coercive. Results of these studied found that democratic leadership was more effective. Management scientist Chester Barnard, working in the 1940s and 1950s, suggested that employees who feel that an order is unreasonable cannot be coerced into complying with it; thus, the success of an authoritarian structure relies on the employee's willingness to follow the order.

Subsequently, new approaches to organization structure were developed that considered human, or psychological, factors; these approaches influenced the development of the Carnegie approach and the Theory Y approach described below.

CARNEGIE APPROACH

The Carnegie approach to organizational structure was developed at the Carnegie Institute of Technology during the 1950s and 1960s by a diverse group of scholars, including James March and Herbert Simon. While acknowledging that the approach of the human relations school improved organizational effectiveness, these scholars focused on the decision-making behavior of individuals rather than on employee satisfaction. They proposed that organizational structure should control how individual decisions are made and that this characteristic would maximize organizational efficiency.

The Carnegie approach focuses on three main aspects of decision making: distribution of information, conflict resolution, and the influence of organizational goals on decision making.

Distribution of information. The classical (bureaucratic) approach to decision making emphasizes responsibility for decision making and lines of authority. The Carnegie approach, in contrast, recognizes that the internal flow of information also affects the decision-making ability of employees at different levels. By appropriately withholding or providing information, organizations can more effectively and less obtrusively dictate who makes what decision. For example, a health care organization considering a change in staffing patterns might determine that this decision should be made by managers at the supervisory level. Information about client, census, staffing patterns, and similar data would be shared with management staff at this level but would not involve employees below that level.

Informal channels of communication and the difficulty deciding at which level information should be withheld make information management a challenge. Lower-level employees may have important input that is not available to management if they are not involved in information distribution.

Conflict resolution. Both classical organizational theory and the human relations school view conflict as dysfunctional. The Carnegie school, in contrast, sees conflict as a natural outgrowth of mutual decision making and as an issue that should be resolved through bargaining, with the involved parties agreeing on a compromise that accomplishes some of the aims of each party.

Organizational goals. In organizations with classical structure, upper-level managers are responsible for goals and design tasks and train employees to accomplish these goals. Organizations with a structure based on the human relations model recognize that employee satisfaction plays a role in achieving goals by promoting or inhibiting goal attainment. With the Carnegie approach, however, goals are set by both employees and managers through bargaining processes that recognize both organizational and individual goals.

Theory Y approach

Behavioral scientist Douglas McGregor was among the first to explore the potential conflict between organizational requirements and individual goals. In his influential book, *The Human Side of Enterprise* (1960), he compared two approaches to organizational design, which he identified as the Theory X and Theory Y approaches. Theory X is the classic bureaucratic approach; Theory Y advocates democratic participation of employees (participative leadership) and less job specialization; participative leadership allows employees to share in decision making and is an important motivator of employee effort.

McGregor suggested that different assumptions underlie Theory X and Theory Y approaches to organizational structure. Theory Y assumes that employees want to perform at an optimal level and do not avoid work. Consequently, the basic approach to employees differs from that of the Theory X organization. Theory Y organizations allow employees to analyze the structure of their jobs and to suggest changes— not only in their own responsibilities but also within the organization as a whole. In a Theory Y organization, the focus of management is to promote and support; in a Theory X organization, the focus is to control and police.

The Theory Y organization assumes that employees as are imaginative, creative, and ingenious as managers. Therefore, its structure allows employees to contribute to management decisions, greatly increasing the pool of ideas and solutions. The Theory X organization, in contrast, assumes that employees would rather be told what to do.

Scanlon organizations are examples of the Theory Y approach in practice. Joseph Scanlon, associated with the steelworkers' union movement and later with the Massachusetts Institution of Technology, worked for collaborative union-management approaches to problems. The approach that he developed during the 1940s sought to integrate the goals of both employees and the organization in a way that promoted the interests of both parties. The organizational structure based on Scanlon's approach recognizes that indi-

THEORY X AND THEORY Y ASSUMPTIONS

Theory X and Theory Y are based on different assumptions of people as human beings and as workers. Theory X emphasizes the need to control individuals; Theory Y, the need to encourage and support them.

THEORY X ASSUMPTIONS	THEORY Y ASSUMPTIONS
Human beings dislike work	Work is natural
Human beings avoid responsibilities	Human beings seek responsibility, are creative, and are underutilized
Workers must be coerced and policed	Workers are self-directed and self-motivated

vidual and organizational goals are more likely to be accomplished when employees have a high investment in meeting their own goals for self-advancement and achievement and when the organization's objectives include meeting these employee goals.

Two hallmarks of Scanlon organizations are cost-reduction sharing and group contribution to organizational effectiveness. Cost-reduction sharing programs encourage employees to devise ways for the organization to save money—either by altering work processes or by making changes in consumables (items consumed in production). In a health care setting, for instance, an employee might suggest a change in reporting forms that could reduce redundancy and save time or identify a cheaper, dependable substitute for routinely used supplies. All employees share in the savings resulting from the changes on a monthly basis.

This differs in several ways from the practice of awarding bonuses to individual employees who make cost-saving suggestions. It lets all employees share equally in any successful cost-reduction, eliminating the need for secrecy and promoting idea sharing; also, it allows employees to reap monetary benefits on a continuing monthly basis.

The second feature of Scanlon organizations is the formation of groups or committees to identify ways to enhance productivity and efficiency and to contribute to cost reduction. Based on the view that all employees are innovative, creative, self-disciplined, and willing to assume responsibility, these groups include employees from every level and section of the organization. In a health care setting, for instance, staff nurses from the medical unit might collaborate with pharmacists, physicians, laboratory technicians, and managers to examine ways to reduce the cost of caring for a specific type of client treated on the medical unit. The resulting cost reductions would be shared by all employees in the facility.

This use of all components of the structure to evaluate and suggest changes to the organization as a whole can lead to other changes as well. Bringing together employees from all hierarchical levels changes relationships among those at different levels. Interdependence of individuals and departments is appreciated more readily and respect for all forms of work is enhanced. Managers more readily solicit and accept suggestions from employees and are less likely to be seen as having all the answers. The Scanlon approach also helps employees develop a sense of competence and self-control and lets them see their input reflected in organizational change.

CONTINGENCY APPROACH

In contrast to the classical and human relations schools, which propose characteristics of an ideal organizational structure, the contingency approach suggests that the ideal structure may vary—or be contingent—on many variables.

English industrial sociologist Joan Woodward was among the first to demonstrate the effect of one important variable—technological complexity—on organizational structure. Working with English companies, Woodward identified structural differences related to the level of complexity involved in production.

Woodward described three complexity levels—small-batch, large-batch, and continuous-process technology. Custom furniture production is an example of small-batch technology; a commercial bakery is an example of large-batch technology; and an oil refinery is an example of continuous-process technology. Woodward discovered a direct relationship between technological complexity and organizational structure, suggesting that "one particular form of organization was most appropriate to each system of production" (Woodward, 1965).

The impact of technology on nursing and health care is obvious. As use of technology increases, health care facilities must develop policies regarding the proper use of technology and which people should be permitted to use which forms of technology. Additional management structure is needed to supervise the training and evaluation of staff members designated as appropriate users of a specific technology. Even in less technologically based settings, such as home care and community health care, the increasing acuity of clients has led to a commensurate increase in the complexity of organizational structure. The type of structure adapted by a particular health care agency may depend on the level of complexity of technology.

Other contingency theorists identified additional factors that influence organizational structure, including size and environment. Lawrence and Lorsch (1967) pointed out the importance of size and environment. Large organizations require additional managers, generally arranged in a hierarchical fashion. A small rural community hospital, for instance, is likely to have fewer rules and a more informal approach to operations than a large, metropolitan, corporate-owned hospital. In the community hospital, a small group of managers typically makes most decisions and a small cadre of employees remains with the hospital for long periods. In contrast, the larger facility would typically have policies developed at the corporate as well as local level; while many decisions would be made by on-site managers, often using standard operating procedures, others would be made at the corporate level.

Staff turnover tends to be greater in larger organizations; contributing factors are transfer within the corporation and the ability of larger organizations to tolerate higher turnover.

However, in some cases, high staff turnover results from the perception that the larger organization is insensitive to employee needs.

MODERN SYSTEMS APPROACH

The modern systems approach is based on the work of systems theorist Ludwig von Bertalanffy in the 1950s. Von Bertalanffy described a system as a complex of elements in interaction, comprised of all its subcomponent parts and their properties along with the relationships between those parts (Bertalanffy, 1955).

A system can be closed or open. A closed system is self-contained and exchanges nothing with the surrounding environment. An open system accepts input from the environment; it develops a throughput, or product and sends an output of the product back to the environment. The strength of an open systems approach is its focus on the interaction of component parts operating as a unified whole, exchanging material with the surrounding environment.

A health care facility, which requires the input of clients, staff, and supplies to operate, is an open system. Its throughput is alteration in client health, which it exports back to the environment at the end of the interaction in the form of healthy clients.

The body also is an open system. Taking in food and water, it transforms these substances into other products (throughputs) and exchanges outputs with the environment. Even the process of nursing can be viewed from a systems approach, with client and nurse forming subunits that interact, share energy and goals, and arrive at change.

Systems theory focuses on the various types of systems within an organization, including economic, political, informational, and administrative systems. Systems theorists examine the strategic or most important parts of the system, the nature of the relationships among parts, and the goals that drive the system. Important concepts in systems theory include feedback, steady state, entropy and negative entropy, differentiation, integration, and coordination.

FEEDBACK

Feedback refers to provision of information from the environment that allows the system to regulate itself. In a health care facility, such feedback may include information about trends in consumer activism, the latest surgical equipment, or the shortage of registered nurses. Feedback also refers to information about the operation of the system itself, including how clients perceive their care or how nurses view the facility. Feedback allows the organization to make adjustments in operations to maintain a steady state.

STEADY STATE

Steady state refers to constancy in energy exchange. A system that continually expends more energy than it can take in soon goes bankrupt. Steady state is achieved through self-regulation. A health care facility, for example, tries to hire an appropriate level of staff, buy the necessary amount of supplies, and attract a manageable and profitable number of clients. Excess or deficit in any of these factors throws the system into disarray, such as when a natural disaster creates a large number of casualties requiring treatment or a nursing strike results in an insufficient number of staff.

ENTROPY AND NEGATIVE ENTROPY

Entropy is energy that is "bound," or unavailable for use by the system to do work. Negative entropy, also called negentropy, is energy that can be used by the system. Negative entropy is a measure of the tendency of the system toward order and organization; entropy the measure of the tendency toward disorder (Hazzard, 1971).

Entropy and negative entropy can be examined in several ways. Wasted energy, for example, can be viewed in terms of energy expended by staff members in running errands to the pharmacy to try to compensate for an inadequate transportation system. Energy also can be viewed in a more traditional sense. For instance, if a piece of equipment expends energy in a wasteful manner, this means that the wasted energy also is not available to perform work. An effective system tends toward efficient order, organization, and energy use.

DIFFERENTIATION, INTEGRATION, AND COORDINATION

Differentiation, or development of subgroupings, results from a system's attempts to survive. Systems tend toward growth, differentiation, and specialization. Suppose, for example, that a health care facility works hard to attract new clients. Additional clients create the need for increased staff, which in turn fosters development of differentiated units for specific types of client care.

Other factors—integration and coordination—work to bring the system together so that it operates as a unified whole. For instance, while expanding and developing specialized units, the health care facility also is coordinating and integrating transportation and communication systems that will allow it to function effectively as a whole.

Using the systems approach. To analyze the structure of an organization using the systems approach, we might focus on communication systems within a health care facility. We would examine feedback mechanisms, the steady state, the amount of energy available (negative entropy), the amount of energy unavailable (entropy), and the extent of differentiation and integration. We also would examine the organization's inputs, throughputs, and outputs to the environment.

Consider the case of a nursing unit in the emergency department that has few formally established feedback mechanisms to gauge the effectiveness of its admitting procedures. Suppose the nurses frequently fail to include information about prior admissions when a patient is transferred to the medical floor. Lack of feedback leaves the emergency department staff unaware that this communication deficiency affects the ability of the medical floor staff to admit patients satisfactorily (inputs), assess them and complete admission procedures (throughputs), and export them to the appropriate hospital unit or to the external environment (outputs).

To remedy the situation, emergency department staff could review communications, including admissions processes, in monthly emergency department meetings. To promote more effective communications subsystems, emergency department nurses might incorporate a formal check for previous admission records on the admission and assessment sheet.

McWilliams (1980) describes how systems analysis helped solve a communication problem on a busy 55-bed surgical unit. Nurses had been having trouble relaying messages and passing information to other staff members and patients, and had been wasting time trying to track down information they needed for client care. Using a systems approach to analyze the problem, McWilliams first defined the system and its subparts, then analyzed the unit's current communications system and identified all problem areas. She defined input in the communication subsystem as all the messages, requests, and reports received and processed by the staff members and output as similar messages "transmitted to clients, doctors, visitors and employees on other nursing divisions or in other departments" (McWilliams, 1980).

McWilliams found that the problem area was throughput, where messages were altered, transformed, and made ready for output. She conducted a survey to determine what proportion of time nurses spent on direct client care, indirect client care, and nonoperative time (such as waiting for supplies or people, taking breaks or eating, and attending meetings). She found that the time spent specifically on communications amounted to 8% of the total time of nurses and assistants and 27% of the total time of ward secretaries—a substantial proportion.

After identifying these problem areas, McWilliams devised ways to improve the system. She developed magnetic message boards in centralized locations to list clients' names and room numbers, using a coding system with magnets of different colors and shapes representing common messages (such as to indicate that a urine sample had been ordered or that the client had been transported to the radiology department for X-rays). When the status or location of a particular client changed or a message concerning that client was received, a color-coded magnet was placed next to the client's name. Thus, nurses could tell from a quick glance at the message board whether a client had left for X-rays, had gone to surgery, needed to have a urine specimen taken, or had to be kept on nothing-by-mouth (NPO) status. This information-sharing method made communications on the unit much more effective.

ROLE OF GROUPS IN ORGANIZATIONAL STRUCTURE

A group consists of two or more people who interact, share a common ideology or interest, and consider their relationship a point of uniqueness—that is, they recognize their interaction as a relationship (Reitz, 1987). Groups form for various reasons. As they develop, they become effective or ineffective—from the standpoint both of individual members and the group as a whole. A group may be formal or informal, open or closed.

Groups are important to organizations. Luthans (1985) identifies six ways in which groups affect organizations:

- Groups can accomplish certain tasks that could not be achieved by individuals in isolation.
- Groups have an increased pool of knowledge and skills that can be used to address a task.
- Groups can promote decision-making methods that allow presentation of multiple viewpoints.
- Groups can promote changes in organizational policies and procedures.
- Groups can increase organizational stability and help control employee behavior.
- Groups within organizations also help orient individual members to the organization, provide the chance for group members to learn more about the self, help group members gain new skills and achieve goals they could not achieve on their own, and satisfy the human needs for social acceptance and affiliation.

PRIMARY AND REFERENCE GROUPS

Important types of groups are primary groups and reference groups. Primary groups are groups "characterized by intimate, face-to-face association and cooperation. They are primary in several senses, but chiefly in that they are fundamental in forming the social nature and ideals of the individual" (Cooley, 1911).

Examples of primary groups are the family group and the peer group. Both strongly influence the behavior of group members in developing values and norms. Primary groups are the main agents of socialization, transmitting cultural values, goals, and expectations. An example of a primary group in a health care setting is a group of operating-room nurses who work at the same facility.

Reference groups give individual members a standard for self-evaluation, helping them to determine whether they are functioning at an acceptable level by giving or withholding recognition. Examples of reference groups in a health care setting include a group of experienced critical care nurses in a particular geographic region and a nursing students' clinical group.

According to Reitz (1987), reference groups fulfill two needs. They provide group members with the basis for social comparisons, allowing them to evaluate themselves through comparison with other members; and they provide social validation for the individual's values and beliefs.

Both primary and reference groups help individual members define themselves, their values, and their beliefs and help them determine how successful they have been according to these values, beliefs, and goals.

GROUP FORMATION

Groups form for such reasons as physical proximity, common interests, and mutual benefit of members.

Physical proximity. When members of a potential group have easy access to one another, interaction can take place more easily. The physical structure of an organization can enhance or reduce the likelihood of group formation by encouraging or discouraging interaction. In a health care facility, groups may form within a specific department. If a department is isolated physically, the group may be composed solely of people who work in that department. A good example is the typically close-knit group of operating-room nurses, who are separated from other nurses by physical barriers that reduce traffic and the risk of contamination of their work environment, by schedules that typically differ from those of other nurses, and even by their distinctive clothing.

Common interests. Commonly, individuals who perceive that a group holds values that they share seek to join that group. Common interests can stimulate formation of subgroups within established groups or can lead to the formation of entirely new groups. Whether in settings external or internal to the work environment, common interest enhances group formation.

Membership in groups external to an organization, such as professional organizations, clubs, and churches, may lead to formation of internal groups. For example, volunteers for the American Heart Association may form a subgroup at work to press for increased staff time for cardiac rehabilitation; a church quilting group might meet at lunch to compare and work on handiwork on a quilt commemorating AIDS victims.

Mutual benefit. Groups can bring mutual benefit, such as economic, security, or social benefits. Employees of a particular corporation may form a union that strives to improve wages and working conditions; employees concerned about poor lighting in the company parking lot may join the security committee to press for improved lighting; unmarried employees wishing to interact with other single people may establish an informal lunch group that eats at the same hour.

The desire for status and success also attracts people to groups. A group perceived as having status, being successful, or including members who have status or are successful is more attractive than a group that lacks these qualities. For instance, a weight-loss group whose members have lose weight successfully has more appeal than a group whose members have been less successful.

When deciding whether to join or stay in a group, a person weighs the relative costs and benefits. Obviously, if the benefits of group membership outweigh the costs, that person is more likely to join or stay in the group.

In a formally established group in which membership is expected, however, membership satisfaction plays a major role in group effectiveness in retaining membership. For example, all employees in a particular health care facility may be required to join a certain union. If the benefits associated with union membership (such as equitable wages and safe working conditions) outweigh the costs, the group is likely to persist. If the costs (including dues, required meetings, and expectations for behavior during collective bargaining and strikes) outweigh the benefits, a member may decide to leave the union—even if this means changing jobs.

In some cases, a person is not free to decide whether to remain in a group solely on the basis of satisfaction. Suppose a nurse who belongs to the union at a health care facility is dissatisfied with the union she was forced to join. She does not wish to move to find work elsewhere because she lives in a desirable area and has family members nearby; also, the closest nonunion hospital is 4 hours away. Because relocation is undesirable or impossible, this employee decides to keep her job and remain in the union. Thus, she is dependent on the union (group), despite her dissatisfaction it. Consequently, she may feel less free to voice her concerns and may have less autonomy than she would in a group in which membership is voluntary.

Both satisfaction with and dependence on a group affects how individual members function within a group; this, in turn, affects the larger organization within which the group exists. The more strongly a group shares the organization's goal and the more successfully it promotes the interests of group members and the larger organization, the greater the mutual benefit.

FORMAL AND INFORMAL GROUPS

A group may be formal or informal. Formal groups have officially established goals and responsibilities. An example is an emergency committee of a health care facility, which may be composed of nurses from the emergency department, intensive care unit, and operating room; representatives of nursing management; emergency physicians; and the assistant administrator. Group membership is controlled by policy and responsibilities are laid out formally.

An example of an informal group is a group of nurses who meet weekly during lunch to quilt together. Membership in such a group is established informally and relationships and responsibilities are fluid. Another example is a research interest group composed of any nurse interested in nursing research that meets twice a month to discuss a recently published research article. This group might be slightly more structured than the quilting group; for instance, each nurse might be expected to identify and present an article for discussion once a year, and members might be committed to helping one another gain confidence in interpreting research reports.

OPEN AND CLOSED GROUPS

A group can be open or closed. In a closed group, membership is limited to specific persons or to persons holding specific positions. In an open group, membership is optional and anyone can join, regardless of role or position. Formal groups tend to be closed groups with a static membership.

The benefits of a closed group include stability and continuity, which may allow the group to achieve goals effectively. A drawback is that persons who wish to join a closed group sometimes require a considerable orientation period before they can become fully functioning members. Closed groups also may lack the stimulation of innovative thinking that comes from the contributions of new members.

The benefits of an open group include frequent invigoration with new members and new ideas and the ability of new members to attain status more easily. The disadvantages of an open group is its relative instability, which may hinder achievement of long-term goals.

Developmental Stages of Groups

Groups undergo a developmental process during which members become acquainted; rules and expectations are established, tested, and modified; and the group either coheres or fails to cohere.

During the orientation stage—the initial period after group formation—members typically learn about one another and their orientation to the specified task. Little is done to address the group's specific mission. Anxiety may be high if the group is a formal one or has a timeline to complete a specific task. If a formal leader has not been chosen, one generally emerges during this period. An informal leader is a member who takes over the leadership role to accomplish a task without being appointed formally to that responsibility. Either self-selected or selected by the group, the informal leader emerges because of the need for someone to guide the group's efforts.

The second stage of group formation is marked by conflict as members attempt to resolve differences in opinion about the group's nature and function. At this stage, subgroups representing different viewpoints may form. To make the group effective, members must move beyond this conflict stage to one in which shared values and goals are endorsed.

During the third stage, the cohesion stage, the group perceives itself as a unified body in which members are invested personally. The members are prepared to address appointed tasks and pursue the aims that have been validated jointly.

The fourth stage, maturity, is marked by a shift in attention from the group to the task. Members begin to turn their attention away from the group and toward the external environment. They assess the task to be accomplished and typically go through a period of unrealistic optimism about the group, followed by unrealistic pessimism. Optimism stems from the enthusiasm that follows group formation; pessimism, from the realization that the task at hand will require more effort than the group anticipated. If the group

STAGES OF GROUP DEVELOPMENT

- *Orientation*
- *Conflict*
- *Cohesion*
- *Maturity*

can work through unrealistic optimism and pessimism, it will evolve into a mature group.

According to Reitz (1987), the mature group has four characteristics:

- Individual differences are accepted without being labeled good or bad.
- Any remaining conflict is over substantive issues that are relevant to the group task.
- Decisions are made through discussion that encourages dissent; no attempt is made to coerce unanimity or decision making.
- Members are knowledgeable about the group's processes and their own contribution to the group's functioning.

FUTURE OF ORGANIZATIONAL STRUCTURE

Many innovative structures have been proposed for nursing and health care delivery. The bureaucratic structure traditionally adopted by health care facilities may become less common because it increasingly is viewed as less effective and efficient than other structures.

Reasons for this possible trend include consumer demands for increased access to health care for all persons, the evolution of nursing to full professional status, rapidly accelerating changes in technology and communications, and the growing fiscal crisis in health care. These changes argue for exploration of alternative structures for health care delivery.

CHARACTERISTICS OF SUCCESSFUL HEALTH CARE FACILITIES

One approach to assessing health care organizations and promoting more effective structures stems from Kramer's study (1988) of magnet hospitals—those with reduced staff turnover. Studying how and why these hospitals were able to retain nurses (one of the most important characteristics of a successful health care organization), Kramer found that these facilities had a bias for action, kept the nursing staff close to the client, and promoted autonomy and entrepreneurship.

The bias for action was reflected by decentralized decision making; unlike other hospitals, the magnet hospitals did not require nurses ascend multiple bureaucratic levels to obtain authorization to make changes. Kramer also identified a phenomenon called "chunking," which enhances organizational fluidity and action by breaking tasks into "chunks" assigned to movable teams (often formed on a volunteer basis) with specific tasks. Significantly, magnet hospitals moved nurses in teams, not individually like replaceable parts in the bureaucratic machinery.

Kramer also found that the magnet hospitals kept nurses close to the client (unlike many bureaucratic health care facilities, in which nurses are isolated from clients). In these hospitals, primary care—which maximized interaction with clients—was the major means of nursing care delivery. Nurses gave their clients business cards to help establish a relationship with them. Kramer found a commitment by nurse to provide high-quality care and support of nursing services to give nurses adequate time to provide high-quality care (Kramer, 1988).

Kramer suggested that by promoting autonomy and entrepreneurship, magnet hospitals create an environment that rewards rather than penalizes employee experimentation and risk taking. In contrast to bureaucratic organizations, managers at magnet hospitals expect innovation and creativity from employees at all levels; decentralized decision making allows easier introduction of innovations. Kramer also found that magnet hospitals encourage entrepreneurship (the initiative to develop a new method, approach, or product) and risk taking (such as proposing and obtaining permission to try out new ways of doing things). According to Kramer, the philosophy characterizing many magnet hospitals is that "autonomy includes not only the freedom to act and succeed, but also the freedom to act and fail" (Kramer, 1988).

QUALITIES OF MAGNET HOSPITALS

- *Decentralized decision-making*
- *Emphasis on keeping the nurse close to the client*
- *Promotion of employee autonomy and entrepreneurship*

NURSING CENTERS

Nursing centers, sometimes called community nursing centers or nurse-managed centers, have been hailed by some experts as organizations whose structure gives clients direct access to nursing care. Such centers may be freestanding or associated with schools, health centers, home health agencies, or hospitals. State laws determine whether nurses are permitted to prescribe independently and whether nurses can be reimbursed directly from insuring agencies. Public Law 101-239, passed by the U.S. Congress in 1989, requires states to develop regulation that allows direct reimbursement by Medicaid for certified pediatric nurse practitioners and certified family nurse practitioners when these professionals are legally authorized to act in those states. This is expected to result in clearer regulations at the state level and enhance access to insurers.

Describing nursing centers in rural environments, Barger (1991) states that "using nursing models of health, professional nurses in these centers diagnose and treat human responses to actual and potential health problems, and promote health and optimal functioning among target populations and communities." She describes these centers as client-centered organizations that offer professional, cost-effective care. Such care may include physical assessment, screening, health risk assessment, health teaching, counseling, family planning, prenatal care, and other treatments (including prescribing drugs when authorized).

The advantages of the nursing-center approach to health care include a focus on prevention and education; potential cost-effectiveness; and holistic, client-centered approach. However, such centers continue to battle with insurers, hospitals, and physicians to gain direct reimbursement and the right to function fully within the legally defined nursing role.

EFFECTS OF TECHNOLOGY AND COST

Many traditional health care facilities are reexamining their structures and methods of functioning. According to Strasen (1991), these facilities must adopt several strategies to improve operational efficiency and cost effectiveness to survive

---

ADVANTAGES OF NURSING CENTERS

- *Direct access by clients*
- *Nursing diagnosis and treatment*
- *Client-centered approach*
- *Direct reimbursement of nursing costs*
- *Nursing accountability for client care*
- *Nursing accountability for center operations*
- *Increased nursing autonomy*
- *Increased client advocacy*

in an era of reduced reimbursement and increasing technical complexity. These strategies include flattening the organizational structure, eliminating some management levels, and extending the span of individual managers' control so that no more than four levels of management exist from chief nursing administrator to staff nurse.

Strasen also advocates decentralization of ancillary services and staff (such as radiology transport and laboratory technician staff) to client care units, where they can be cross-trained to provide client care services during down times. Using this strategy, housekeeping, transport, and other technical staff could be responsible for such services as bathing clients and passing dietary trays, in addition to their other duties. Thus, jobs would be redefined, with an emphasis on generalist rather than specialist roles.

Strasen also suggests centralizing supplies in one department, from which they would be transported only once to the point of use. This would eliminate repeated transportation of supplies from receiving points to departments, such as the laboratory or radiology department, followed by retransport to client care areas for use. Thus, supplies would be transported directly from the receiving area to the point of use.

Strasen suggests that budget development include annual staff review to ensure that currently performed tasks are necessary. She advocates a review of the staffing mix and development of staffing formulas that provide appropriate levels of care on a cost-effective basis. Managers would receive a budget based on estimated costs of providing an expected level of service and would be expected to function within that budget.

Strasen points to the cost of increasing technology as a major problem that health care facilities must solve to remain cost-effective. For example, she suggests combining the radiology, computerized tomography, and nuclear medicine departments into one department and decentralizing technicians who transport clients to the client-based unit. This would allow more efficient use of expensive technology, highly trained specialists and technician-level services on the combination unit, and technician-level services on the client care unit.

NURSING'S CALL TO RESTRUCTURE HEALTH CARE

The nursing profession has called for radical restructuring of the American health care delivery system and the organizations that deliver health care. In Nursing's Agenda for Health Care Reform (American Nurses Association, 1991), many major nursing associations, including the American Nurses Association (ANA) and the National League for Nursing (NLN), proposed sweeping changes to address shortcomings of the current health-care delivery system.

Calling for establishment of a core, or basic level, of care, authors of the document recommend the following changes:

- Restructure of the health care system. The restructured system would enhance consumer access by providing primary health care in community-based settings, encouraging consumer responsibility for health care through informed decision making, and promoting use of "the most cost-effective providers and therapeutic options in the most appropriate settings."
- A federally defined standard package of essential health-care services available to all American citizens and residents, provided and financed through an integration of public and private plans and sources. A federally administered health care plan would provide services for the poor. Incentives would be offered to encourage small businesses and persons at risk for insufficient insurance coverage to buy into the plan. At minimum, a private plan would offer the same services as the public plan and could be augmented as a benefit of employment. Employers choosing not to offer private coverage would be required to pay into the public plan.
- Phase-in of essential services. Pregnant women and children would be covered first, along with persons with limited access to health care. Called Healthstart, this program would provide care to the most vulnerable, unprotected population groups.

- Planned change to anticipate health service needs that correlate with changes in national demographics. The authors point out that the traditional approach to health care has been reactive rather than "proactive" and call for research into future health care needs and planning and development of services to meet emerging needs.
- Steps to reduce health care costs. The authors propose required use of managed-care plans, controlled growth of the health care system through prudent planning and resource allocation, development of health care policies based on effectiveness and outcomes research, incentives for consumers to be cost efficient in exercising care options, direct access to a full range of health care providers, and elimination of unnecessarily bureaucratic controls and administrative procedures. (For a discussion of the possible effects of the ANA/NLN document, see Chapter 4, Health care delivery.)

Implementation of these proposed changes would alter the structure of the overall health care delivery system as well as individual organizations within the system. In a typical community, for instance, it might lead to establishment of such innovative structures as nursing centers, in which nurses would provide primary services. Clients would contract with the center on an individual basis; the center would be reimbursed by public or private health care plans. Direct coverage of health care costs would mean that providers would not seek payment at the delivery site. Consumers would have to pay an established deductible amount, beyond which they would not be liable for additional costs of care—even in cases of catastrophic illness.

In acute-care settings, the proposed changes might result in development of collegial health care teams that provide more cost-effective care according to established standards. Thus, restructuring health care services to emphasize prevention and wellness would lead to the emergence of new organizations and delivery systems.

Other consumer and professional organizations also have recommended changes in health care delivery. Although the nature of these changes has not, in all cases, been well defined, the need for change is acknowledged by providers and consumers alike. Restructure of the health care delivery system and health care facilities will provide great opportunities for nurses and the nursing profession to better serve those who currently lack access to the system and those who need more effective access.

SUMMARY

This chapter explored various ways of examining organizational structure. It traced the historical development of the study of organizational structure, beginning with the classical approach, through the human relations school, and the Carnegie approach. It discussed the Theory Y, contingency, and systems approaches to organizational analysis. It examined the role of groups within organizations and discussed proposed innovations in health care delivery, including nurse-managed centers and magnet hospitals. It presented professional proposals for restructuring of health care delivery and implications for health care organizations.

APPLICATION EXERCISE

Analyze the communications component of the organizational structure of a local health care facility. Obtain a copy of the facility's organizational chart. With the assistance of an instructor, arrange to interview several nurses at the management level and the staff nurse level to obtain additional information. Analyze the communications components from the perspective of the systems model. Ask nurses at the staff level and management level to describe the system from their point of view:

1. How are communications carried out within the organization?

2. What types of communication exist?

3. How is communication accomplished from management to staff and from staff to management?

4. What are the perceived strengths of this approach to communication?

5. What are the perceived weaknesses of this approach to communication?

6. What changes in the communication process (if any) are desired by nurses at the management and staff levels?

Based on your research, describe the communication subsystem as follows:

1. What are the components of the subsystem?

2. What are the inputs, throughputs, and outputs of the subsystem?

3. How do the components of the subsystem interact?

4. Are interaction methods effective?

5. Is the subsystem effective?

6. What strengths and weaknesses does the subsystem exhibit from the viewpoint of nurses at both the staff and management levels?

REVIEW QUESTIONS

1. What are the advantages and disadvantages of the classical bureaucratic approach to organizational structure?

2. What are the assumptions underlying the Theory X and Theory Y approaches, as described by McGregor?

3. What are the similarities and differences between M-form organizations and Scanlon organizations?

4. What are the advantages and disadvantages of using a systems approach to study organizational structure?

5. What are the developmental stages that groups undergo?

REFERENCES

American Nurses Association. (1991). "Nursing's agenda for health care reform." (Supplement to the *American Nurse.*) Washington, D.C.: Author.

Barger, S. (1991). "The nursing center: A model for rural nursing practice." *Nursing and Health Care,* 12(11), 290-294.

Barnard, C. (1938). *Functions of the Executive.* Cambridge, MA: Harvard University Press.

Cooley, C. (1911). *Social organization.* New York: Scribner.

Fayol, H. (1949). *General and industrial management.* (Translated by C. Stors). London: Pittman.

Hazzard, M. (1971). "An overview of systems theory." *Nursing Clinics of North America,* 6(3), 385-393.

Kramer, M. (1988). "Magnet hospitals: institutions of excellence." *Journal of Nursing Administration,* 18(1), 13-24,

Lawrence, P., and Lorsch, J. (1967). *Organization and environment.* Boston: Harvard University.

Luthans, F. (1985). *Organizational behavior* (4th ed.). New York: McGraw-Hill.

McGregor, D. (1960). *The human side of enterprise.* New York: McGraw-Hill.

McWilliams, C. (1980). "Systems analysis can solve nursing management problems." *Supervisor Nurse,* 11(5), 17-26.

Ouchi, W. (1984). *The M-form society: How American teamwork can recapture the competitive edge.* Reading, MA: Addison-Wesley.

Reitz, J. (1987). *Behavior in organizations* (3rd ed.). Homewood, IL: Irwin, Inc.

Robey, D. (1986). *Designing organizations* (2nd ed.). Homewood, IL: Irwin, Inc.

Strasen, L. (1991). "Redesigning hospitals around patients and technology." *Nursing Economics,* 9(4), 233-238.

Sullivan, E., and Decker, P. (1988). *Effective management in nursing.* Menlo Park, CA: Addison-Wesley.

Taylor, F. (1911). *The principles of scientific management.* New York: Harper and Row.

Von Bertalanffy, L. (1955). "General systems theory." *Main Currents in Modern Thought,* 11, 75-83.

Woodward, J. (1965). *Industrial organization.* London: Oxford.

RECOMMENDATIONS FOR FURTHER STUDY

Alexander, J., and Mark, B. (1990). "Technology and structure of nursing organizations." *Nursing and Health Care,* 11(4), 194-199.

Manthey, M. (1991.) "Empowering staff nurses: Decision on the action level." *Nursing Management,* 22(2), 16-21.

Sovie, M.D. "Hospital Culture—Why Create One?" *Nursing Economics,* 11(2):69-74, March/April 1993.

Van Slyck, A. (1991). "A systems approach to the management of nursing services, part I: Introduction: The art of management." *Nursing Management,* 22(3) 16-19.

Weinbart, M. (1991). "Commercially managed healthcare: An experience." *Nursing Management,* 22(1) 40-41.

Wood, C. (1991). "Health care rationing: The Oregon experiment." *Nursing Economics,* 9(4), 239-243, 262.

4

HEALTH CARE DELIVERY

OBJECTIVES

After studying this chapter, the reader should be able to:

1. Describe the development of public health in the United States.

2. Identify the three systems of health care delivery.

3. Discuss current problems in health care delivery.

4. Discuss the impact of acquired immunodeficiency syndrome (AIDS) on the health care system.

5. Describe the Centers for Disease Control recommendations for the practice of human immunodeficiency virus (HIV)-positive health care workers.

6. Describe recent changes in health care settings and personnel.

7. Identify reasons for spiraling health care costs.

8. Describe the American Nurses' Association proposal for health care reform.

INTRODUCTION

Chapter 3, How organizations are structured, discusses the growing need for restructuring the health care system and its means of delivery in the United States. Although the country has developed and implemented a number of health care innovations, the system itself remains inaccessible to many people. The reasons for this are many and complex. In 1991,

60 million Americans, many of whom were elderly, were either uninsured or underinsured (American Nurses' Association, 1991), resulting in a waste of both human and health care resources. Furthermore, the lack of prenatal care and readily available childhood immunizations eventually leads to illnesses and expensive demands on the health care system that might otherwise have been prevented.

An inaccessible health care system has resulted in other inequities related to life expectancy and infant mortality. Roemer (1986) states that, because of inadequate health care access, "[b]lacks suffer disadvantages in virtually every condition affecting health; their life expectancy at birth is 69.5 years compared with 75.1 years for whites." The infant mortality rate is higher in the United States than in 15 other industrialized countries, including several with lower per capita incomes. In many of these poorer countries, citizens have access to proper care through a national health care system.

The state of the U.S. health care system is not the result of under-expenditure. Health care currently amounts to 12% of the gross national product, or approximately $756 billion. (American Nurses' Association, 1991). Rather, the system's problems seem to stem from the fact that "much of the excellent health service of which the nation is capable has not been made accessible to everyone" (Roemer, 1986).

This chapter begins by tracing the development of the U.S. health care delivery system and explaining its present structure. It then discusses changes in the types of health care personnel and settings and explores problems facing the health care system. The chapter then covers factors that influence health care costs and concludes with a discussion of reform proposals.

HISTORICAL BACKGROUND

Health care delivery has changed greatly over the past 200 years. Midway through the 19th century, clients received home visits by nurses or physicians, or they came to the physicians' offices. Few hospitals and clinics existed. During this time, the responsibility for health care rested principally upon the individual and family. Whereas a physician or other practitioner might visit a client's home to treat a specific illness-related episode, individuals or their families were expected to provide basic acute illness care as well as necessary long-term health care measures. Only indigent people and people without family or community support went to a hospital.

Toward the end of the century, as urbanization increased and public and private transport became more reliable, client care shifted from the home to clinics, hospitals, and physicians' offices. The era of extensive hospital building also began. The number of hospitals, the majority of which were general county hospitals, increased from 178 in 1873 to 4,400 by 1910. As health care technology developed, centralization of its related services followed. Now, instead of being available at many places, technology-related services were offered at central locations, namely, hospitals and clinics. The centralization of technological services lowered costs for providers and clients.

The early 1900s also saw the establishment of school nursing programs, voluntary health agencies, and public health service programs. With the development of these institutions and agencies, health care teaching and disease prevention measures began.

As urbanization has continued, families typically have become widely separated. Increasingly, family members cannot participate in health care decisions or care for other members during illness. As a result, physicians make more and more important health care decisions for their clients, and care for acutely and chronically ill clients has moved from the home into hospitals.

PUBLIC HEALTH CARE

Health care delivery in the United States has evolved into three specific systems: public, private, and military. The public health care system involves governmental agencies at the local, state, and national level. It comprises local health care departments and large federal programs such as that administered by the Centers for Disease Control (CDC). Roemer (1986) describes the changes in public health care as occurring in five stages (see *Public health development*, page 118).

During the initial stage, from 1800 to 1870, the individual and family provided most of the health care for family members. The public became involved when epidemics broke out. Typically under such circumstances, the local government would form a commission that would issue recommendations for environmental measures. For example, in 1798, a yellow fever epidemic broke out in New York City. Over the next several years, a local board of health took measures to drain swamps and improve other environmental conditions. An appointed health inspector enforced quarantine and isolation regulations. The board and health inspector, however, had no responsibilities beyond those concerning the yellow fever epidemic. Only after the Civil War did state boards of health assume more responsibility than the immediate handling of acute threats to public health.

The second period, from 1870 to 1910, was characterized by increasing urbanization and immigration. The National Quarantine Act, passed in 1878, sought to bar the immigration of individuals infected with communicable diseases.

Also during this period, scientific developments influenced health care planning and delivery. Surgeons and other health care practitioners began using antisepsis, which further supported the centralization of medical services into hospitals and larger clinics. The public could receive diphtheria immunization by 1883 and typhoid vaccination by 1898. Other new technologies helped in disease diagnosis. The thermometer and ophthalmoscope were in use by 1860; the sphygmomanometer followed in the 1880s, although initially only physicians could use it. The roentgen ray (X-ray) was discovered in 1895.

As technology and the centralization of its related treatments increased, more and more clients of all economic classes came to hospitals for diagnostic tests and treatment. To care for the growing client population, hospitals increas-

PUBLIC HEALTH DEVELOPMENT

Stage 1: 1800 to 1870
- *Focus on individual and family*
- *Treatment in the home*
- *Short-term boards of health*

Stage 2: 1870 to 1910
- *Urbanization: shift to hospitals, physicians' offices*
- *Technologic, medical advances*
- *Health care legislation (National Quarantine Act 1878, first Bureau of Child Hygiene 1908)*

Stage 3: 1910 to 1935
- *Workplace health care focus (workers' compensation, worksite safety inspections)*
- *Continued urbanization*

Stage 4: 1935 to 1960
- *Social legislation (Social Security Act of 1935)*
- *National Health Survey, 1935 to 1936*
- *Health care legislation (Hill-Burton Hospital Construction Act, 1946, National Mental Health Act, 1946)*

Stage 5: 1960 to Present
- *Health Professions Education Assistance Act, 1963*
- *Social legislation (Economic Opportunity Act, 1964, Title XVIII, Medicare, 1966, Title XIX, Medicaid)*
- *Spiraling health care costs (decreased access by poor and indigent people, implementation of Prospective Payment (DRGS) systems, calls for system reform)*

(Source: Roemer, 1986)

---

ingly relied on student nurses and medical residents to provide care as part of their training and apprenticeship. As a result, the education and training for physicians and nurses became more structured.

At the turn of the century, health department responsibilities began to extend beyond infectious diseases. In 1908, under the auspices of the New York City Health Department, the Bureau of Child Hygiene was established. Child Hygiene nurses visited tenements and provided education and care for poor mothers and their children. Other agencies that provided care for specific illnesses and conditions followed; one of these was the Society for Social and Moral Prophylaxis, whose responsibility it was to reduce the spread of sexually transmitted diseases.

The third period of public health service development, from 1910 to 1935, focused on prevention. Agencies were formed to ensure workers' compensation for work-related injuries and to assume responsibility for safety inspections. In addition to the hospitals and clinics that were focused on acute illness care, a separate public health system devoted to injury and illness prevention and health promotion began to emerge.

The fourth period of development, 1935 to 1960, witnessed the passage of important health-related legislation, including the Social Security Act of 1935. This landmark legislation provided for maternal and child services and the diagnosis and treatment of handicapped children, responsibilities that expanded the role of the public health service beyond that of prevention.

In 1935 and 1936, the government conducted the National Health Survey, which produced recommendations calling for reforms in the Social Security Act and the establishment of a national workers' health insurance. The passage of appropriate legislation was precluded by the onset of World War II.

After World War II, the 1946 Hill-Burton Act provided for the subsidization of hospital construction in rural areas. Also in 1946, the National Mental Health Act established mental health clinics within and external to public health service agencies. The National Institutes of Health (NIH), an agency within the U.S. Public Health Service, was also expanded, although NIH research continued to focus on treatment rather than prevention and grants were made almost exclusively to physician-researchers.

Since 1960, the public health service system has changed considerably. The 1963 Health Professions Education Assistance Act provided funds to colleges and universities for health care worker education. Neighborhood health centers were established under the 1964 Economic Opportunity Act. These centers, controlled by the local community, offered a full range of preventive and restorative treatments for poor citizens. In 1973, President Nixon terminated the program and shifted the health care responsibilities to the public health service.

In 1966, two amendments to the Social Security Act were passed: Title XVIII, Medicare, and Title XIX, Medicaid. Under these two amendments, the federal government assumed responsibility for the care of elderly people and most indigent citizens. These two programs are discussed later in this chapter.

High medical costs characterize the final stage in Roemer's scheme. As more and more citizens received health care at diverse institutions, medical costs rose alarmingly. Few incentives existed to limit services or to control costs. In the 1980s, the federal government implemented measures to limit costs, introducing a plan for financial reimbursement according to diagnosis-related groups (DRGs). The plan limits reimbursement for Medicare to an amount deemed appropriate for a particular diagnosis, regardless of the actual treatment cost. The allotted reimbursement may be more or less than the actual cost. If the cost exceeds the amount designated by the DRG category, the health care provider must bear the burden, thereby encouraging the provider to find cost-effective yet adequate care delivery.

Recognizing potential abuses of the DRG system, such as inadequate care delivery and premature discharge, Medicare established peer review organizations (PROs) in each state. PROs develop guidelines for hospital admission and treatment and monitor hospitals to ensure that proper care is provided.

THE CURRENT STRUCTURE

One could reasonably argue that health care in the United States does not represent a "system." A system implies a coordinated whole with an identified mission and interrelated parts with specific functions. Too often health care seems composed of unrelated, competing, and sometimes hostile parts, each with a different idea about what should be done by and for the client.

To the degree that health care systems do exist, the United States has three—a private health care system; a public, or Medicare/Medicaid, system; and a military system—and a person may come in contact with all or only one during a lifetime. The basic services provided by the public health service underlie all three systems. These services include water monitoring, sewage disposal, and air pollution control.

PRIVATE HEALTH CARE

Private health care includes all services paid for by the client or the client's private insurance. It also includes care provided by preferred provider organizations (PPOs) and health maintenance organizations (HMOs). Individuals, in many cases through employment benefits, establish a network of health care agencies and providers to use principally during acute illnesses. The following example illustrates use of the private health care system:

> Mary Smith is a computer programmer for a large corporation. She and her family are covered under an insurance policy carried by her company. The coverage allows Mary and her family to choose care from any physician or hospital. When Mary or a member of her family becomes ill, they go to the physician they have selected. The physician receives direct payment at the time of service. Hospitalization is handled in a similar way, with Mary selecting the hospital, and payment going directly to it at the time of service. Mary's insurance plan has a deductible that must be met each year before coverage begins. After the deductible is met, Mary's insurance covers 90% of the health care costs.

Under this system, the client's choice of health care provider may be limited by the type of coverage. The client may also change providers within the parameters described by the coverage. Employer and employee contributions usually finance this type of health care.

MEDICARE AND MEDICAID

Established in 1966 as Titles XVIII and XIX of the Social Security Act, the public health care programs Medicare and Medicaid provide insurance for other client groups. Medicare principally serves the needs of elderly clients.

To access Medicare, a client must, in most cases, be 65 years old. Medicare benefits provide for care by physicians, chiropractors, and other health care providers. Medicare also provides for hospital care, including a semiprivate room, medications, tests, operating room and intensive care services, and occupational and physical therapy. It may also cover home health care, outpatient rehabilitation, and psychiatric care. Despite Medicare's various benefits, a client should always confirm that an anticipated service is covered. Although Medicare may nominally cover a particular service, some agencies and practitioners do not accept Medicare clients because of the reimbursement level.

One deficit of Medicare is its failure to cover some services that, if provided, would allow clients to remain in their homes and independent. For example, it does not cover home health aides, Meals on Wheels, or housekeeping services. Also not included in Medicare coverage are hearing aids, eyeglasses, and most preventive health care measures. As a result, a Medicare client may not receive the early care that could forestall a more serious and much more expensive illness or injury.

When caring for a Medicare client, nurses should be aware of the client's possible resentment about the service level available, or about treatment by other health care providers who may have communicated that a client is of less value if covered only by Medicare benefits and has no other private insurance. Having been refused service or having been made to feel that incomplete reimbursement is being offered, a Medicare client may be sensitive to perceived slights or oversights.

Medicare clients should carry their cards at all times and confirm coverage of any planned services. A booklet titled *Your Medicare Handbook* (Department of Health and Human

Services, 1987), available through the Department of Health and Human Services, explains how to use the Medicare system.

Medicaid, unlike the federally administered Medicare program, has a state component and its implementation varies from state to state. It covers eligible low-income and disabled citizens, providing for physician care, acute and long-term hospital care, laboratory and other tests, and some outpatient services. In some states, Medicaid covers dental and eye care as well as drugs. It also covers dependent children of eligible families. Individuals at a certain income level are eligible for Medicaid and Medicare benefits.

Nurses should encourage Medicaid clients to carry their cards with them and to confirm coverage of any proposed service. The nurse should also ensure that the client does not feel discriminated against because of his or her Medicaid status. Regarding all clients as individuals and helping to identify appropriate providers can prevent misunderstandings and delays.

MILITARY SERVICES

Military service personnel and their families receive care from a well-coordinated health care system that focuses on preventive care. They have immediate access to clinics, hospitals, and dispensaries throughout the world at no cost. Military clients, however, have no choice about the physician or health care provider who will render services. The Civilian Health and Medical Program of the Uniformed Services covers their dependents.

A network of Veterans Administration hospitals provides health care services for retired or disabled veterans, emphasizing long-term care and rehabilitation. Unlike health care services provided for the active military and their families, those for retired or disabled veterans do not focus on preventive care.

The military system forms an interesting contrast to the private health care system, which most people use. Although they have no choice of provider, military members have, in

CHANGES IN HEALTH CARE PERSONNEL AND SETTINGS

- *Increased number of nurses*
- *Growing independent nursing practice*
- *Greater articulation between levels of nursing education*
- *Proliferation of technological specialties*
- *Shift to home and community settings*
- *Innovative systems and settings for health care delivery*

principle at least, direct and easy access to free and all-inclusive health care when it is needed. Furthermore, in the well-integrated military system, a single client record tracks the person from one caregiver or institution to another. Despite recent criticism about the care level provided to veterans, the system has many attractive features.

CHANGES IN HEALTH CARE PERSONNEL

Kelly (1987) identifies several categories of primary care providers, including chiropractors, medical doctors, doctors of osteopathy, nurse midwives, and nurse practitioners. Medical physicians represent the greatest number, but the number of nurses is increasing. Despite physician resistance fueled by potential revenue loss or concern for client care level, this trend will probably continue. Other recent changes have affected the number and types of health care personnel. In the wake of the 1989 Omnibus Budget Reconciliation Act, which requires direct Medicaid reimbursement for pediatric and family health care providers, many states are introducing legislation that would provide direct reimbursement to certified nurses in these categories. Such legislation, combined with an increasing emphasis on service and cost-effective care, should effect an increase in the number of nurses.

Registered nurses account for the largest group (about 1.4 million) of nursing personnel, with licensed practical nurses and certified nursing assistants each accounting for about 800,000 (Kelly, 1987). Nursing educators are working to enhance the articulation among the different nursing levels and to create educational ladders that promote access.

In California, for example, a joint task force composed of associate degree and baccalaureate degree educators has worked for years to develop an articulation framework that will enhance movement from associate degree– to baccalaureate–level nursing programs and minimize duplication of courses. The group's model recognizes a basic core of content taught at both levels and additional content provided only at the baccalaureate level. These articulation plans should encourage nurses to pursue higher-level educational degrees.

Kelly (1987) lists 32 other categories of health care services personnel, ranging from music therapists to hospital administrators. The number of categories related to health care technology, such as nuclear medicine technologists and radiologic technicians specializing in mammography, is increasing.

As the number of professionals and allied health workers increases, finding the appropriate health care provider becomes more problematic. The isolation of the different health care systems (public and private, for example) and the frequent lack of any coordinated approach to health care delivery, on either an individual or a societal basis, only aggravates the problem.

The difficulty can be seen with the onset of a health concern. Should the client consult a medical physician? A chiropractor? A podiatrist? A family nurse practitioner? Which conditions is the primary care provider trained to treat, and what methodologies and treatments are available? Which services are covered by the client's insurance? What support services and referral services should be available? Where is treatment available (work, clinic, hospital, home)? Nurses should understand that clients may be confused by the inevitable proliferation of health care personnel categories.

INSTITUTIONALIZED ELDERLY CLIENTS

The U.S. General Accounting Office has estimated that 20% to 40% of elderly people in institutions are there simply because they have inadequate external support that would allow them to remain at home. Ironically, the institutional care provided by the nation's health care system costs more than care that would support the elderly client's independence.

CHANGES IN HEALTH CARE SETTINGS

Greater emphasis is being placed on care provision in the client's home and community. Jamieson (1990) describes one innovative approach to delivering health care to a population generally underserved. The Block Nursing program was established in 1982 in St. Paul, Minnesota, to serve the St. Anthony Park community of 6,969 residents, 12.5% of whom are elderly people. The program was developed to help elderly clients with health needs remain in their homes rather than being institutionalized at greatly increased cost.

Under the Block Nursing program, paid professionals, a network of volunteers, and a community sensitized to the needs of its elderly citizens provide the health care services. The nurses are employees of the Ramsey County Public Health Nursing Service, and all participants live in the area. In addition to nursing care, Block Companions provide home health and homemaker services. Volunteers trained in a 30-hour course provide support and peer counseling. Biweekly care conferences are held to coordinate services. According to Jamieson (1990), the total cost of the program is 24% less than the minimum cost of placing clients in nursing homes, where 85% of the clients served by the Block Nursing program would otherwise be. In addition to being cost-effective, the program promotes prevention and recovery, effective integration of services, and greater family and community involvement.

Changing health care delivery settings are also evident in relation to indigent clients. As states deal with unprecedented fiscal crises, the burden of caring for indigent citizens is being shifted to the local community. This approach has forced communities to reexamine the needs of their indigent populations and to reallocate available dollars. One result has been that the California Nurses Association has advocated:

- support for evening clinics
- provision of perinatal and well-baby care as a priority
- collaboration among diverse public programs to provide care for indigent people, to coordinate services to save monies, and to increase access
- emphasis on early rather than late intervention.

Changes in health care settings are important steps in meeting the growing and complex needs of our diverse society.

HEALTH CARE PROBLEMS

Many problems affect the delivery of health care in the United States. They range from increasing numbers of elderly clients to the impact of a major epidemic such as acquired immu-

---

U. S. HEALTH CARE PROBLEMS

- *Growing elderly population*
- *Increased drug and alcohol use*
- *Spread of the AIDS epidemic*
- *Decline in rural health*
- *Escalating health care costs*

nodeficiency syndrome (AIDS). Underlying these problems is the basic difficulty of handling increased health care costs.

THE ELDERLY POPULATION

The ratio of American citizens over 65 to those under 65 is 1:9. This ratio will increase by 2030 to 1:5. According to the U.S. Senate Special Committee on Aging, half the aging population will be 75 or older (U.S. Senate Special Committee on Aging: 1987).

As people age, the incidence of chronic health care problems increases and the need to provide care for chronic conditions becomes more acute. This need for chronic care occurs just as the elderly person's ability to meet the escalating costs of health care is declining. According to the Special Committee on Aging, 12.4% of people age 65 or older already fall below the poverty level, with the most impoverished being age 85 or older. Most of these citizens have only minimal resources with which to maintain health and to deal with chronic health care problems, such as coronary artery disease, hypertension, and vision difficulties. This state of affairs suggests that additional services and personnel will be required to meet the elderly population's needs and that costs necessary to provide such care will become a societal responsibility.

The cost of institutionalizing elderly people who can no longer care for themselves can be enormous. Strumpf and Knibbe (1990) state that "[with] annual nursing home costs of $22,000 or more per person per year, with little coverage under public programs, and with no significant private insurance coverage available, chronic illness can emotionally and financially destroy thousands of American families each year. Many people are destitute within 13 weeks of entering a nursing home."

The type of health care many elderly clients receive is another major problem. Because of inadequate finances or insurance coverage, preventive needs are, in many cases, neglected until the individuals can access acute care. This lack of preventive health care allows more serious conditions

GLOBAL INCREASE OF ELDERLY POPULATION

The percentage of the global population age 65 or older will increase from 10% in 1975 to nearly 20% by the year 2030

to develop. These conditions usually are more difficult and expensive to treat. The result is increased cost.

Rivlin and Wiener (1988) suggest that three changes must be made to adequately address the problem of caring for elderly clients. The client's uncertainty and anxiety about payment for long-term care must be addressed; measures that will allow elderly people to remain in their own homes as long as possible must be instituted; and a greater coordination of care must occur as care quality improves. How to accomplish these changes is a matter for debate. For example, a system of national health care might ensure that long-term care costs for elderly people be included in a basic form of social insurance. Coverage for in-home care by relatives or others might be expanded to allow elderly people to remain at home for longer periods. Finally, a coordinated care that provides services monitoring could be instituted. Other proposals call for expanding private insurance coverage.

INCREASING DRUG AND ALCOHOL USE

Drug use is widespread and not limited to the adult population (see *Drug misuse*). Some studies estimate that two-thirds of American high school seniors have used illicit drugs, and people from all socioeconomic levels use cocaine. Illicit drug use impacts the health care system in many ways. Not only does drug use itself produce harmful physical effects, but the social disruption—thefts, assaults, and territorial disputes—caused by illicit drug traffic drains time, money, and energy that could otherwise be available for other health care initiatives.

Pregnant drug abusers represent a significant health care problem. Studies have clearly documented the suffering of "crack babies" and the impact of drug abuse on the unborn child. How best to provide health care for mother and child, however, is difficult to determine. On the one hand, societal values would allow that individuals choose their own health care and decide whether or not to seek prenatal care. On the other hand, decisions made by a pregnant woman also affect the unborn child, whose compromised health may become

DRUG MISUSE

Drugs range from prescription medications, such as Valium and Halcion, to street drugs, such as crack cocaine and marijuana. Misuse of legally prescribed drugs can cause health deterioration just as illicit drug misuse can. Sometimes substances, such as nicotine, caffeine, and alcohol, are classified as drugs and sometimes as lifestyle components. Regardless of their classification, drugs that are misused or abused can have a decidedly adverse effect on health.

the financial responsibility of society. At issue are reproductive rights as well as health care rights. Some people have suggested that known drug abusers should be required to use birth control measures until they undertake and satisfactorily complete therapy. Deciding who should make such health care decisions is a type of ethical dilemma discussed in Chapter 7, Ethical implications for nursing practice.

Kelly (1987) estimates that one-third of the deaths attributable to heart disease, cancer, strokes, accidents, and pulmonary disease might have been prevented by decreasing the risk factors of hypertension, smoking, and alcohol abuse. Although smoking and alcohol abuse are not usually considered as serious as cocaine or heroin use, they contribute substantially to the nation's health problems. As with other drugs, the use of tobacco or alcohol during pregnancy compromises the health of both mother and child. Also, the use of tobacco or alcohol by children and young adults will effect future health and productivity.

AIDS

About 8 to 10 million people worldwide are infected with AIDS. Of these, about 30% are women, who constitute one of the fastest-growing affected groups (World Health Organization, 1991). Because many of these women are uninsured or underinsured, they have reduced access to health care and rely on public assistance for care. Furthermore, evidence seems to indicate that because of their reduced access to health care, women with AIDS are diagnosed late in the course of the disease. Ellice Parker, a member of the board of directors of the Women's AIDS Network in San Francisco, states that "The average time from diagnosis to death for women with AIDS is five months; that's partly because they are diagnosed so late." ("World AIDS Day," 1990).

The *San Francisco Chronicle* ("AIDS Toll Rising," 1990) reported that AIDS will shortly become one of the five leading causes of death in women of childbearing age. This statistic has ramifications not only for women but also for children exposed to the virus in utero; one-third of the babies born to women infected with the human immunodeficiency virus (HIV) subsequently develop pediatric AIDS ("World AIDS Day," 1990).

AIDS also affects other minority groups that historically have received less than optimal health care. Black and Hispanic women account for more than 70% of the total of American women between ages 25 and 34 infected with HIV (CDC, 1990). Other high-risk populations include intravenous drug users and sexually promiscuous individuals, many of whom may have only minimal contact with traditional health care delivery settings. Because they may be the only health care providers who contact these people, nurses in urban clinics and neighborhood shelters must learn to screen clients for AIDS-related infections.

AIDS affects not only the people who contract the disease and bear its physical, emotional, and financial burdens but also the professionals responsible for delivering health care. Like other catastrophic diseases, AIDS magnifies concerns for personal safety; nurses, physicians, and ancillary staff worry about the risks to their own health, even though the low risk of contracting the disease in a work setting is well documented.

The care of AIDS clients is made more complex in the United States by prejudices toward the male homosexual and intravenous drug user populations initially affected. Because of this prejudice, many people hold people with AIDS responsible for their condition, whereas they do not feel the same way toward people with other diseases, including lung cancer and coronary disease, that also have a lifestyle component. One study found that nurses considered clients with AIDS more responsible for their condition than were patients with other diagnoses (Kelly, et al., 1988).

This problem may diminish as people become aware that AIDS affects a broad spectrum of people from all walks of life. The announcement in 1991 that basketball star Earvin Magic' Johnson was infected with HIV and was retiring from the game provoked an unprecedented number of telephone calls to local health departments and to the CDC in Atlanta. Nevertheless, nurses and other health care workers must learn to separate the illness from other considerations that should not influence the giving of professional health care.

Nurses share the responsibility for ensuring that all appropriate safeguards for their own and other clients' safety are provided in each work setting. The nurse should follow guidelines for universal precautions, and necessary supplies and equipment should be readily available. Nurses should also support AIDS education for colleagues. Such education helps to dispel myths and misconceptions about the disease and helps personnel to deal with feelings about clients who follow different lifestyles. The nurse should remember that "Health care workers are expected to provide care to patients with HIV infection and AIDS. The American Nurses' Association (ANA) believes that nurses have a moral duty to provide such care" (Viens, 1990).

An environment needs to exist in which health care workers can provide care safely and confidently for AIDS clients. Efforts are under way to make AIDS testing of health care workers and the disclosure of HIV-positive clients to health care personnel mandatory. Opponents argue that neither requirement is appropriate because neither contributes to halting the spread of the disease. Proponents hold that both health care workers and clients should be informed if they will be in contact with an HIV positive individual, regardless of the risk. The ANA House of Delegates rejected mandatory testing and disclosure of HIV status because "they will not

CENTERS FOR DISEASE CONTROL RECOMMENDATIONS FOR HEALTH CARE WORKERS AND AIDS

- *Adherence to universal precautions*
- *No restrictions on noninvasive procedures by HIV-positive workers*
- *Workplace definition of exposure-prone procedures*
- *Guidelines for exposure-prone situations:*
  - *– health care workers to know own HIV status*
  - *– local panel to advise on performing exposure-prone procedures*
  - *– possible notification of affected clients*

From American Nurse, September 1991

prevent the transmission of HIV disease and are therefore not warranted" ("ANA Members Say No," 1991).

In July 1991, the CDC released their formal guidelines for the prevention of blood-borne diseases, including hepatitis B virus (HBV) and AIDS (see *Centers for Disease Control recommendations for health care workers and AIDS*). Legislation that would require states to mandate compliance with the new CDC guidelines has been proposed. Interestingly, the guidelines do not mandate AIDS testing or HIV status disclosure. Provisions include the following:

- All health care workers should adhere to universal precautions. Those with exudative lesions should refrain from all direct patient care. Proper equipment disinfection and sterilization should be accomplished.
- No basis exists for restricting the practice of health care workers with HIV or HBV, provided these workers follow universal precautions and recommended disinfection and sterilization and do not perform invasive, exposure-prone procedures, that is, those during which the opportunity for exposure to the virus is significant.
- Exposure-prone procedures should be identified in each health care setting.

- Personnel performing exposure-prone procedures should be aware of their HIV or HBV status and should not perform such procedures until they have been counseled by an expert review panel. The panel will establish the circumstances in which the personnel may continue to perform such procedures and, if deemed necessary, notify involved clients of their health care provider's positive HIV or HBV status (Morbidity and Mortality Weekly Report, 1991).

Recognizing that they will interact with many clients who will not have been tested for HIV, nurses should ensure that proper precautions and safeguards are always available. They should consider blood and body fluids potentially contaminated, whether by HIV, HBV, or other pathogens, and deal with them appropriately.

The Occupational Safety and Health Administration (OSHA) developed mandatory standards for dealing with infectious material, as defined by the CDC, including blood; semen; vaginal secretions; cerebrospinal, synovial, pericardial, pleural, peritoneal, and amniotic fluids; saliva in dental procedures; any body fluid contaminated by blood; and all undifferentiated body fluids (Pugliese, 1992). The OSHA mandatory standards comply with the CDC voluntary guidelines for universal precautions and apply to every employee who may reasonably be expected to come into contact with blood or body fluids. The new OSHA requirements include the following:

- development of a written infection control plan
- employee training in risk-reduction techniques and infection-control protocols
- observance of universal precautions by all personnel
- availability of HBV vaccine free of charge to all exposed workers
- provision of counseling, prophylactic treatment, and monitoring of any employee with "mucous membrane, non-intact skin, or parenteral contact" with blood or other potentially infectious fluid (Pugliese, 1992).

Under these new guidelines, employers must provide appropriate equipment, such as self-sheathing needles, gloves, gowns, and masks. They must also train employees in the use of the equipment. When an employee sustains a needle stick or other exposure, the hospital must test the client for HIV, hepatitis, or other infection. Whether such testing requires client consent varies with the laws of the state involved.

The impact of AIDS on the health care delivery system will be enormous. In addition to the cost of caring for 150,000 identified AIDS patients, there is the cost of caring for at least 150,000 persons infected with HIV. Because AIDS is perceived as a hazard in the workplace, the recruitment of health care workers at all levels probably will decline. Dealing with the AIDS epidemic will be one of the most significant challenges of the next century.

HEALTH CARE COSTS

By the year 2000, if conditions remain the same, health care costs will increase to 15% of the gross national product (Haddon, 1990). During the second half of the 1980s, health care inflation increased at more than double the national inflation rate. Physicians' fees and hospital costs have significantly attributed to this cost increase.

Physicians' fees have risen steadily since the 1950s because of the lack of competition for the delivery of primary care services and the lack of controlling regulations for fees or insurance reimbursement (Grace, 1990). Several factors are changing this situation. First, the nation no longer suffers a shortage of physicians. This has lead to increased competition among physicians. In addition, the public has begun to view other health care providers, including nurse practitioners, as cost-effective alternatives to routine physician-based care. As the number of states that authorizes third-party reimbursement to nurses increases, competitive pressures will result in greater efficiency and cost-effectiveness. For example, if one practitioner can delivery a well-baby checkup for a lower fee, other competing practitioners will have to consider offering a similar service at a comparable cost.

Hospitals have also contributed to health care inflation. Between 1970 and 1980, hospital care costs more than tripled. The fee per hospital day rose from $15 in 1950 to $245 in 1980, equivalent to a 450% increase when adjusted for inflation (Rubin, 1983). Reasons for rising hospital costs include burgeoning technology, medical specialization, the threat of consumer litigation, the expense of conforming to governmental and private insurance requirements, and the nursing shortage of the 1980s.

New medical technologies have also had an effect. To remain competitive and to attract both physicians and clients, hospitals have had to introduce expensive new technologies and equipment. Many clients expect that these new techniques and procedures will be available to them, without regard to cost. The ethical dilemmas of when to use new technologies, who should pay for them, and how to expend health care dollars for the general good have yet to be adequately defined, let alone resolved. Chapter 7, Ethical implications for nursing practice, discusses these problems.

Specialized health care also inflates medical costs. As the number of medical specialists grows, public pressure to access them intensifies. People also tend to believe that insurance coverage should extend to specialist care.

At the same time that they are expecting additional access to complex technology and specialist care, clients seem more and more willing to undertake litigation against health care providers and facilities. To avoid costly suits and resultant negative publicity, many physicians practice "defensive medicine" by ordering extensive tests and hospitalization. Such measures add to care costs when less expensive technology in an outpatient setting might have been adequate. Until the government and the health care community delineate what the individual can expect from health care services and decide who shall bear the financial burden for such care, controlling the costs of "defensive medicine" will remain difficult.

The nursing shortage that began in the mid-1980s and that probably will continue into the 21st century is the result of major societal changes. Women have moved into the occupational mainstream, where they compete successfully in medical, legal, and other traditionally male-dominated

REASONS FOR RISING HEALTH CARE COSTS

- *Increased physicians' fees*
- *Increased hospital fees*
- *Increased technology costs*
- *Medical specialization*
- *Litigation costs*
- *Nursing services costs*

professions. Because women now have many more professional opportunities, few have pursued the traditional nursing preparation.

In addition to having a greater number of professional choices, women now pursue occupations that will give them greater independence and greater financial reward. Because most opportunities for nurses remain centered in the traditional hospital setting and because women view this setting's paternalistic, bureaucratic approach to management and leadership as a liability, women are choosing other occupations.

Finally, because the overall number of students entering college is declining, fewer people are choosing from among the competing professional opportunities. This diminished student population is reflected by the decreasing number of people entering nursing school.

The nursing shortage, coupled with new opportunities for nurses in non-hospital settings, has produced a long overdue rise in nursing salaries. Lippman (1991) reports that salaries for nurses working full-time in acute-care hospitals rose 17% from 1989 to 1991. The average annual nursing income is now reported at $36,100. Wage compression—the absence of wage hikes as experience is gained—is also being rectified; Lippman reports that during 1991, the hourly rate for experienced registered nurses (RNs) rose twice as much as that for new nurses. These wage increases, however well-deserved, have contributed to the rising costs of health care services.

Grace (1990), in her analysis of escalating medical care costs, includes, among other factors, the health care consumer's passive role. She charges that until consumers become educated to understand the difference between preventive health care and care that attempts to cure illness after the fact, they will continue to pay exorbitant fees for health services. Grace also claims that when selecting treatment options, "the consumer is purposefully kept ignorant, and therefore, the decision-making control is in the hands of the provider. As a result, the most costly form of treatment is usually that provided" (Grace, 1990).

Grace states that nurses have a crucial role in promoting change and helping to reduce costs. She advocates that nurses educate consumers about moving from medical care focused on illness to a more preventive health care system. "Ultimately, a revolution of the citizenry is the only force to create change in a democracy. Nursing has the capacity to educate the consumer to create such changes" (Grace, 1990). She also believes that nurses must cease being passive "co-conspirators with hospitals and physicians in maintaining the current medical care system" and that they can accomplish this by informing clients of the unnecessary, expensive, and potentially harmful and invasive tests and treatments routinely performed.

PROPOSALS FOR REFORM

This chapter has covered the development of American health care, the different health care delivery systems, changes in personnel and settings, the major problems confronting the system, and the reasons behind burgeoning health care costs. The remainder of the chapter explores strategies for reforming the health care delivery system and describes the forces impelling us to a more equitable structure.

Historically, movements to provide any socially supported system of health care have met with opposition, not just in the United States but in other countries as well. Roemer (1986) points out that "the attitude of the medical profession as a whole toward social measures to increase the economic access of patients to medical care has ranged from indifferent to cool to bitterly hostile." Disputes between physicians and insurers have occurred in Australia, France, Germany, Britain, Japan, and even Canada. In 1962, when national health insurance reforms were introduced in Canada, physicians in Saskatchewan withheld all but emergency services for 23 days after the Medical Care Insurance program was enacted in that province. Despite this opposition, a comprehensive national health care system was enacted, and similar legislation now provides health care coverage for all provinces.

Physicians are not alone in opposing forms of socialized medicine, which implies governmental control of basic health care services available to the citizenry at large. Many advocates for minority and indigent populations oppose such reform, claiming that it will result in second-rate care to targeted groups. Other, financially independent people have ready access to a higher standard of privately purchased care and feel no need for system reform.

The movement toward some form of health insurance that provides basic care for all citizens is gaining momentum. Advocates recognize that such a system cannot avoid some inequity; wealthier clients will continue to be able to buy care exceeding that provided by the basic program. Nevertheless, most people realize that the current system is simply too inefficient and costly to maintain. Curtin (1991) describes several situations that have made the public realize the necessity for change. She tells about a friend raising money for a neighbor whose insurance money had run out before he could have his last two chemotherapy treatments. She describes an elderly man who robbed a bank for $17 to pay for medication that his insurance would not cover. By contrast, she describes how a public-interest group obtained a court order to maintain an irreversibly comatose client on life support, contrary to the wishes of his family and at a cost of $1,000 per day.

Other proposals urge that the United States adopt a health care delivery system similar to Canada's. Haddon (1990) states that "[although] the quality of health care in the U.S. is comparable to that of Canada, there is a tremendous difference in health care costs; in the U.S., it typically costs 67% more to repair a broken leg than in Canada." One reason for this cost discrepancy is the level of physicians' incomes. Malloy (1988), in comparing physicians' incomes in the two countries, states that American physicians have, on the average, a 70% higher before-taxes income than Canadian physicians.

Not only do U.S. citizens pay more for health care, they also, Haddon charges, receive less comprehensive care. All **Canadians are covered by national health insurance, which** is principally financed by tax revenues. Although the provinces administer the care, the national government sets the basic care standards. Malloy (1988) states that Canada's national health insurance covers all costs except those of a few limited procedures, such as cosmetic surgery. Furthermore, the Canadian system does not limit consumer choice of health care facilities or physicians.

Some Canadians unwilling to undergo long waits for elective treatment or surgery have come to the United States to obtain services. In other cases, American technology may not be available for routine use in Canada, again prompting individuals to seek medical care in the United States. Nevertheless, if the basic care of all citizens is the principal requirement for a national health system, the Canadian system should certainly be investigated as a potential model.

The ANA, supported by many other health care organizations, has proposed a health care reform plan (see *ANA proposal for health care reform*, page 140) that calls for the following:

- restructure of health care settings to include enhanced consumer access to services through the primary health care delivery in community settings; enhanced consumer responsibility for personal health and informed decision making in selecting health care services; support for using the most cost-effective providers and therapeutic options in the most appropriate settings
- identification of a standard health care package that will provide services to all citizens and residents, to be financed through combined public and private plans
- a public plan covering the poor, based on federal guidelines and eligibility requirements
- a private plan offering at minimum the nationally standardized package of essential services; increasing the coverage could be an employment benefit of employment; employers not offering private coverage must pay into the public plan for their employees
- a phase-in of essential services, beginning with pregnancy and child coverage; a "Healthstart" plan to address needs of vulnerable populations

---

A.N.A. PROPOSAL FOR HEALTH CARE REFORM

- *Health care delivery system restructuring*
- *Universally available standard health care package*
- *Phase-in of services: initial emphasis on pregnancy and children*
- *Changes to reflect changing national demographics*
- *Decreased health care costs by required use of managed care, incentives to support managed care, control over system growth, cost-effective health care options, systemwide policy development, direct access by consumers to providers*
- *Case-managed health care*
- *Long-term care coverage*
- *Insurance reform*
- *No point-of-service pay; no balance billing*
- *System review and evaluation*

- planned change to accommodate shifting national demographics, including changes in population, ethnicity, age, socioeconomic status
- reduced health care costs as a result of required managed care in public and private plans, consumer and provider incentives to use managed-care approaches, control of health care system growth through planning and resource management, incentives to use cost-effective health care options, development of health care policies based on effectiveness and outcomes research, direct consumer access to the full range of qualified health care providers
- case management for continuing health care needs
- long-term care provisions, including short duration and extended-care services, and an increased emphasis on the individual's responsibility to plan for long-term care
- insurance reform to ensure coverage access and to protect insurers and individuals against excessive costs
- access to services without payment at point of service and elimination of balance billing (for uncovered amounts) in private and public plans
- public and private sector review of the system to determine resource allocation, cost-reduction approaches, allowable

insurance premiums, and reimbursement levels for providers; the reviewing system would operate under federal guidelines and would include consumers, providers, and payers. (ANA, 1991).

The philosophy underlying the ANA plan is that all citizens and residents of the United States should have equitable access to a core of health care services. The health care consumer becomes the focus of the system and assumes increased responsibility for personal care and how it should be provided. The ANA proposal also emphasizes preventive care and an efficient use of resources to provide cost-effective care. The ANA has urged state nurses' associations to pursue implementation of those elements in the Agenda for Health Care Reform that are best suited to the political climate in each association's state.

Gaffney and Mikulencak (1993) point out the importance of formulating a national health care policy that addresses the need for restructuring the health care delivery system, rather than simply focusing on high costs and financing. Without restructuring, they argue, an ineffective system will continue to leave many clients unable to access or pay for services.

HEALTH CARE REFORM UNDER THE CLINTON ADMINISTRATION

With the election of William Clinton as President of the United States in 1992, old and new proposals for health care reform were scrutinized by the Interagency Task Force on Health Care, headed by Hillary Rodham Clinton. The administration's proposals were originally expected to be released in May, but the complexity of the undertaking delayed both release of the proposal and action upon it.

The main features of the Clinton administration's health care reform proposal include: access to care by those who are uninsured; standard benefits; delegation of responsibility to states to set up alliances of consumers and employers that will develop agreements with pools of insurers regarding the delivery of health care. (*Time,* May 1993)

Basic care, as envisioned, would include mental health care, dental care, hospitalization, outpatient care, physician visits, prescription medications, and more preventive care. More importantly, basic care would be "portable," moving with the insured client from one job to another, and no one would be denied insurance on the basis of preexisting illness.

During the first months of the Clinton administration, other important developments in health care occurred. The cost of prescription medications came under sharp attack, with the release of information that drugs developed with federal support were being marketed by private drug companies at exorbitant rates of up to $350,000 per year for treatment with such drugs as Ceredase (*Time,* March 1993). The prospect of price controls on prescription drugs caused pharmaceutical companies to voluntarily reduce some prices and to engage in extensive public relations campaigns to justify the costs of medications.

Another early Clinton administration aim was to decrease the number of unimmunized children. While the costs of the vaccines were cited as one cause, a more substantial problem appears to be a shortage of immunization clinics and their limited hours of operation. New national standards for pediatric immunization were developed, with the aim of communicating to families the importance and availability of childhood immunizations (Clinton, 1993). The Clinton immunization initiative has been threefold: it earmarked $300 million to make immunization services more available to those who need it; it directed Department of Health and Human Services Secretary Donna Shalala to "negotiate aggressively with drug manufacturers to insure that states can get the vaccines they need at affordable prices" (Clinton, 1993); and it called for inclusion of a childhood immunization program as part of the national health care package.

As the Clinton administration's health care proposal developed, various states also began proposing changes in the way health care is administered. Some states have established comprehensive insurance associations designed to cover high-risk clients. In Florida, for example, a newly enacted state law will require that all state residents have access to medical insurance by the end of 1994. This will be accomplished through the establishment of 11 health care alliances which will negotiate with insurers for coverage.

In New Jersey, efforts to standardize coverage have been undertaken; insurance companies are now required to offer individuals and groups of up to 50 the choice of a standard managed-care plan or one of five other plans. The least expensive option is expected to cost approximately $1,000 per year.

In California, which failed to pass a flawed state health care plan in 1992, individual companies have begun to make changes in employee insurance. Burgeoning health care costs have resulted in a move to managed care; The oil company Chevron, for example, has phased out its traditional open-choice plan and now requires employees to choose between an HMO (Kaiser-Permanente) or a PPO (HealthNet).

As national and state health care policies continue to evolve, the inherent conflict between the need for cost containment and the need to provide basic health care will continue to be a major issue. The success of state and national policies depends on the institution of cost-effective health care, which includes full utilization of nurses in health care delivery.

SUMMARY

This chapter traces the historical development of health care delivery in the United States. It then describes the major health care delivery systems—private, public, and military. It explores problems in health care delivery, including care provision for elderly and AIDS-infected clients and drug users. The chapter also discusses recent changes in health care personnel and settings and analyzes the reasons for spiraling health care costs. It concludes with a comparison of proposed health care delivery reforms.

Developing an equitable, affordable health care delivery system will be one of the most important tasks confronting the nation during the next decade. By understanding the health care system's historical development and being aware of its shortcomings and problems, nurses can make valuable contributions to the provision of cost-effective care for all citizens.

APPLICATION EXERCISE

Choose a client population that traditionally has had difficulty obtaining health care (homeless clients, indigent clients, working uninsured clients, retired elderly clients). After consulting with your instructor, arrange to interview appropriate health care personnel in a local setting and ask the following questions:

1. If a client (from the identified underserved group) came for emergency treatment at your facility, how would this client's request for health care be handled?

2. How would the client's request be handled in a nonemergency situation?

3. To which public services do you refer such clients?

4. To which voluntary community services do you refer such clients?

5. What difficulties do you have in providing services for these clients?

ALTERNATE APPLICATION EXERCISE

Identify a local agency or hotline that provides resource information for indigent clients. Request information on the types of services and costs of services available to indigent clients in your community.

REVIEW QUESTIONS

1. How has the burden of responsibility for health care changed since the late 19th century?

2. What legislation has affected the development of public health care?

3. What problems make obtaining adequate care from the health care system difficult?

4. How are clients and health care workers protected by the new CDC recommendations for HIV-positive workers?

5. What populations are served by Medicare and Medicaid coverage? Which services are covered? What problems related to Medicare and Medicaid service exist?

6. Contrast the private health care system with the military health care system. What are the advantages and disadvantages of each system?

7. What factors have contributed to the rise in health care costs?

8. Describe the major components of the ANA proposal for health care reform.

REFERENCES

"AIDS Toll Rising among Childbearing Women," *San Francisco Chronicle,* July 11, 1990.

"ANA Members Say No to Mandatory AIDS Testing," *American Journal of Nursing* 91(8):68-69, August 1991.

American Nurses' Association "Nursing's Agenda for Health Care Reform," Supplement to *The American Nurse*, June 1991.

Centers for Disease Control, *HIV/AIDS Surveillance Report,* September 1990, pages 1-18.

Curtin, L.L. "Rube Goldberg and the Great American Healthcare System," *Nursing Management* 22(5):9-11, May 1991.

Deloughery, G.L. *Issues and Trends in Nursing.* St. Louis: Mosby Inc., 1991.

Gaffney, T., and Mikulencak, M. "Restructuring Health Care Includes Discussing Options," *The American Nurse* 25(2):18, February, 1993.

Grace, H. "Can Health Care Costs Be Contained?" *Nursing and Health Care* 11(3):125-130, March 1990.

Haddon, R.M. "An Economic Agenda for Health Care," *Nursing and Health Care* 11(1):21-26, January 1990.

"Indigent Health Care Decisions now in Local Hands," *California Nurse* 87(9):1-3, October 1991.

Jamieson, M.K. "Block Nursing: Practicing Autonomous Professional Nursing in the Community," *Nursing and Health Care* 11(2):250-253, May 1990.

Kelly, J.S., et al. "Nurses' Attitudes towards AIDS," *The Journal of Continuing Education in Nursing* 19(2):78-83, 1988.

Kelly, L.Y. *The Nursing Experience: Trends, Challenges and Transitions.* New York: Macmillan Publishing Co., 1987.

Leddy, S., and Pepper, J.M. *Conceptual Bases of Professional Nursing,* 2nd ed. New York: J.B. Lippincott Co., 1989.

Lindberg, J.B., et al. *Introduction to Nursing: Concepts, Issues, and Opportunities.* New York: J.B. Lippincott Co., 1990.

Lippman, H. "Nurses Are Worth More Than Ever," *RN* 54(10):50-56, October 1991.

Malloy, M. "Health, Canadian Style," *The Wall Street Journal,* April 22, 1988.

McCloskey, J.C., and Grace, H.K. *Current Issues in Nursing,* 3rd ed. St. Louis: C.V. Mosby Co., 1990.

Morbidity and Mortality Weekly Report (No. RR-8) 40, 1991.

Pugliese, G. "Universal Precautions: Now They're the Law," *RN* 55(9):63-69, September 1992.

Rivlin, A.M., and Wiener, J.M. *Caring for the Disabled Elderly.* Washington, D.C.: Brookings Institution, 1988.

Rubin, R.J. "Proposal for National Solutions; The Administration's Perspective," in "New York Academy of Medicine: Struggle for the Assurance of Access to Health Care," *Bulletin of the New York Academy of Medicine,* January-February 1983.

Roemer, M.I. *An Introduction to the U.S. Health Care System,* 2nd ed. New York: Springer Publishing Co., 1986.

Strumpf, N.E., and Knibbe, K.K. "Long-Term Care: Fulfilling Promises to the Old Among Us," in *Current Issues in Nursing,* 3rd ed. McCloskey, J.C., and Grace, H.K. (eds.), St. Louis: Mosby, Inc., 1990.

U.S. Department of Health and Human Services. *Aging America: Trends and Projections.* Washington, D.C.: Senate Special Committee on Aging, 1987.

U.S. Department of Health and Human Services. *Your Medicare Handbook.* Pub. No. HCFA 10050. Baltimore: Health Care Financing Administration, 1987.

Viens, D.C. "AIDS Ethics," *California Nurse* 86(10):10, November/December 1990.

"World AIDS Day: Women and AIDS—A Growing Epidemic," *California Nurse* 86(10):1-9, November/December 1990.

World Health Organization. *World AIDS Day Newsletter*, No. 1, June/July 1991.

RECOMMENDATIONS FOR FURTHER STUDY

Clinton, H.R., "Nurses in the Front Lines," *Nursing and Health Care, 14,* 6: 286-288, June 1993.

Grimaldi, P.L. "Medicare Reduces Targets for Physician Payments," *Nursing Management* 22(3):14-15, March 1991.

Jonas, G. "Nurses in the Gulf," *RN* 54(10):38-41, October 1991.

Rogers, M., et al. "Community-based Nursing Case Management Pays Off," *Nursing Management* 22(3):30-34, March 1991.

Selby, T. "RNs Oppose Mandatory HIV Testing," *The American Nurse* 23(8): 2, September 1991.

Strasen, L. "Redesigning Hospitals Around Patients and Technology," *Nursing Economics* 9(4):233-238, 1991.

Wood, C. "Health Care Rationing: The Oregon Experiment," *Nursing Economics* 9(4):239-243, 1991.

5

CULTURAL IMPLICATIONS FOR NURSING PRACTICE

OBJECTIVES

After studying this chapter, the reader should be able to:

1. Describe values held by members of dominant American culture.

2. Identify ways in which culture can affect health.

3. Describe cultural barriers to client care.

4. Identify prerequisites for culturally respectful care.

5. Discuss how culture affects communication and space needs.

6. Explain how time perceptions (temporal perspective, tempo, and importance of punctuality) might vary from culture to culture.

7. Describe the various family configurations.

8. Discuss alternate health care practices and how they might affect client care in traditional settings.

9. Describe how to assess an individual from a different cultural group.

INTRODUCTION

Cultural factors are playing increasingly important roles in all aspects of American health care, from individual interactions between nurse and client to larger-scale health care planning for a community or the nation as a whole. This is partly the result of demographic changes, which reveal a growing number of ethnic minorities in the United States. With new immigrants from Vietnam, Laos, Cuba, and Hong Kong living among established and encultured immigrant groups from Western and Eastern Europe, the Philippines, China, and Mexico, our society has become amazingly diverse.

Culture does not refer simply to ethnicity or national origin. It is, according to British anthropologist Edward Tyler, "that complex whole which includes knowledge, belief, art, morals, law, custom, and any other capabilities and habits acquired by man as a member of society" (Boyle and Andrews, 1989). Arnold and Boggs (1989) believe that culture includes the following components:

- religious beliefs
- rituals or ceremonies
- health practices
- language
- family interactions
- time orientation
- space orientation
- nonverbal communications customs
- nutrition and food preferences
- child-rearing practices
- values systems.

People's perceptions and actions related to these components define and express their culture, and these can vary widely. For example, a middle-class, professional African American will probably express the various cultural components in ways quite different from a poor, recent immigrant from Haiti. The cultural understandings of the *Sansei*, third-generation Japanese Americans, may differ from *Issei*, or first-generation Japanese immigrants. White Seventh-Day Adventists will have cultural beliefs and patterns different from white Roman Catholics.

Cultural understanding is critical to health care. Assessments and interventions that do not consider cultural components may not succeed and, in some cases, may cause negative consequences. A nurse unfamiliar with the communication behaviors of a certain ethnic group may assume that a client understands the instructions the nurse has given when in fact the client may only be showing politeness. As a result, the client may take external medications internally or may neglect or inaccurately perform treatments. Unfamiliarity with cultural norms can cause other difficulties. For example, a nurse whose own cultural values include showing concern through touch may offend a client to whom touch is inappropriate except with close family members.

Boyle and Andrews (1989) point out that "nursing interventions that are culturally relevant and sensitive to the needs of the client decrease the possibility of stress or conflict arising from cultural misunderstandings." Such nursing, which seeks to understand and assist clients as members of diverse cultural groups, is referred to as transcultural nursing. It requires that nurses know the clients' health beliefs, lifestyle, and health practices as well as their own. Nurses who are aware of their own cultural beliefs and values can avoid imposing them upon clients and in the process avoid ethnocentrism, or the belief that one's own values and beliefs are superior to all others.

Nurses preparing to practice in a certain locality should acquaint themselves with the different cultural groups with which they will interact. Familiarity with cultural needs and values, family patterns, common health problems, and, if possible, the language will enable nurses to provide more effective care and help clients make decisions about health care. A list of resources about various cultures appears at the end of the chapter.

CULTURE IN THE UNITED STATES

The dominant culture in the United States remains that of the white, Anglo-Saxon Protestant majority. This culture values work, frugality, conformity, and stability. Its members tend to be materialistic and to follow the nuclear family model. Within this group, however, younger members are developing values and practices that diverge from the norm. They enjoy life; they follow alternate family models; they accept individuality and change; and they are more informal than older members.

Many people in the United States, including those in the Anglo-Saxon majority, want to master a situation rather than passively accept it. This cultural orientation can cause frustration when events preclude such an outcome. For example, a client oriented toward active mastery might be intensely frustrated by a terminal cancer diagnosis. On the other hand, people from cultures that emphasize acceptance of life's experiences may find unalterable situations, such as the cancer diagnosis, easier to deal with. Misunderstandings can occur between clients and caregivers who hold different values. A caregiver who cannot passively accept unalterable conditions may think that a client who passively (and peacefully) accepts a terminal diagnosis is simply giving up.

The dominant white culture values external, material things rather than internal matters involving contemplation. As a result, group members become attached to objects and their accumulation rather than focused on internal processes. They frequently emphasize the need to accumulate possessions—homes, cars, clothing—even when such accumulation requires a highly stressful work schedule that leaves little time for contemplation and relaxation.

White Anglo-Saxons also emphasize a rational approach to life and consider tradition and custom less important in determining behavior than empirical evidence. People from other cultures may more highly value traditional wisdom and behavior. For example, they may treat diseases with herbs or acupuncture even when these practices cannot be scientifically confirmed as effective. White Anglo-Saxon Americans might use acupuncture for something like anesthesia but probably only after the practice has been rationally explained to them or demonstrated to be effective.

U.S. VALUE *ORIENTATIONS*

- *Active mastery*
- *Material possessions*
- *Rational, empirical analysis*

DEMOGRAPHIC CHANGES

Americans are exposed to many cultures, within the country and without, and this contact affects our knowledge of other people and their values. Every year, U.S. citizens travel abroad in large numbers, and immigration to the United States from many locations continues. In 1988, 4,006,700 Americans traveled abroad; most visited Canada (447,300), Mexico (601,800), West Germany (491,1000), the United Kingdom (284,800), and the Philippines (273,400) (U.S. Department of Commerce, 1990). The immigration rate was at a low in 1970 with only 373,000 immigrants arriving. The rate has increased, with 643,025 immigrants arriving in 1988 and 1,536,483 immigrants arriving in 1990. In 1990, 112,400 immigrants arrived from Europe; 338,600 from Asia; 975,600 from Canada, Mexico, the Caribbean islands, and Central America. An additional 85,800 came from South America; 35,900 from Africa; and 6,300 from all other countries (U.S. Department of Commerce, 1992).

Within the United States, the populations of most races are growing, with certain groups growing more rapidly than others. In 1980, the total white population was 188,372,000; in 1990, it was 199,686,000. This represents an increase of 6%. In 1980, the African American population was 26,495,000 and grew to 29,986,000 in 1990, representing an increase of 13.2%. The population of Hispanic citizens was 14,609,000 in 1980 and 22,354,000 in 1990, a 53% increase. Native American citizens numbered 1,420,000 in 1980 and 1,959,000 in 1990, a 37.9% increase (U.S. Department of Commerce, 1992).

States experience changing demographics differentially. Certain states have higher percentages of citizens from other countries and ethnic backgrounds. California, for example, has experienced a sizable influx of both legal and illegal Mexican immigrants and of Asians from Vietnam, Laos, Cambodia, and other Southeast Asian countries. Within the next two decades, California will probably become the first state to have no cultural group in a majority.

All these demographic changes indicate to the nursing community that nurses will soon be treating more clients with different beliefs and values, different approaches to health, and different ways of dealing with illness and death.

CULTURE AND HEALTH

In the past, workers in many disciplines assumed that their responsibilities included the modification of others' beliefs and behaviors to conform with those of Western culture. Following this philosophy, educators bused Native American children to schools where the children's cultural beliefs and values could be replaced with more modern, "scientific" ideas. Health care workers encouraged Native Americans, for example, to abandon traditional treatments and healers and to adopt scientific, Western approaches to illness and disease. Society expected immigrants to become "regular" Americans, assimilating and identifying with the dominant culture.

Total assimilation was never accomplished. Ethnic and cultural groups developed effective methods for transmitting their culture to their youth, and many people continued to rely on the health practices traditional to their culture and avoided contact with Western medicine. If they did use Western health care, they usually did so only after other, traditional remedies had failed.

Deloughery (1991) suggests several ways in which culture affects health: Culture determines a person's role and status in the family; it influences the availability of social, material, and professional supports. In addition, the way in which particular cultures view health and illness—especially chronic illness—affects the way members of that culture deal with symptoms, including pain and discomfort. This in turn influences people's decisions about when and how to seek health care and how they view health care in general.

A person's family role and status can strongly determine the quality of that person's health care. For example, in some Eastern societies that undervalue women, women and female children may receive little or no health care. Even in societies that view women mainly as child bearers, prenatal and delivery care may be minimal.

Robinson (1991) describes experiences in a Canadian mission hospital in Pakistan. The hospital's clients are women and children who come there because the government-sponsored hospital is overcrowded and unable to accommodate

CULTURAL FACTORS AFFECTING HEALTH

- *Family roles and reponsibilities*
- *Type and availability of support systems*
- *View of health and illness*
- *View of health care systems*

them. Health care is in effect rationed, and "women and children come last." Maternal mortality is nearly 1,000 out of 100,000 compared with 4 out of 100,000 in Canada. Women begin bearing children at early ages, and most births occur at home.

Personnel at the hospital's clinic regularly treat urinary fistulas, breast infections, diarrheal infections, and dietary deficiencies. Because most women marry soon after their initial menstruation, women who come to the hospital for prenatal care are very young. The nurses teach methods to prevent illness, reinforce helpful culturally based practices, and attempt to modify harmful health practices, such as putting cow dung on the infant umbilical cord.

Social, material, and professional support also influences a person's health. The accuracy of this theory is demonstrated in the United States, where income level practically determines health care access and the way in which health care is provided. The number of Americans without health insurance now exceeds 30 million (Sundwall and Tavani, 1991). Uninsured people usually do not or cannot use the health care system for basic and preventive care. As a result, they are denied access to important early measures that promote and retain health. They may also neglect childhood immunizations and prenatal care.

The definitions of health and illness vary from culture to culture. Hughes (1979) discusses North Amazonian Indians who believe that the disfigurement brought on by endemic dyschromic spirochetosis, an infection caused by various ubiquitous spirochetes, is a sign of normalcy; individuals unmarked by the disease are considered unhealthy or abnormal, and they are unable to arrange marriages. Boyle and Andrews (1989) similarly report that the African Mano consider primary and secondary yaws a normal condition rather than a disease, probably because the condition is so widespread.

Most cultures think of health as something more than simply the absence of disease. Societies that value personal development and growth may consider a person's ability to reach his physical and mental potential a sign of true health.

Societies that emphasize group contribution may focus on the individual's contributions to the group through work rather than on the individual's personal growth.

People's varying perceptions of proper body weight provide a good example of how cultural norms influence the definition of health. American culture values thinness and considers people who are heavier than average unhealthy or unattractive. Another society may consider obesity a sign not only of health but also of high economic and social status. In such a society, thinness may be a liability that could render an individual unable to contract marriage or work.

What a culture considers illness may or may not involve disease. Disease, as defined by Western medicine, represents the biological manifestation of an abnormal condition. Illness, on the other hand, is the subjective experience of feeling unwell. Cultural groups with few health care resources may expect individuals to cope with disease as part of life. Such cultures may not recognize illness until the individual becomes unable to perform normal work and social functions. In our own culture, individuals with chronic disease, such as diabetes, may not consider themselves ill once they have adapted their lifestyles to accommodate the disease. Similarly, individuals who have undergone coronary bypass surgery and rehabilitation for coronary artery disease may consider themselves healthy despite evidence that their health remains compromised.

How a cultural group regards chronic illness affects the way its members treat people with such illnesses. Some cultures provide support for families who must care for chronically ill members. This is especially true if the ill family member is elderly. In such cultures, the family caregivers usually do not think of their positions as particularly burdensome. People from other cultures may consider caring for chronically ill family members a tremendous burden that should be borne by society rather than by the family.

Families from cultures that do not provide adequate support for chronic illness care may become emotionally, physically, and financially exhausted and have the ill relative institutionalized. The phenomenon of "Grannie dumping,"—

abandoning an elderly relative, usually female, in a hospital emergency room—is a recent development in our own culture.

Culture also partly determines how people perceive and deal with pain and discomfort. Some cultures, including those of many Asian countries, emphasize a stoic response to pain; individuals from such cultures may loathe reporting discomfort or even extreme pain. In Latin cultures, responding openly to pain may be an expected illness behavior. A nurse working in an obstetric unit with laboring women from Asian and Latin cultures should not consider overt responses a necessarily accurate indication of the clients' pain level. Skillfully eliciting information during physical and cultural assessments can help nurses identify the presence of pain and alleviate it in a manner respectful of cultural values and expectations.

HEALTH IN APACHE CULTURE

Traditional Indian medicine (TIM) as practiced by the Apache, "involves the healing interaction of the mind, body, and spirit" (Kimbrough and Drick, 1991). Traditionally, the Apache believe that disease results from an imbalance in mind, body and spirit, and that healing is the process of reestablishing that balance. Whereas Western medicine views disease as something caused by external agents, such as germs, stress, or environmental hazards, TIM looks internally at the person's emotions and state of mind. TIM "does not discount the presence of microbial viruses and disease-causing organisms. It does hold that the body always follows the mind" (Kimbrough and Drick, 1991).

Ceremonies conducted by a medicine man who follows a strict ritual help the Apache deal with illness. The medicine man first cleanses the area in which a ceremony is to be held. He may do this by waving a smoking sage in different directions and asking the Great Spirit to cleanse the area. Through various ceremonies, the medicine man may minimize obstacles and strengthen the ill person's healing processes, but he cannot actually make an ill person well. That must be accomplished by the ill person. (Kimbrough and Drick, 1991)

The Apache believe that illness dissipates a person's positive energies, or "aura," and that during illness, a person is vulnerable to negative energies that can aggravate illness. As a result, they consider the doorway to the ill person's room an important barrier to negative energies.

A nurse working with an Apache client in a typical health care setting should try to incorporate the client's cultural health care beliefs with institutional expectations. Recognizing and accommodating traditional Apache practices are important first steps. Projecting a positive attitude, assisting with ceremonies while acknowledging institutional needs, and showing respect and care for the client can further enhance health care.

CULTURAL BARRIERS

Many factors can inhibit effective relations between nurses and clients from different cultures. These factors include lack of knowledge about other cultures, cultural stereotyping, ethnocentrism, and prejudice and discrimination.

THE RESULTS OF IGNORANCE

Many immigrants to the United States quickly learn the customs and expectations of our dominant culture. Others, particularly elderly people, may remain isolated in ethnic enclaves. Nurses should not expect such clients to understand the traditions and practices of Western medicine. Similarly, although nursing curricula are beginning to cover different cultural health beliefs, many nurses do not understand their clients' values and practices. A nurse ignorant of such may approach a client paternalistically and unintentionally dismiss the client's cultural beliefs by suggesting that Western medicine "knows what is best." Such misunderstandings can lead to confusion and antagonism.

Other problems can result from cultural ignorance. Boyle and Andrews (1989) discuss the problems associated with hospital food service. Nurses who lack cultural sensitivity may not realize that a client cannot decipher the hospital menu or that the client may have specific reasons for not wanting to follow the typical "American" diet. Nurses should be aware of clients with lactose intolerance, more common among Black and Asian clients, and not urge them to drink milk; they should also be aware of those with religious prohibitions against specific foods.

CULTURAL STEREOTYPING

Assuming that all members of a religious, ethnic, social, or racial group are alike also creates barriers to health care. Although cultural assessments presume certain similarities among individuals of a cultural group, the nurse must take particular care to identify the individual client's needs, beliefs, and values. For example, thinking that a member of a particular religious group does not drink alcoholic beverages or practice birth control may be erroneous.

ETHNOCENTRISM

As it relates to health care, ethnocentrism presumes that the only valid health care beliefs and practices are those of one's own culture. Although nurses should educate clients about their illnesses and treatments, they must also recognize that other ways of viewing and promoting health exist. A transcultural point of view allows nurses to value their own beliefs and practices while respecting clients' beliefs and values.

Nurses should also understand that although many ethnic and religious cultures have comfortably combined Western health practices with their own traditional health practices, other groups remain unable to do so. These groups may be uncomfortable with or antagonistic toward the idea of developing a bicultural point of view with the dominant culture. By recognizing ethnocentrism in themselves and in client groups that they serve, nurses can participate with clients in a joint, transcultural approach to health.

PREJUDICE AND DISCRIMINATION

Denigrating any cultural group and ascribing negative traits to all its members has as little place in health care as in any other facet of life. Nurses who stereotype black families as poor, undereducated, and lacking in cohesion as well as those who think of all white clients as affluent and without problems face the danger of delivering discriminating, possibly inadequate care to these groups. For example, a nurse who sees a black child in the emergency department and assumes that the child comes from a home that lacks knowledge about health care and insufficient resources to provide adequate care may improperly assess the child's condition, alienate the family, and jeopardize the child's health status. In the same manner, clients from the dominant culture may have health care needs that are not met because a nurse may assume that people who belong to the dominant culture do not have a particular health problem.

DEALING WITH CULTURALLY DIFFERENT CLIENTS

Just as specific cultural barriers exist, specific activities and actions that can help the nurse and client overcome such barriers also exist. As a first, perhaps most important step toward dealing with culturally different clients, the nurse should acquire knowledge about the cultures most frequently encountered. The nurse can accomplish this by reading, attending workshops and classes, and talking to people from different cultures. Two special reference sections appear at the end of this chapter (see "Recommendations for further study," pages 185 and 186). These sections list works about different cultural groups and works by writers belonging to these groups.

When confronted with diverse interpretations not only of health and illness but also of life itself, many people feel unsettled or disturbed. This reaction is known as culture shock. Many tourists in foreign countries experience a form of culture shock, which may cause them to return home feeling alienated and resentful. Student nurses may experience culture shock when they move from school to a work setting. Most immigrants will readily testify that culture shock contributes much to the stress of adapting to their new country.

After the initial culture shock subsides, some people may become converts to the new way of thinking and denigrate their previous beliefs and values. Nurses should understand that exposure to a different culture does not require that they abandon or feel guilty about their own. Sometimes young members of immigrant families are ready converts to the new values and beliefs they encounter. These young people may lose respect for the traditions of their cultural group, thereby causing cultural clashes within themselves and their families. Nurses should realize that such clashes may exist within families for which they are caring.

Nurses can further enhance care for culturally different clients by dealing with the clients both as members of their ethnic, racial, or religious group and as individuals with particular needs, values, and beliefs. Doing so helps prevent stereotyping and prejudice. When performing assessment, the nurse should affirm cultural beliefs and values and determine if divergent needs exist.

Most codes of ethics and bills of patients' rights state that nurses are expected to provide safe and competent care to all individuals. State boards of registered nursing support this expectation. The California Board of Registered Nursing "Statement on Delivery of Health Care to Patients with Communicable Disease" (1986) stipulates that

> The Board of Registered Nursing supports the right of all consumers to receive dignified and competent health care as set forth in the California Administrative Code, Section 1443.5. ... Although the nurse is not expected to take life-threatening risks in caring for clients, it is not acceptable to abandon any client based on age, religion, gender, ethnicity or sexual orientation.

Developing a professional philosophy that acknowledges client worth and client responsibility for health-related decisions should help nurses to become more comfortable in caring for culturally different clients.

As discussed in Chapter 1, Communication and interpersonal relations, how nurses and clients share information and interact with each other profoundly affects their relationship and client care. Communication techniques are as important to the nurse as other essential skills, such as medication administration and physical assessment.

Giger and Davidhizar (1991) suggest specific approaches to culturally different clients that should help to establish and ensure effective communication between nurse and client.

- Assess beliefs held by culturally different clients. (see "Performing a cultural assessment" later in this chapter).
- Assess communication variables and alter communication strategies to meet cultural needs. Nurses should assess the degree to which they will be affected by cultural differences. For example, if because of her culture, a female client refuses to answer questions about her own health, to whom should the nurse address the questions?
- Base care on the needs communicated by clients, taking their cultural background into account.
- Show respect for clients and their culture by respecting communication from them.
- Use a nonthreatening approach to communication. Take time to establish a relationship, allow the client to become comfortable before asking for personal information, and include family members when culturally appropriate.
- Confirm communication. Don't assume that information has successfully been communicated. Even when using translators, be alert to indications that the client does not understand.
- Recognize and respect client reluctance to discuss sexual matters, especially with strangers.
- If the client speaks an unfamiliar language, adopt special approaches. Use simple terms, avoid abbreviations and jargon, and consider pictures and drawings as useful adjuncts. If used, interpreters should communicate the substance of the information and show respect for clients and their culture.

Certain actions can minimize cultural conflicts. Caregivers can provide holistic care that recognizes the

ELEMENTS OF CULTURAL ORIENTATION

- *Communication patterns*
- *Space needs and expectations*
- *Time orientation*
- *Membership in groups*
- *Biological variation*

interrelatedness of individuals and their environment. Resources can be provided for nurses in the form of bicultural staff, translators, and information about different cultural groups. Developing a culturally relevant role for the client's family can also enhance care. Nurses can identify and incorporate appropriate nontraditional resources, including alternate health care practitioners as well as herbs and other treatments. Finally, health care institution policy should promote cultural pluralism and support nurses and clients in their efforts to work together.

CULTURAL ORIENTATION

Cultures can be distinguished on the basis of several criteria. Some of the more important criteria relate to concepts of communication, space, time orientation, and membership in groups. Each criterion reveals values and beliefs significant to particular cultures. (The concept of communication as a criterion is discussed above.)

CONCEPTS OF SPACE

How people perceive and think of space determines in part how they define territory, maintain privacy, communicate intimacy, and show authority. Understanding how different cultures use space can help the nurse communicate more effectively with a client. In some cultures, individuals closely associate their identity with a particular space and live their lives in one location and one dwelling. Traditional Navajos, for example, feel direct connection with ancestral lands, and having to leave historical homelands can produce feelings of severe loss and disorientation. Individuals from the dominant American culture typically move more frequently and easily, and nomadic bedouins may establish no permanent homes but instead carry those things that mean home with them as they wander.

The space a person requires for comfort when interacting with another varies from culture to culture. In some Arab cultures, for example, people are accustomed to close contact with others; such contact may make a person from another culture uncomfortable. Nurses should be aware of the ways in which clients define their "personal" space. They may use overbed tables or a drawn curtain to obtain a sense of privacy. They may place personal objects in a closet or on a chair to suggest possession. Nurses can show respect for a client's spatial definitions by asking permission to pass through a closed curtain or to move a bathrobe from a chair.

When moving a new client into a double room that has been occupied for some time by only one person, the nurse can help redefine personal spaces by introducing the two clients and orienting the new client to the room. The nurse can explain hospital policies concerning telephone and television use so that both clients understand expectations. If one client's family is going to visit at a certain time, the nurse might arrange for the other client to go to the cafeteria or to sit outside on a patio during that time, or the nurse might shift the location of the family visit.

TIME ORIENTATION

Time is another culturally influenced concept that can affect health care. People of the dominant U.S. culture are preoccupied by time. They are concerned about being on time, about wasting time, and about having "quality time" for important life activities. Many other cultures do not share this preoccupation with time. Western European cultures display different concepts of time. Swiss and German cultures show great concern for punctuality and timely observances. Historically, French culture has not placed such value on punctuality. According to Stoetzel (1953), 21% of the French population do not feel impelled to be on time; nor do they experience the feeling of wasting time. These people do not relate the value of time to accomplishing specific activities within a certain period, and they do not feel a social or interpersonal pressure to arrive for appointments on time.

These differing concepts of time can cause tension and conflict between individuals. In the hospital, for example, if the caregiver values punctuality and the client does not, they will probably not have the same understanding about ap-

TIME ORIENTATION

Time orientations affect an individual's perception of punctuality and tempo, or the pace at which life is lived. They also partly determine how the individual emphasizes past, present, or future experience.

- *Punctuality*
- *Tempo*
- *Temporal perspective (past, present, future)*

pointments and time activities. Nurses can help by not assuming that clients automatically understand the importance of arriving at a specific time for tests or treatments. Explaining to clients why a designated time is required may help. If possible, the nurse could identify a general time frame, such as morning or afternoon, for the client's appointment.

Tempo, or the pace at which life is lived, also varies from culture to culture. The tempo in urban Los Angeles is different from that in rural areas that are just a few miles away. Individuals transplanted from a slow-paced to a fast-paced environment may become stressed and feel as if they are unable to keep pace with everyone else. Moving from a fast-paced culture to a slower-paced one can also produce stress. The transplanted individual may feel that accomplishing anything is difficult, or that others are lazy or irresponsible about time. Nurses caring for clients accustomed to a slower pace can prevent stress by carefully explaining medication and treatment schedules. They can also give clients a greater sense of control in such situations by allowing them to help make decisions about when activities will occur.

Societies and individuals may be predominantly present-oriented, past-oriented, or future-oriented. These different time orientations can further affect health care. For example, undereducation, unemployment, or feelings of powerlessness may make some individuals feel trapped in a downward spiral. They will probably not be future-oriented because needs have overwhelmed them, and they will probably have little expectation that things will change. Their present-time orientation may hamper them in focusing on future health risks and current health-related behaviors that could either reduce or enhance risks to self or others. For example, a poor family living without housing in Chicago may be concerned only with the need to find food for the day and shelter for the night. Long-term health practices, such as childhood immunization, may be beyond their consideration.

In most cultures, one time orientation dominates; the other two orientations exist but in minor roles. American middle-class culture is heavily future-oriented: Parents enroll infants in preschools at birth, young adults invest for retirement, and people plan their funerals and buy burial plots well in advance. On the other hand, among the Navajo, present-time orientation predominates (Hall and William, 1960). Religious beliefs may contribute to this orientation: "Death and everything connected with it is repulsive to the Dineh [Navajo] and dead humans are buried as quickly as possible. Traditional Navajos have no belief in a glorious afterlife" (Locke, 1989).

Time orientation can influence client receptivity to health care strategies. For example, future-oriented cultures may more easily appreciate the advantages of preventive health care. In dealing with clients whose time orientation differs from their own, nurses must take care not to make improper assumptions. Late appointments or failure to plan for future health care does not mean that an individual is lazy, uncaring, or irresponsible. The problems associated with time orientation, however, do pose challenges to caregivers who would assist clients to achieve a better health care level in the present and future.

MEMBERSHIP IN GROUPS

Most people belong to several types of groups. The most common include groups based on family, religion, ethnicity, community or special interest. In addition to considering ethnic groups (the focus of this chapter so far), health care professionals must take particular interest in family and religious groups.

FAMILIES

Families significantly affect health care. Family members may provide direct care, decide on medical treatments, and encourage client participation in the healing process.

The typical nuclear family in the United States was once thought to be headed by a father, the principal wage earner, who provided for a mother who stayed at home to raise children. This family image now coexists with many versions, some more easily recognizable than others. The typical nu-

GROUP TYPES THAT AFFECT HEALTH CARE

- Family
- Religious
- Ethnic
- Community
- Special interest

clear family must now join a list of family types that includes blended, extended, single-parent, and nontraditional families.

Blended Families. When divorced people with children re-marry, they form a blended family, bringing with them the members from each former family and adding to that any new children born. This arrangement creates complex relationships, especially for children who may have two separate homes and sets of parents as well as natural siblings, step-sib-lings, and half-siblings.

Blended families potentially increase the number of peo-ple who may want to be involved in health care decisions. Like all other families, the blended family may be cohesive and helpful in health care situations, or it may be fragmented and its members at odds with one another. The nurse dealing with a client from a blended family must be sensitive to the different allegiances and feelings present. If, for example, a child has two sets of parents, the nurse needs to know which set will be making the health care decisions. Once this has been settled, the nurse may then schedule visits to allow each couple time with the child. The nurse may also have to clarify roles and the decision-making structure for all involved adults.

Extended Families. An extended family includes parents, grandparents, aunts, uncles, cousins, and may include close family friends. The presence or absence of an extended family can be important to client treatment and recovery. In the past, when families were less mobile and family members lived closer together, more people could be involved in post-hos-pital client care. If an elderly client required help after discharge, several members of the extended family would share care responsibilities. The long distances that frequently separate family members today make this type of support difficult. In the case of an elderly client, care may become the sole responsibility of the other spouse or of a single child who lives nearby. The nurse can help the client and family by assessing the care needed and determining the need and availability of outside assistance. The nurse might also help determine if the client requires an extended care facility.

A client's extended family can include friends who take on family responsibilities when traditional family members are unavailable. Through sensitive inquiry, the nurse can determine the client's support system and how it can be integrated into the post-discharge care process.

Single-parent families. The increase in the number of divorces over the past generations has left a number of families headed by single parents, usually female. To help the one adult responsible for giving care, the nurse can identify possible support sources, including the formal or informal extended family. In a case of serious illness, the other parent may become involved. Depending on how the parent/child unit feel about the other parent, this involvement may be stressful or helpful.

If the primary parent does not want involvement from the nonparticipating parent, the nurse must be guided by legal requirements, which may include prohibiting the nonparticipating parent from seeing the child. The nurse may, however, inform the parent about the child's condition and progress. Nursing care that recognizes the needs of all concerned individuals will best assist family members to support the ill child.

Nontraditional families. Nontraditional families include homosexual couples with or without children, alternative families, and communal families. The nurse should extend members of such families the same respect granted traditional family members.

Homosexual partners today may have had marriage ceremonies and consider themselves as much a unit as a traditional couple. Such couples may have children borne to one or both partners or by adoption. Regardless of the nurse's personal feeling about homosexuality, support of the individual client and those involved in care of the nontraditional family is important. Members of such families should receive the same respect accorded to members of traditional families.

Alternative families are composed of heterosexual couples, with or without families, who live together and consider themselves families without the legal sanction of marriage.

FAMILY TYPES

Understanding the different family types, their strengths and limitations, is an important step in planning for effective inclusion of family members in the health care process.

- *Traditional*
- *Blended*
- *Extended*
- *Single-parent*
- *Nontraditional*

Many states recognize a legal union when two individuals have lived together for a specified time. The people involved in these common-law marriages have the same rights and responsibilities as formally married spouses.

A communal family is a type of extended family composed of unrelated individuals who choose to live together for support or because of shared beliefs. The commune may or may not have established criteria for accepting new members and may contain traditional family units within it. Generally, communes identify and assign duties to each member. In Israeli kibbutzim, for example, certain members care for the children by either living in the children's houses or teaching in the schools.

In dealing with a communal family, the nurse may interact with a traditional set of parents supported by an informal extended family or with a communal leader who makes health care decisions for all members. By respecting the client's wishes concerning consultation and decision-making, the nurse can assure the client and communal family of support.

FAMILY CONSIDERATIONS

In dealing with any family type, the nurse must attend to certain general considerations. These include communication patterns among family members, family member roles, and the family's overall functioning level. The nurse must also assess whether the family will support or impede client recovery. Good family communication, well-defined and accepted roles, and a high functioning level will make client support easier to achieve.

RELIGIOUS GROUPS

A client's religious involvement may range from nominal church membership, characterized by a sense of identity with the group but not by active participation, to intimate daily participation in religious activities. In times of illness and incapacitation, many clients turn to religious groups for support. A client who has been inactive in the group for many years may find reestablishing such a relationship difficult. Through assessment, the nurse can determine if a client wants assistance contacting religious leaders or obtaining religious materials, books, or emblems.

Although many nurses and nursing students may have a general idea of the major religions' main tenets, they should also familiarize themselves with less well-known religious groups with which they may interact. To illustrate how religious information can help the nurse better support clients, this section discusses two less common religious groups and the health care implications associated with each.

Church of Jesus Christ of Latter-day Saints. A rapidly growing organization, the Church of Jesus Christ of Latter-day Saints, which also is known as the Mormon Church, remains small when compared with other religious groups although it now counts more members than such traditional churches as the Presbyterian church and the Episcopal church. Founded in 1830 by Joseph Smith, the church moved from the East across the plains to Utah. There, in 1847, Brigham Young established the church, which today has about 7 million members throughout the world ("Update," 1988). Each year, between 4 million and 5 million travelers visit Temple Square in Salt Lake City, where the church's headquarters and home of the Mormon Tabernacle Choir is located.

Smith set forth 13 articles of faith that represent the tenets central to Mormon belief:

We believe in God the Eternal Father, and in his Son, Jesus Christ, and in the Holy Ghost.

We believe that men will be punished for their own sins, and not for Adam's transgression.

We believe that through the Atonement of Christ, all mankind may be saved, by obedience to the laws and ordinances of the Gospel.

We believe that the first principles and ordinances of the Gospel are first, Faith in the Lord Jesus Christ; second, Repentance; third, Baptism by immersion for the remission of sins; fourth, Laying on of hands for the gift of the Holy Ghost.

We believe that a man must be called of God, by prophecy and by the laying on of hands, by those who are in authority to preach the Gospel and administer in the ordinances thereof.

We believe in the same organization that existed in the Primitive Church; apostles, prophets, pastors, teachers, and evangelists.

We believe in the gift of tongues, prophecy, revelation, visions, healing, and interpretation of tongues.

We believe the Bible to be the word of God as far as it is translated correctly; we also believe the Book of Mormon to be the word of God.

We believe all that God has revealed, all that He does now reveal, and we believe that He will yet reveal many great and important things pertaining to the Kingdom of God.

We believe in the literal gathering of Israel and in the restoration of the Ten Tribes; that Zion will be built upon this, the American continent, that Christ will reign personally upon the earth, and that the earth will be renewed and receive its paradisiacal glory.

We claim the privilege of worshiping Almighty God according to the dictates of our own conscience, and allow all men the same privilege; let them worship how, where or what they may.

We believe in being subject to kings, presidents, rulers and magistrates, in obeying, honoring and sustaining the law.

We believe in being honest, true, chaste, benevolent, virtuous and in doing good to all men; indeed we may say that we follow the admonition of Paul – We believe all things, we hope all things, we have endured many things, and hope to be able to endure all things. If there is anything virtuous, lovely, or of good report or praiseworthy, we seek after these things.

The Mormon Church is organized into wards composed of up to 800 members in the same geographic area. A bishop assisted by two counselors heads each ward. Wards compose larger units called stakes, each of which is headed by a stake president. The Office of the First Presidency, located in Salt Lake City, is responsible for central administration.

No paid ministers exist within the church, but all worthy men can hold a priesthood and can administer blessings. A Mormon client may request such blessing. The nurse need make no special arrangements other than providing a quiet environment and privacy. Usually, several individuals will give the blessing.

The Mormon Church has a strong social support network, usually coordinated through the office of the bishop and the women's auxiliary, the Relief Society. Through this network, the church consistently provides considerable client assistance after discharge. The nurse can help the client by identifying support needs and offering to contact the appropriate individuals.

The Mormon Church urges all members to stock a 2-year supply of food, clothing, and personal necessities as a personal safety net; however, needy members can contact the Church for support during economic distress or long-term illness. In addition, the church maintains an active welfare system coordinated through the ward bishop's office.

Church members who have gone to temple and received endowments (blessings) wear special undergarments to remind them of the blessings and covenants they have entered into. Members consider these undergarments a source of comfort and protection and usually wear them at all times. Finally, Mormons follow a dietary code called the Word of Wisdom, which prohibits smoking and the drinking of alcohol, tea, or coffee. It further encourages a limited meat intake. Mormons generally fast on the first Sunday of the month, beginning after the last meal on Saturday and ending Sunday evening. Although Mormons abstain from all food and drink during a fast, they will take medications. Ill church members are released from the obligation to fast.

When dealing with a Mormon client, the nurse should identify support personnel within the church, provide the opportunity for blessings and prayers, and obtain copies of scriptures, including the Bible and the Book of Mormon. The nurse should also establish dietary preferences and allow endowed members to wear their special garments as possible. As with all clients, showing respect and consideration helps to establish a therapeutic relationship.

Jehovah's Witnesses. Initially known as the International Bible Students, Jehovah's Witnesses was established in 1931 by Charles Taze Russell. Joseph Franklin Rutherford succeeded Russell and founded the Watchtower Bible Society.

Today, Jehovah's Witnesses has congregations in 100 countries and missionaries in 250 countries. Watchtower publications are published in more than 110 languages

The Jehovah's Witnesses faith includes the following beliefs:

> The one true god is Jehovah God, whose Witnesses from Abel to the present testify to His rule's establishment on Earth.
>
> The concept of the trinity (God the Father, Son, and Holy Ghost) is an error promulgated by Satan (Watchtower Bible and Tract Society, 1953, *Let God Be True* (rev. ed.) Brooklyn, New York: Author.) Jesus is conceived of as the perfect man whose sacrifice atones for the life that Adam forfeited in the Garden of Eden. Jesus was sent by God, but is not God.
>
> The second coming of Jehovah God is imminent, before which a great battle, Armageddon, will be fought against the forces of evil.
>
> During the final battle in which Jesus Christ will lead the righteous, the wicked will be destroyed. There is no Hell, because the wicked will be eliminated in this final battle. Christ will return as a spirit rather than as a resurrected human.
>
> During the millennium to follow, Jesus will rule with the resurrected, righteous dead and the Witnesses. At the end of the 1000 year period, Satan will be briefly loosed before he is destroyed and Paradise is established on Earth.
>
> Jehovah's Witnesses believe that eating blood is against God's will and that those who do are cut off from God.
>
> Jehovah's Witnesses do not serve in the armed forces and do not salute national flags or observe holidays, including Christmas.
>
> Jehovah's Witnesses do not drink liquor, do not smoke, and disapprove of divorce. They consider the Bible a book of prophecy, and most members are excellent scriptorians.

When caring for Jehovah's Witnesses, nurses should clarify the client's dietary needs and desires because of the religion's prohibitions. Because of their belief, Jehovah's Witnesses will probably refuse blood transfusions, even in life-threatening circumstances. This refusal can prove difficult for family members who may not be of the same faith and for caregivers with contrary principles. The courts have consistently supported adults in their right to refuse treatment; however, the courts have usually ruled that transfusions cannot be withheld from minors.

Nurses should also respect client beliefs about national symbols and holiday observances. They should not expect or urge Jehovah's Witnesses clients to participate in preparations for national holidays or Christmas. Nurses should also communicate respect for the client's pacifist beliefs.

Nurses and other health care providers can use an ethical decision-making structure to decide how to deal with such issues. This structure helps the nurse determine how such decisions should be made, who has the authority to make them, and what obligation each individual has toward supporting the decision. Chapter 7, Ethical implications for nursing practice, discusses such dilemmas and related problem-solving strategies.

ASSESSING RELIGIOUS GROUPS

When gathering information on religious beliefs and their potential impact on health care, nurses should include in their assessments the following considerations:

- What are the client's principal beliefs and religious practices, including holy days and special ceremonies?
- What dietary restrictions apply, including fasting practices?
- What restrictions related to treatments or procedures (biopsies, amputations, drug and blood product use) apply?
- How does the client view illness and death and issues such as organ donation and autopsy?
- What religious supports are available to the client?
- How can the nurse help the client obtain desired religious support?

ALTERNATIVE HEALTH CARE PRACTICES

A knowledge of alternative, or nontraditional, health care practices can help the nurse better care for clients who are combining these with traditional Western practices. Com-

ALTERNATIVE
HEALTH CARE

• *Homeopathy*
• *Osteopathy*
• *Chiropractic*
• *Naturopathy*
• *Chinese medicine*
• *Faith healing*

mon practices include homeopathy, osteopathy, chiropractic, naturopathy, Chinese medicine, and faith healing.

Although we think of Western health care practices as being scientifically and empirically sound, early applications of these practices were, in many cases, more harmful than helpful. During the "heroic" age of traditional medicine, roughly the period from 1780 to 1850, many approaches to illness that now seem unscientific, even bizarre, were in vogue. These included bleeding, during which blood, sometimes by the pint, was withdrawn, and intestinal purging with strong substances, such as mercury chloride or calomel. Clients took antimony salts as emetics and endured blistering with a heated glass. Many nontraditional approaches emerged, often introduced by traditionally trained doctors, in reaction to these aggressive and harmful treatments.

HOMEOPATHY

Samuel Hahnemann developed homeopathy in the late 1700s. Having been trained in traditional medical approaches, Hahnemann believed that physicians should not use treatments that had not been validated. He noted that many successful cures, including the use of the cinchona bark for malaria, produced the same symptoms as the disease, including fever and perspiration. He contended that administering substances that would produce such similar body responses would promote healing. As a result, he advocated administering minute, diluted doses of remedies that would produce symptoms of the disease being treated. He called his system homeopathy, meaning treatment "similar to the disease." Hahnemann also advocated using diet, along with remedies, to treat illness and suggested that remedies be shown to be effective for both men and women.

Hahnemann's system can be summarized by three laws. The Law of Similars refers to the practice of using remedies that produce symptoms resembling those of the disease being treated. The Law of Infinitesimals refers to Hahnemann's contention that as remedies were diluted, they became more efficacious in treating the disease. This principle extends to solutions that are diluted to such a degree that they contain no molecules of the original substance. Homeopathic practitioners contend that such remedies retain the essence, or active principle, even if the original substance is no longer present in the solution. Hahnemann's Law of Chronic Disease proposes that chronic illness results when harmful interventions suppress symptoms. Hahnemann believed that many traditional treatments hindered the body's own efforts to deal with the pathologic condition.

Western medicine today recognizes many of the issues raised by homeopathic practitioners, including supporting the body in its efforts to heal itself and not introducing potentially harmful treatments before they have been demonstrated to be effective. The nurse dealing with a client incorporating homeopathic approaches should be aware that the client's homeopathic remedies might interact with prescribed medications. By thoughtfully and sensitively asking the client about the homeopathic treatments and remedies being used, the nurse will be able to design an appropriate care plan. Realizing that the client may have reservations about traditional medications and treatments will enable the nurse to plan more effective client teaching concerning prescribed drugs and their importance for treatment.

LAWS OF HOMEOPATHY

- *Law of Similars*
- *Law of Infinitesimals*
- *Law of Chronic Illness*

OSTEOPATHY

Andrew Still developed the osteopathic approach during the late 1880s. Still, like Hahnemann, had been trained in the traditional Western medical tradition, but he became disenchanted with the use of drugs that he believed were often harmful to clients. Still believed a misalignment of the bony structure interfered with blood flow and with the nervous system, resulting in illnesses. He advocated manipulating the bony structure to restore balance of affected systems. During the 20th century, osteopathic physicians began using certain drugs as they were determined to be beneficial and safe. Today, osteopathic training and licensure is considered comparable to traditional medical preparation.

CHIROPRACTIC

Chiropractic, or "medicine by hand," was developed by David Daniel Palmer during the late 19th century. Palmer believed that spinal misalignment caused illness and disease. Treatment consisted of spinal manipulation to correct the misalignment. A schism arose between what were termed "straight" practitioners and "mixers," who combined spinal manipulation with other treatments, including diet and physical therapy. Today, chiropractors are licensed in all states.

As with clients using homeopathic approaches, nurses caring for clients also consulting a chiropractor should discover which chiropractic interventions and treatments are being used. They should conduct their inquiry so that clients do not feel denigrated for their beliefs.

NATUROPATHY

The naturopathic approach evolved from the European spa movement of the 18th and 19th centuries. Benedict Lust established the first College of Naturopathy, and he is credited with its early development. Treatment consisted of clients being sent to health resorts, or spas, for relaxation and treatment. Naturopathic practitioners believe that healing is promoted by removing clients from the environment in which they became ill and by using natural cures, including massage, diet, manipulation, and restful environment. Many European countries still use this therapy, which also forms the basis of the "retreat" practiced in the United States. Naturopathic practitioners are less commonly licensed than are other nontraditional practitioners; about 25% of states grant licenses.

Nurses should be aware that some naturopathic practitioners use hair shaft analysis to determine chemical imbalances within the client and that such analysis may not be accurate. Although a hair shaft analysis will identify what a client's hair lacks, this may not correspond to a deficiency in the client's body. Therefore, remedies prescribed on the basis of hair shaft analysis may lead to harmful excesses. For example, the prescription of additional vitamins, minerals, or metals may lead to harmful effects or overdose.

CHINESE MEDICINE

"Chinese medicine" refers to the practice of applying a specific philosophical system to the health and healing process. Practitioners believe that health represents a balance of energy, Chi. Excess or deficit energy leads to illness. In this system, energy is considered to be a five-stage process based on the characteristics of five substances, or "elements," including wood, fire, earth, water, and metal, arranged in a hierarchy. Wood, for example, controls earth because trees grow in the earth, and metal controls wood because trees can be felled with metal implements. Practitioners associate each of the five elements with different organs or organ systems.

Treatment involves identifying imbalances and restoring natural balance between yang, the positive element, and yin, the negative element. Yang is associated with openness, bigness, maleness, light, "outside," and with the hollow and secreting organs. Yin is associated with darkness, smallness, femaleness, "inside," and with solid organs. Practitioners may use acupressure and acupuncture, both believed to increase or decrease energy amounts received by a particular part of the body. Other treatments include massage and herbal and diet therapy based on yin and yang and the five elements.

Long disregarded by Western medicine, these approaches are now receiving closer examination. Exchanges between Western and Eastern countries have illustrated the efficacy of acupuncture in inducing pain relief and anesthesia, and combined approaches to client care are becoming more frequent. Nurses should assess clients for the use of nontraditional treatments in a supportive and respectful manner. This should include identification of dietary, activity, and treatment regimens because they may affect the selection of other medications or treatments.

FAITH HEALING

People from many religious denominations believe in faith healing. Its forms may vary from simple prayer to prescribed rituals and ceremonies that must be precisely followed to be effective. Roman Catholic clients, for example, may undertake a journey to Lourdes, France, where 2 million visitors go each year. Lourdes is the site of a spring at which a peasant girl received a vision of the Queen of Heaven. People believe that the spring water has healing properties. Clients from certain Protestant denominations believe that certain designated individuals may effect a cure by the "laying on of hands." Certain Native American groups believe that the invocation of a Great Spirit through specific ceremonies can help people cure themselves.

During assessment, nurses should determine how a client feels about faith healing and whether the client desires the support and services of a priest, congregation member, or other appropriate figure. The nurse must always be careful to respect the client's beliefs and make efforts to provide for requested ceremonies, prayers, or other interventions. Knowing the requirements of such interventions enables the nurse to anticipate conflicts and to find acceptable accommodations. For example, if the chanting of a curative ritual will disturb other clients, the nurse can make arrangements to hold the ceremony or ministration in another area or when the other clients are absent.

BIOLOGICAL VARIATION

Clients from different cultures also exhibit biological variation, a particularly important concept for nurses who may have learned assessment techniques using the Caucasian client as the norm. Caucasian biology is also frequently used as the norm for calculating laboratory values and drug regimens. Normal physical variations among clients from different cultures may present difficulties during assessment if the nurse uses an approach based on Caucasian clients.

The potential problem can be illustrated by an obvious biological difference among cultural groups—skin color. When caring for people of color, the nurse must determine normal skin color, texture, and turgor for an individual and must also determine what suggests abnormality. The nurse can establish a baseline color in good light, relying on least pigmented body surfaces, usually the palms, soles, and abdomen. Having identified a normal baseline, the nurse can more easily detect deviations.

For some populations, the nurse can use the oral mucosa and the conjunctiva to assess skin changes; however, the nurse should know that hyperpigmentation may occur on the tongue and oral mucosa of dark-skinned people as a normal phenomenon and that pigmented spots may exist on the sclera. Nevertheless, the nurse can usually use the conjunctiva to assess pallor and cyanosis once a baseline color has been established. Some people suggest that in dark-skinned clients, the lips, buccal mucosa, and tongue are best for assessing central cyanosis and the nails and extremity skin are helpful in identifying peripheral cyanosis.

Nurses should know that biological variations can account for atypical test results that are in fact normal for certain individuals. Boyle and Andrews (1989) note that the normal hemoglobin level for African Americans is lower than that for other groups and that evidence exists that Asian Americans and Mexican Americans have higher hemoglobin and hematocrit values than do Caucasians. These differences could affect the diagnosis and treatment of conditions such as anemia. Recognizing that individuals from different cultures have different health risks, different physical assessment needs, and different reactions to drugs and tests is part of good nursing.

PERFORMING A CULTURAL ASSESSMENT

Several cultural assessment formats and models exist, and the nurse should use the model appropriate to the situation at hand. A nurse in the emergency department of a busy urban hospital may need a different format than one working in a physician's office or in a home-care setting. The nurse must evaluate the workplace constraints and needs as well as the client's immediate and long-term needs to determine how to make a cultural assessment.

Deloughery (1991) suggests obtaining data on three basic cultural points: religious preference, family makeup and functioning patterns, including dietary customs, and health care patterns. Following this and depending on the circumstances, the nurse questions the client about the specific health care problem. Does the client understand the cause of the problem and its onset? How does the client view the problem's seriousness? Is the problem recurrent? How has the client dealt with the problem in the past? What family and community support does the client think is necessary?

Boyle and Andrews (1989) suggest a more complex approach that helps the nurse understand a cultural group as a whole. Their approach comprises eight major categories:

- brief history of the cultural group's origin
- value orientation, including ethics code, behavior standards, and world view (also included are attitudes toward time, work, money, and other significant values)
- interpersonal relations, including family and child rearing, ways of showing respect and assertion, roles/relationships
- communication, including how language, arts, music, and literature are used
- religious beliefs, rituals, needs
- social systems, including economic, political, and educational
- dietary habits and needs
- beliefs related to health and illness.

Regardless of the approach used for an initial cultural assessment, the nurse should ask the following questions:

- What does the client think about the nature of the illness? What does the client believe to be its cause? How does the client usually deal with the problem? How can others help?
- What support systems are available to the client? Is support from family, religious, community, or ethnic groups available to the client during and after treatment? Does the client need assistance contacting these individuals?
- What treatments is the client using to maintain health and treat illness? Are nontraditional healers involved? What remedies or treatments are ongoing or under consideration? What assistance will be needed from the health care institution or staff to accommodate a combined approach to the problem?

- What biological and social factors should the nurse consider when planning client care? What health care risks and individual needs characterize the client's culture? What communication problems might occur?
- What does the client want from traditional medicine? What problems are foreseeable? What decisions can be anticipated? How might any legal or ethical problems be addressed?

As the client answers these questions, the skillful nurse will identify other concerns and issues that can be sensitively queried. By communicating to clients a desire to understand their values and beliefs and by demonstrating respect and consideration for cultural differences, nurses can enlist client support in obtaining information vital to the treatment course.

SUMMARY

Culture is a broad concept that includes social, spiritual, and biological variables. Culture influences the way people view health and illness and the way they respond to health care problems. To provide efficacious treatment, health care personnel must recognize different cultural patterns and needs and respect the client's right to make treatment decisions. Nurses should acquire knowledge about the health beliefs and practices of those cultural groups with which they most often interact. They should learn about the different cultures' orientation to issues such as space and time; they should become informed about various religious beliefs and practices; they should learn about any alternative health care practices used by clients; and they should recognize biological differences among races.

Nurses must understand that respect—for the individual and for values and beliefs that may be differ from their own—is essential to successful care of culturally different clients.

APPLICATION EXERCISE

Develop and perform a cultural assessment of someone of your choice. Depending on circumstances, the person may be an actual client, a fellow student, or an acquaintance. Conduct the assessment in a quiet environment and ensure the person that all responses will remain confidential. To illicit characteristics and needs, develop and ask questions that address the following areas:

1. Principal Cultural Group
- identified or described by client

2. Communication and Interpersonal Relations
- language used at home
- communication difficulties with health care personnel
- time perceptions (punctuality, tempo, temporal orientation)
- space interpretations
- potential barriers to care in traditional settings

3. Definitions of Health and Illness
- preventive practices
- effects of illness on dietary preferences
- views of traditional health care system
- barriers related to accessing the traditional care system

4. Alternate Health Care Practices
- methods used, practitioners involved
- treatments or medications used
- barriers in the traditional health care setting that hamper practice of alternate health care
- overcoming or minimizing barriers

5. Religious Needs
- religious affiliation
- degree of religious involvement
- barriers in the health care setting to accommodating religious needs
- overcoming or minimizing barriers

6. Family and Other Support Systems
- family members who might be involved in care
- family expectations during illness
- other support systems (community, religious, ethnic) available
- integrating support systems in care plan

7. Value Orientation
- client's value system compared with values of dominant U.S. culture (mastery of situations, materialism, rational approach to problems)
- minimizing barriers related to different value system

8. Biological Variation
- implications related to the client's culture
- discrepancies from traditional norms and values possible in laboratory and other data
- precautions needed to account for any biological variations

9. Nursing Self-assessment
- feelings about caring for a client from this cultural group
- knowledge possessed and needed about this group
- concerns about communications, life style, religious preference, values, and health care practices
- support available for dealing with the client effectively and sensitively

Alternate Application Exercise

1. Identify a culture about which you have little knowledge. Then choose one of the cultural assessment topics listed in the Application Exercise. Concentrating on the topic, gather information related to the culture you have chosen. Summarize the information you find in a short paper, describing how the cultural information you found could affect health care delivery. (See 'References on ethnic groups' and 'Works by ethnic writers' under "Recommendations for further study" below).

2. Read one book from the 'Works by ethnic writers'. What health care barriers related to the culture portrayed in the book might a nurse anticipate?

Review Questions

1. What family groupings exist today?

2. What support systems do clients usually access during illness? How can a lack of support affect client care?

3. What roles do families and other groups play in caring for members? How does cultural orientation affect these roles?

4. Briefly define cultural stereotyping, ethnocentrism, and prejudice and discrimination.

5. What problems exist in dealing with clients whose time sense differs from that of the dominant culture?

6. Identify one alternate health care approach. What problems should the nurse anticipate in caring for a client using both traditional and alternative health care approaches?

7. How can nurses accommodate clients using alternative health care approaches in a traditional setting?

8. Why is a cultural assessment important? What difficulties would you anticipate during a cultural assessment of your clients?

REFERENCES

Arnold, E.A., and Boggs, K. *Interpersonal Relationships: Professional Communication Skills for Nurses.* Philadelphia: W.B. Saunders Co., 1989.

Boyle, J.S., and Andrews, M.M. *Transcultural Concepts in Nursing Care.* Glenview, Ill.: Scott, Foresman/Little, Brown College Division, 1989.

Deloughery, G.L. *Issues and Trends in Nursing.* St. Louis: Mosby Inc., 1991.

Giger, J.N., and Davidhizar, R.E. *Transcultural Nursing: Assessment and Intervention.* St. Louis: Mosby Inc., 1991.

Hall, E., and William, F. "Intercultural Communication: A Guide to Men of Action," *Human Organization* 19:7-9, 1960.

Hughes, C. "Medical Care: Ethnomedicine," in *Health and the Human Condition.* Edited by Logan, M., and Hunt, E. Belmont, Calif.: Wadsworth, 1979.

Kimbrough, K.L., and Drick, C.A. "Traditional Indian Medicine: Spiritual Healing Process for All People," *Journal of Holistic Nursing* 9(1):25-29, January 1991.

Locke, R.F. *The Book of the Navajo.* Los Angeles: Mankind Publishing Co., 1989.

Massey, M. "What You Are Isn't Necessarily What You Will Be" (video). Magnetic Video Corporation, Farmington, Mich.

Ortiz, A. "Through Tewa Eyes: Origins," *National Geographic Magazine* 18(4):6-13, October 1991.

Robinson, K.R. "Canadian Nurse in Pakistan," *The Canadian Nurse* 87(2):26-29, March 1991.

Stoetzel, J. "The Contribution of Public Opinion Research Techniques to Social Anthropology," *International Social Science Bulletin* 5:494-503, 1953.

Sundwall, D.N., and Tavani, C. "The Role of Public Health in Providing Primary Care for the Medically Underserved," *Public Health Reports: Journal of the U.S. Public Health Service* 106(1):2-5, January-February 1991.

Tripp-Reimer, T. "Research in Cultural Diversity: Directions for Future Research," *Western Nursing* 6(2):253-255, 1984.

"Update," in *Ensign: The Ensign of the Church of Jesus Christ of Latter-day Saints* 80, March 1988.

U.S. Department of Commerce, Bureau of the Census. *Statistical Abstract of the United States*, 110th ed. Washington, D.C.: U.S. Department of Commerce, Bureau of the Census, 1990.

U.S. Department of Commerce, Bureau of the Census. *Statistical Abstract of the United States*, 112th ed. Washington, D.C.: U.S. Department of Commerce, Bureau of the Census, 1992.

RECOMMENDATIONS FOR FURTHER STUDY

References on ethnic groups

Billingsley, A. *Black Families in White America.* Englewood Cliffs, N.J.: Prentice-Hall, 1968.

Bullough, V.L., and Bullough, B. *Health Care for the Other Americans.* East Norwalk, Conn.: Appleton-Century-Crofts, 1982.

Hashizume, S., and Takano, J. "Nursing Care of Japanese American Patients," in *Ethnic Nursing Care: A Multicultural Approach.* Edited by Orque, M., et al. St. Louis: C.V. Mosby Co, 1983.

Mayor, V. "The Asian Community: the family bereavement and dietary beliefs." *Nursing Times* June 6, 1984, pages 40-42.

Mills, S.C. "Saudi Arabia: An Overview of Nursing and Health Care," Focus on Critical Care, 13(1):50-56, 1986.

Tom-Orme, L. and Hughes, C.C. "Health beliefs about diabetes mellitus in an American Indian tribe," in Carter, M. (ed.), Proceedings of the 10th Annual Transcultural Nursing Conference. Salt Lake City: Transcultural Nursing Society, 1985.

Tong, A. "Food habits of Vietnamese immigrants." *Family Economic Review* 2:28-30, 1986.

Works by ethnic writers

Acuna, R. *Occupied America: A History of Chicanos.* New York: Harper & Row Publishers, 1981. (Hispanic)

Bulosan, C. *America is in the Heart: A Personal History.* Seattle: University of Washington Press, 1973. (Filipino-American).

Douglass, Frederick. *Life and Times of Frederick Douglass.* New York: Carol Publishing Group, 1983. (African American)

Ellison, R. *Invisible Man.* New York: New American Library, 1952. (African American)

Garcia Marquez, G. *One Hundred Years of Solitude.* New York: Avon Books, 1971. (Hispanic)

Hong Kingston, M. *The Woman Warrior: Memoirs of a Girlhood Among Ghosts.* New York: Vintage International, 1989. (Chinese American)

Hurston, Z. N. *Their Eyes Were Watching God.* New York: Harper & Row Publishers, 1990. (African American)

Morrison, T. *Sula.* New York: New American Library, 1982. (African American)

Neihardt, C. *Black Elk Speaks.* Lincoln: University of Nebraska Press, 1979. (Native American)

Ortiz, S.J. *From Sand Creek.* New York: Thunder's Mouth Press, 1981. (Native American)

Rivera, T. *Y No Se Lo Tragó La Tierra: And the Earth Did Not Devour Him.* Translated by Vigil-Piñón, E. Houston: Arte Público Press, 1987. (Hispanic)

Silko, L.M. *Ceremony.* New York: Penguin Books, 1986. (Native American)

Singer, I.B. *The Collected Stories.* New York: Farrar, Straus and Giroux, 1990. (Jewish)

Wright, R. *Black Boy: A Record of Childhood and Youth.* New York: Harper & Brothers, 1945. (African American)

6

LEGAL IMPLICATIONS FOR NURSING PRACTICE

OBJECTIVES

After studying this chapter, the reader should be able to:

1. Describe the origins of common, statutory, and constitutional law.

2. Distinguish between public law and private law.

3. Discuss the four components of credentialing, including licensure, registration, certification, and accreditation.

4. Identify the components required to demonstrate nursing negligence or malpractice.

5. Identify usual reasons for client suits and describe measures to avoid them.

6. Describe the judicial process, from the filing of a complaint to the rendering of a decision or verdict.

7. Explain how to prepare for being a court witness.

8. Identify how advance directives impact nursing practice.

9. Understand nursing expectations related to informed consent.

INTRODUCTION

This chapter discusses the relation between law and nursing. Beginning with the historical development of law, the chapter identifies the traditional division of constitutional, statutory, and decisional branches. It next explains how law affects client and nursing rights and discusses nursing credentialing and regulation, professional nursing standards, and contracts. Next, the chapter defines negligence and malpractice and identifies areas of specific risk. It describes legal proceedings, including depositions, testifying, and court conduct, and identifies nursing areas that are prone to legal action. Specific areas of concern, such as orders not to resuscitate, living wills, and durable power of attorney, also are discussed. The chapter then explains how nurses can reduce the risk of legal action (conforming to professional practice standards and using risk management techniques and quality assurance activities) and concludes by discussing malpractice insurance.

LAW AND NURSING: RECENT DEVELOPMENTS

In the past, nurses were considered both by the law and by the health care profession to be dependent practitioners who could not be held accountable for their actions. Instead, the physician, hospital, or clinic assumed legal responsibility for nurses' acts. As nursing practice has become more autonomous, however, nurses have increasingly been held responsible for their actions.

The legal and societal emphasis on individual rights over social responsibility is also contributing to change within the nursing profession. Individuals have the right to make decisions about their own health care. This right is generally observed, even though it may increase the societal burden of caring for those who cannot provide for themselves because of earlier health care choices. As a result, many groups (clients' rights organizations, the consumer movement, the women's movement, and others) are working to create structures that promote individual responsibility while recognizing society's obligation to provide a minimum care standard.

Clients' rights organizations have demanded greater opportunities for clients to consent or to decline treatments. Consumer rights advocates have demanded increased access to cost-effective health care as well as the right to safety, the right to be informed, the right to choose, and the right to be heard. The women's movement, by enfranchising a population that has historically been ill-treated by the health care and legal systems, has called for far-reaching reforms, including the redistribution of health care resources and the development of a system that not only safeguards consumers' legal rights but also regulates litigation and related monetary awards.

COMMON, STATUTORY, AND CONSTITUTIONAL LAW

U.S. law is a combination of common and statutory law, which is supported by the concepts embodied in the U.S. constitution. Common, or decisional, law has evolved from the pronouncements of kings, who decreed and ruled by Divine Right, and the decisions of judges, who based their rulings on the decisions of their kings and other judges. Statutory law results from legislation developed and passed by Congress, state legislatures, and city councils.

In 1215, King John of England issued the Magna Charta, which inhibited the rights of kings to dictate law and granted citizens certain individual and property rights. Many historians consider this document to be the cornerstone of constitutional law, which finds its fullest expression today in the U. S. Constitution. This document establishes the basic law of the land and grants certain powers to the federal government and others to the individual states. Each state in turn has its own constitution, which further defines authority. Federal and state constitutional law underlies all common and statutory laws.

Within the bounds of constitutional law, then, federal and state legislatures provide the statutory law to which citizens, associations, and corporations are subject. Federal statutes are referred to as U.S. Codes. Title VII of the Civil Rights Act, which makes discrimination against someone on the basis of race, sex, religion, or country of origin an offense, is a federal statute. States establish similar statutes, such as education codes regulating the conduct of schools and penal

THE ORIGIN OF U.S. LAW

- *Common law: court decisions*
- *Statutory law: legislatures*
- *Constitutional law: constitutions*

TYPES OF LAW

Public law
- Criminal law
  (misdemeanors,
  felonies)

Private law
- Contract law
- Tort law
  - intentional torts
  - unintentional torts
    (negligence,
    malpractice)

codes regulating the conduct of state prisons. An important state statute for nurses is the Worker's Compensation Act, which ensures compensation for work-related injuries.

As times change, some laws need revision. To meet this need, specified public agencies have been established to monitor and adjust certain aspects of the laws through rules and regulations, which then have the force of law. Administrative agencies with regulatory responsibilities include the U.S. Department of Health and Human Services and the U.S. Food and Drug Administration.

In areas where constitutional and statutory law do not provide guidance, the principles of common law continue to be applied. The concept of "stare decisis" is followed, in which the court affirms the intent to "stand by things decided" or to follow established precedent. In this manner, the court follows the same rules and principles in deciding cases in which the conditions are similar to cases already decided. If conditions are different, and a different decision is reached, an expansion of common law results.

PUBLIC LAW AND PRIVATE LAW

Laws can be classified as public and private. Public law applies to the relationship of the individual to federal, state, or municipal government. Private law covers the relationship between individuals and consists of contract law and tort law. Contract law governs agreements between individuals for services and remuneration. In cases for which no contract exists, tort law determines individual rights and responsibilities. The word tort, derived from a Latin word meaning "twisted," refers to an act of wrongdoing. Tort law governs wrongdoing between individuals without formal contracts.

Like all individuals, nurses are subject to public law. Related crimes are categorized as felonies and misdemeanors. Felonies are serious offenses punishable by imprisonment or, in some states, death. Nursing felonies might include mercy killing—an intentional act—or causing client death by accidentally administering drugs to which the client was allergic. In these cases, the severity of the charge would depend on the nurse's intentions. Misdemeanors are less serious offenses usually punishable through fines and short-term imprisonment. Nursing misdemeanors might include taking chocolates from a client's nightstand without permission or failing to turn in change found in a client's clothing.

Like public law, private law distinguishes between intentionally committed wrongs and those committed accidentally. As it applies to nursing, private law could cover intentional torts, such as libel and slander, and unintentional torts, such as negligence and malpractice. Later sections in this chapter discuss these issues.

NURSING LAW

The first laws governing nursing practice were enacted in the early 1890s. These laws, termed "permissive" laws because they included no constraints on the practice of nursing, stated that the registered nurse title could be used only by individuals who had been registered and who had paid the requisite fee. In 1903, North Carolina became the first state to register nurses. Other states followed, and by 1923, all states had nurse registration laws.

New York State passed the first mandatory nurse practice act in 1938. This act divided nursing practice into registered nursing and practical nursing and stipulated that only licensed individuals could practice. By 1952, all states had nurse practice acts, the majority of them being mandatory. In 1955, the American Nurses' Association (ANA) formulated the first definition of nursing practice. In 1973, the ANA amended its original definition to eliminate the prohibition against nursing diagnosis, a recognition of nurses' growing responsibilities.

The formulation of standards related to client care and nursing practice has further defined nursing. Client care standards include those developed for Medicare and Medicaid clients, which describe the type and level of care that a client can expect. Initiated by clients' rights groups, other legislation has been passed to protect the rights of elderly and terminally ill clients. The Joint Commission for Accreditation of Healthcare Organizations (JCAHO) also has developed accreditation standards that ensure certain types and levels of care. ANA standards of nursing practice define expected nursing behaviors in a broad context. The American Hospital Association has published a patient's bill of rights. (See *A patient's bill of rights.*) Other standards apply to maternal-child care, geriatric clients, and community health settings.

Institutions have also devised and implemented standard care plans that describe expected nursing performance for clients with various problems. For example, a hospital may have a standardized care plan for clients undergoing laminectomy. The care plan could be modified to fit the individual client while ensuring an overall standard of care.

CLIENT RIGHTS, NURSING RIGHTS, AND NURSING DUTY

An appreciation of inherent individual rights informs the concept of client rights. A right is a claim or privilege to which one is entitled. As individuals, clients are entitled to respectful treatment. The nurse should also respect the client's choices regarding treatment and care. Client rights may or may not be protected by law. For example, although the American Hospital Association states that patients should be informed about the relationship between the hospital and other health care and educational institutions, formal laws imposing penalties for hospitals that fail to provide such information may not exist.

When statements of rights do exist, as they do for elderly, disabled, and dying clients, they may not only describe rights due or owed to someone but also suggest the responsibilities, or duties, of others to safeguard these rights. For example, most statements regarding clients' rights to competent and respectful care suggest that the caregivers must maintain knowledge of current developments in their field, display competence in all required skills, and use a respectful approach. Chapter 7, Ethical implications for nursing practice, further discusses the concepts of duty, value, and rights.

A PATIENT'S BILL OF RIGHTS

1. The patient has the right to considerate and respectful care.

2. The patient has the right to . . . relevant, current, and understandable information concerning diagnosis, treatment, and prognosis. Except in emergencies when the patient lacks decision-making capacity and the need for treatment is urgent, the patient is entitled to the opportunity to discuss and request information related to the specific procedures and/or treatments, the risks involved, the possible length of recuperation, and the medically reasonable alternatives and their accompanying risks and benefits. Patients have the right to know the identity of physicians, nurses, and others involved in their care, as well as when those involved are students, residents, or other trainees. The patient also has the right to know the immediate and long-term financial implications of treatment choices . . . .

3. The patient has the right to make decisions about the plan of care prior to and during the course of treatment and to refuse a recommended treatment or plan of care to the extent permitted by law and hospital policy and to be informed of the medical consequences of this action. In case of refusal, the patient is entitled to other appropriate care and services that the hospital provides or transfer to another hospital. . . .

4. The patient has the right to have an advance directive (such as a living will, health care proxy, or durable power of attorney for health care) concerning treatment or designating a surrogate decision maker with the expectation that the hospital will honor the intent of that directive to the extent permitted by law and hospital policy. Health care institutions must advise patients of their rights under state law and hospital policy to make informed medical choices, ask if the patient has an advance directive, and include that information in patient records. The patient has the right to timely information about hospital policy that may limit its ability to implement fully a legally valid advance directive.

5. The patient has the right to every consideration of privacy. Case discussion, consultation, examination, and treatment should be conducted so as to protect each patient's privacy.

6. The patient has the right to expect that all communications and records pertaining to his/her care will be treated as confidential by the hospital, except in cases such as suspected abuse and public health hazards when reporting is permitted or required by law. The

(continued)

A PATIENT'S BILL OF RIGHTS (continued)

patient has the right to expect that the hospital will emphasize the confidentiality of this information when it releases it to any other parties entitled to review information in these records.

7. The patient has the right to review the records pertaining to his/her medical care and to have the information explained or interpreted as necessary, except when restricted by law.

8. The patient has the right to expect that, within its capacity and policies, a hospital will make reasonable response to the request of a patient for appropriate and medically indicated care and services. The hospital must provide evaluation, service, and/or referral as indicated by the urgency of the case. When medically appropriate and legally permissible, or when a patient has so requested, a patient may be transferred to another facility. The institution to which the patient is to be transferred must first have accepted the patient for transfer. The patient must also have the benefit of complete information and explanation concerning the need for, risks, benefits, and alternatives to such a transfer.

9. The patient has the right to ask and be informed of the existence of business relationships among the hospital, educational institutions, other health care providers, or payers that may influence the patient's treatment and care.

10. The patient has the right to consent to or decline to participate in proposed research studies or human experimentation affecting care and treatment or requiring direct patient involvement, and to have those studies fully explained prior to consent. . . .

11. The patient has the right to expect reasonable continuity of care when appropriate and to be informed by physicians and other caregivers of available and realistic patient care options when hospital care is no longer appropriate.

12. The patient has the right to be informed of hospital policies and practices that relate to patient care, treatment, and responsibilities. The patient has the right to be informed of available resources for resolving disputes, grievances, and conflicts, such as ethics committees, patient representatives, or other mechanisms available in the institution. The patient has the right to be informed of the hospital's charges for services and available payment methods.

Nursing students also have rights. In 1985, the ANA House of Delegates articulated the following student rights:
- the right to qualified instructors
- the right to evaluate teacher performance
- the right to a relevant curriculum in which they have input.

Nurses' rights have also been formally stated. Fagin (1975) identifies the following rights of all nurses:
- the right to find dignity in self-expression and self-enhancement through their special abilities and educational background
- the right to recognition for their contribution through the provision of a proper environment for practice and appropriate remuneration
- the right to a work environment that minimizes physical and emotional stress and health hazards
- the right to determine what constitutes professional practice within the limits of the law
- the right to set nursing standards of excellence
- the right to participate in policy-making affecting nursing
- the right to social and political action on behalf of nursing and health care.

The first three rights primarily address the employer's obligation to provide appropriate pay and a safe professional environment in which work can be performed with dignity. The remaining statements go beyond the individual and suggest certain rights of the profession in general. The right to define professional performance places nursing on a level with the legal and medical professions, thereby enhancing the stature of the individual nurse and the nursing profession.

REGULATION AND CREDENTIALING

Fiesta (August 1990) states that "the legal basis for licensure rests on the government's responsibility to protect the health, safety and welfare of the public." In accordance with this, federal agencies mediate the credentialing and regulation of nursing practice. Credentialing comprises licensure, registration, certification, and accreditation. Regulation is accomplished by enforcing the provisions of licensure, registration, certification, and accreditation.

LICENSURE AND REGISTRATION

Licensure "establishes standards for entry into the practice, defines a scope of practice, and allows for disciplinary action" (Fiesta, August 1990). State nursing boards grant licensure to individuals who have completed an approved program of study, passed at a stipulated level the National Council Licensure Examinations of the National Council of State Boards of Nursing, and paid a required fee. Nurses registered in one state may receive licensure by endorsement from another state, depending on recognition of educational preparation and sufficient national test scores. Licensure by endorsement is complicated by the fact that some states now require the baccalaureate degree for licensure as a registered nurse. As a result, a nurse who is registered in one state but who does not hold a baccalaureate degree in nursing may not be eligible for licensure by endorsement in a state requiring the baccalaureate.

In the United States, licensure to practice as a registered nurse is mandatory, with the following exceptions:

- practice in an emergency situation
- practice while a student in a registered nursing program offered by an accredited nursing school
- practice as a nurse employed by the federal government, for example, in Veterans Administration hospitals (nurses employed by the government must be licensed but not necessarily in the jurisdiction in which the facility is located).

State nurse practice acts define what constitutes the scope of practice and, by extension, what constitutes unauthorized practice. Some states, contrary to ANA recommendations, also define advanced nursing practice for nurse midwives, practitioners, and nurse anesthetists, rather than defer to professional association definitions. The ANA views this as an infringement of organized nursing's right to determine the scope of advanced practice. If a state's nursing practice act does not delineate advanced practice, such as nurse mid-wifery, the professional association can do so. In addition to the nurse practice acts, state-mandated rules and regulations and rulings by the board of registered nurses or the board of nurse examiners further define the scope of nursing practice.

Nurse practice acts frequently seem vague to nurses who desire explicit statements about expected conduct in specific circumstances. Although they describe broad grounds for disciplinary action, the practice acts cannot describe all legally allowed or unallowed actions in which registered nurses might engage. Because of the expanding scope of nursing practice the general descriptions of responsibilities provided by the nurse practice acts allow for easier modification as responsibilities change.

Grounds for disciplinary action by state boards of nursing and the courts include obtaining a license through deception, falsifying school records, fraud, criminal acts, substance abuse, and incompetent and unprofessional conduct. (See "Negligence and Malpractice" and "Intentional Torts" in this chapter for further discussion of these offenses.) When a board receives a complaint, an investigation begins. A hearing takes place at which the nurse may cross-examine witnesses, bring defense witnesses, and have individual counsel present. The accused nurse also has the right to a record of the proceedings and to judicial review of the action.

CERTIFICATION

Certification usually involves additional education, either formal or informal, and the passing of an examination. It represents professional recognition by a nursing organization, such as the ANA or other nursing specialty organizations, of advanced achievement in a specific area of practice. One certification developed jointly by the ANA credentialing center and the American College Health Association recognizes nurses with expanded knowledge and skill in college health.

Similar certification is available in emergency nursing, operating room nursing, and medical/surgical nursing. Thirty organizations oversee nurse credentialing, the largest being the American Nurses Credentialing Center, and 200,000 nurses hold certification. ("Sixteen Thousand RNs," November/December 1991).

ACCREDITATION

As individuals are licensed and certified, nursing schools are accredited as confirmation that the education provided meets specific standards set forth by law or by state boards. Each state's board of nursing or board of nurse examiners defines the basic requirements for that state's nursing schools. Those schools that meet these minimum requirements are legally accredited to provide student instruction.

The NLN also accredits schools. Whereas state accreditation is mandatory, NLN accreditation is voluntary and attempts to provide standards that exceed those defined by the state. For this reason, schools seek NLN accreditation as an indication of their program's professional quality. NLN accreditation is available for associate degree programs, baccalaureate or higher-degree programs, diploma programs, and vocational or practical nursing programs.

Most colleges and universities also require accreditation by a regional accrediting body. Such accreditation examines the school's overall functioning, including governance, financial resources, faculty education, and physical plant adequacy. One such regional accrediting body is the Western Association of Schools and Colleges, which accredits schools in the western United States.

State, professional, and regional educational accreditation work together to ensure that the education offered by a school meets legal requirements as well as those established by educational and professional organizations. How this combined effort affects students might be illustrated by the following example.

> Nursing student John Smith attends California State University at Fresno. He is confident that his school will provide him with the knowledge and experience necessary to sit for the national licensure examination and to practice professionally as a registered nurse. The university is

accredited by the Western States Association of Schools and Colleges, and his nursing school is accredited by the California State Board of Registered Nursing as well as the Council of Baccalaureate and Higher Degree Programs of the NLN. His instructors are all licensed registered nurses, and many hold advanced degrees and certification in their specialty areas. John himself practices under the nurse practice act provisions that allow students enrolled in an accredited school to undertake nursing duties, supervised by an instructor approved by the board of registered nursing.

CONTRACTS

A contract is an agreement between two parties for one to render a specific service for a specific compensation. Contracts provide the basis for understanding the obligation that exists between the nurse and an employer, client, or fellow health care provider. Federal employment laws that affect contracts and help to protect nurses include Title VII of the Civil Rights Act and the Equal Pay Act. These statutes provide for "equal pay for equal work." State employment laws govern worker's compensation, protect against health care discrimination in selected circumstances, such as the refusal to assist with abortion, and protect individuals reporting violations to appropriate personnel or agencies.

Contract law governs the responsibilities of nurses, both as independent practitioners and as employees. Contracts may be written or unwritten, expressed or implied. A nurse, for example, may have a written agreement with a hospital to provide vacation relief for emergency department staff. In this instance, the written contract between the nurse and the employer would describe the employment period, duties to be undertaken, and the remuneration amount.

Nurses also have contracts with clients in their care and with other health care providers who may be sharing responsibility for care. For example, nurses have an implied, unwritten contract with clients that competent care will be given. The nurse also has an implied contract with the physician and other health care practitioners that they will provide timely and accurate information so that the nurse may effectively care for the client.

*V*ALID CONTRACTS

- *are for legal acts*
- *are between competent parties of age*
- *have mutual agreement*
- *have mutual obligation*

Valid contracts are legal and exhibit mutual agreement and obligation. To be legal, the contract must not require either party to do anything illegal, and both parties must be of legal age and competency. Mutual agreement refers to the agreement between nurse and employer concerning employment terms. Mutual obligation implies that both parties are bound, or obligated, by the contract's terms. Many institutions expect nurses to float from one department to another, and this expectation is usually stated in the contract. If nurses are assigned to an area for which they are improperly trained and oriented, the terms of such a contract are not being honored. For example, if a nurse hired to work in the emergency department is unexpectedly assigned to the operating room, the contract between the nurse and the institution would be invalid.

Although contracts can be written or oral, written contracts provide more security. If a nurse signs a written contract to work the three summer months from June through August, the employer cannot unilaterally discharge the nurse in July. Many nurses work with contracts that do not specify the employment period. Such contracts give nurses flexibility in terminating service but fail to protect the nurse if the employer should decide to lay off staff. As an alternative, nurses should negotiate an agreement that termination will occur only for just cause and only on reasonable notice. The conditions of a written contract can only be changed in writing; verbal agreements to alter a written contract are not valid. The nurse should also understand that contractual obligations are not obviated by personal inconvenience. Just because a nurse experiences difficulty in getting to work because of transportation difficulties or family problems, this does not absolve the nurse of the responsibility to report for duty.

Nurses have other legal obligations to the physician, hospital, or clinic for whom they work. Whereas the employer must provide a safe, appropriate working environment and remuneration according to agreement, the nurse, in addition to fulfilling the duties contracted, must uphold the good name of the physician or hospital and not unjustly criticize.

Although the hospital or physician must assume responsibility for employees under the doctrine of respondeat superior, or "let the master answer," nurses remain liable for their own incompetent or illegal actions. If a nurse decides to administer drugs to a cardiac client without first performing an adequate assessment, the nurse would be personally liable for actions that a reasonable and prudent nurse would not have taken.

NEGLIGENCE AND MALPRACTICE

An earlier section (see "Public and Private Law,") differentiated public from private law. Public law governs the relationship between individuals and governments as well as criminal case proceedings involving felonies and misdemeanors. Private law deals with relationships between individuals and consists of contract law and tort law. Torts, or wrongdoings, can be intentional or unintentional. Negligence and malpractice fall into the latter category.

Negligence can result from the omission of an action that a reasonably prudent person could be expected to take or the commission of an action that a reasonably prudent person would not take. Malpractice is a form of professional negligence. Suppose, for example, that a nurse leaves a side rail down on an elderly, confused client's bed and the client falls, incurring a head injury. The unconscious client is taken to the emergency department. The same nurse starts an I.V. as ordered but fails to set the rate appropriately, causing inordinate fluid infusion, which results in further client injury. In failing to raise the side rails of the client's bed, the nurse failed to exercise care that could be expected of a reasonable and prudent person; in this instance, the nurse is guilty of negligence. The nurse then compounded the problem by exhibiting professional negligence in failing to set the infusion rate as a reasonable and prudent professional would; in the second failure, the nurse is guilty of malpractice.

For malpractice to occur, several conditions must be present:

- The nurse had a responsibility to the client (responsible for appropriately setting the I.V. rate).
- The nurse failed to carry out this responsibility (neglected to set the appropriate I.V. rate).
- The client suffered harm (result of the fluid overload occasioned by the unregulated I.V. infusion).
- The cause of client harm—the proximate cause—was the result of the nurse's action or inaction (the rapid I.V. infusion, the result of the nurse's failure to appropriately regulate the I.V.) (Grippando and Mitchell, 1989).

Distinguishing between negligence and malpractice is not always easy, and the terms are frequently used interchangeably. Malpractice usually refers to actions involving professional competence and scope of practice.

Conditions and situations that may lead to negligence or malpractice claims typically involve burns, foreign objects, falls, medications, mistaken identity, equipment defects, and loss of or damage to client property. Other circumstances include the nurse's failure to observe, communicate, or act and failure to take reasonable precautions against client elopement, or unauthorized leaving. Nurses can protect themselves and their clients against unintentional torts by being aware of conditions and situations that give rise to them.

BURNS

Clients most likely to incur burns are those with reduced communication abilities and reduced sensitivity to heat or cold. These include anesthetized, comatose, and very old or very young clients. Hot solutions (including hot food and drink), hot equipment (hot-water bottles, heating pads, radiators, surgical instruments), and chemicals improperly administered or in inappropriate concentrations can cause burns. Common sense as well as professional knowledge can help prevent burns. A nurse who allows a client to enter a bath without first checking the temperature may be guilty of negligence. A nurse who administers a caustic drug in an inappropriate concentration may be guilty of malpractice.

The nurse can best protect clients against burns by always checking and double-checking drug concentrations, operation of any machinery, and the temperature of anything to be applied or given to the client.

FOREIGN OBJECTS

Any procedure that requires inserting a sponge, needle, or other piece of equipment into a client may result in injury if the object is not appropriately removed. During surgery, nurses perform sponge, needle, and instrument counts to check that all equipment has been recovered. If a sponge or needle is missing, an X-ray is taken to ensure that it has not been inadvertently left in the client. Despite such care, failure to remove foreign objects from the body is a frequent cause of negligence and malpractice suits. Nurses can help prevent such injuries by using radiopaque strip sponges and by rigorously accounting for all needles and equipment.

FALLS

Those most at risk of falling include clients recovering from anesthesia as well as sedated, elderly or confused, and visually impaired clients. Typically, clients fall out of beds, off stretchers, while ambulating, and while being transported by wheelchair. The prudent nurse can help prevent falls by assessing the risk in such circumstances. If a client has in the past experienced dizziness during ambulation, the nurse might arrange to have someone standing by with a wheelchair. If a client has been sedated, the nurse should ensure that the bed's side rails are up. Crib rails should not be left down at any time if a nurse or responsible parent is not at the bedside. Most hospitals have specific policies governing side and crib rail use and the supervision of confused or sedated clients. Such policies can become factors in determining whether or not the nurse exercised reasonable and prudent care.

SOURCES OF NEGLIGENCE OR MALPRACTICE CLAIMS

- *Unintentional Torts*
  - *Burns*
  - *Foreign objects*
  - *Falls*
  - *Medication errors*
  - *Mistaken identity*
  - *Equipment defects*
  - *Property damage*
- *Intentional Torts*
  - *Assault*
  - *Battery*
  - *Fraud*
  - *Libel*
  - *Slander*

MEDICATION ERRORS

Administering the wrong medication or dose, using the wrong route, and giving medications at the wrong time or to the wrong client can constitute nursing negligence and malpractice. At high risk are pediatric clients, those taking many medications, and clients taking irregularly scheduled medications. Nurses should never fail to ignore one concrete safeguard against medication errors: the clients themselves. If a client states that the morning pill is always small and white rather than large and red like the one being given, a reasonably prudent nurse will recheck the order, the client's arm band, and the medication dose before proceeding.

Preparing drugs when pharmacy department assistance is unavailable can also place a nurse in jeopardy. Nurses, such as night supervisors, who are expected to prepare such medications should be properly trained and provided with proper equipment. Without such preparation, a nurse should not agree to assume drug preparation responsibilities. Nurses who attempt to give care for which they are untrained are not protected by the hospital against liability.

Finally, the nurse should never administer drugs against the rational client's wishes. Such actions are better characterized as intentional torts—in this case, battery—which are described in more detail later in the chapter (See "Intentional Torts").

MISTAKEN IDENTITY

Mistaken identity can result in medication errors or a client's undergoing the wrong operation. It can also result in a client's being prematurely discharged or given the wrong infant to take home at discharge. The nurse can help prevent identity errors by seeing that all clients have name tags or other approved identification forms and always checking identity before beginning any treatment or procedure. Again, listening to clients who claim that they are not scheduled for an X-ray or enema or that they are to go home today can help the nurse avoid a costly mistake.

EQUIPMENT DEFECTS

To ensure competency, nurses must know about the equipment they must use. Failure to check for equipment defects can result in claims against the nurse and the agency that owns the equipment. Safeguards against equipment-related injuries include ensuring regularly scheduled testing and maintenance and having sufficient backup equipment. Nurses should tag malfunctioning equipment when they discover it so that it is not forgotten.

CLIENT PROPERTY LOSS OR DAMAGE

Nurses should take reasonable measures to guard against client property loss or damage. Helpful measures include sending home valuables with family members, putting items in the hospital safe (if available to clients), and keeping client property in appropriate containers, drawers, and closets. Nurses should also see that watches and eyeglasses are not accidentally transported loose with clients to laboratory or radiology departments because they may be left on a gurney or treatment table. Dentures, wrapped in a napkin or left on the bathroom sink, are perhaps the client property most often lost or damaged.

Nurses should see that clients place their dentures in an appropriately labeled container to prevent loss or damage. Glasses and hearing aids can be kept in cases when not in use. Nurses must use personal judgment to decide if a client is alert enough to use glasses, dentures, or a hearing aid.

FAILURE TO OBSERVE, COMMUNICATE, AND ACT

A nurse who fails to observe a client and take appropriate action may be guilty of negligence or malpractice. Observation may confirm that no communication or action is necessary; ignoring a client complaint about pain, shortness of breath, extremity numbness, or increasing dizziness may result in otherwise preventable client harm. High-risk clients, including incompetent, unconscious, elderly, and young clients, may find communication difficult. The nurse may develop nonverbal forms of communication and observation for these clients.

The nurse who takes some action but fails to communicate it to the physician may also be liable. Hesitating to call a physician intolerant of late-night calls does not relieve the nurse of the responsibility for communicating a change in client condition. Continuing education on how to communicate client information effectively by telephone and on how to deal with hostile physicians can be helpful to nurses.

ELOPEMENT

Elopement occurs when a client leaves the hospital without authorization. It becomes a more serious problem when the client subsequently comes to harm through accident, self-injury, or suicide. Nursing precautions against elopement are complicated by legal restraints that forbid keeping mentally competent clients from leaving the hospital, even without medical approval. Restraining or threatening to restrain a competent client who wants to leave can lead to an assault or a battery charge. Locking a client in a room may be viewed as false imprisonment. Detaining a client is only legally permissible when to do otherwise may cause harm to the public or client. As a result, the nurse must individually assess each situation and document the circumstances. The reasonably prudent nurse should be familiar with the appropriate standard of care and with institutional policies and procedures regarding client leave-taking.

INTENTIONAL TORTS

Intentional torts, which can result in negligence and malpractice, also fall under private law. Intentional torts related to nursing include assault and battery, fraud, libel, slander, and failure to protect client confidentiality, leading to privacy loss.

ASSAULT AND BATTERY

Threatening or actually touching a client in a legally impermissible way can lead to assault and battery charges. Simply making a motion as if to slap a client's hand can constitute assault because the gesture suggests that battery may be done. Battery may or may not involve physical damage to the client; it may simply involve inappropriate touching of clients, their clothing, or belongings they are holding. To be liable for battery charges, the nurse must have touched the client without client permission. The issue can become complicated with a client wavering between competent and incompetent states, as might be the case as a client emerges from an anesthetic. The nurse could appropriately restrain a postsurgical client who is attempting to remove an I.V. while not fully awake. On the other hand, the nurse cannot legally restrain a competent client who declines a treatment—regardless of the physical effects. Nurses should be aware of hospital policies governing client treatment in such circumstances and should document such situations meticulously.

FRAUD

Misrepresenting facts to gain advantage constitutes fraud. Most nurse practice acts address the issue of obtaining licensure by fraud, including work or school record falsification. Fraud in obtaining licensure or employment represents a serious offense, and is grounds for disciplinary action, suspension, or nursing license revocation.

LIBEL AND SLANDER

Libel can occur when false or injurious information is communicated in written form. Slander involves verbal communication of such information. Nurses may libel or slander clients, coworker, or employers, either intentionally or unintentionally. A nurse who communicates rumors about a physician's incompetence to another nurse commits intentional slander. A nurse who communicates to coworkers in writing her suspicion that a client may be infected with the human immunodeficiency virus may have committed unintentional libel.

Although adequate and appropriate health care requires personal client information, the law states that such information will be provided only as professionally necessary. The nurse must take care to disclose factual client information appropriately, or the client's right to confidentiality may be breached.

LOSS OF CONFIDENTIALITY AND INVASION OF PRIVACY

The law provides for the disclosure of personal client information only as it is necessary for proper assessment and treatment. Inappropriately disclosing information, even when it is true and not slanderous or libelous, may be unlawful. For example, a nurse may communicate true information to a coworker about a client's stay in an alcohol rehabilitation center but do so in a setting that enables a hospital visitor to overhear. The disclosure may in turn injure the client's community standing and make the nurse liable for damages.

Nursing students should discuss client-related experiences only in appropriate places and with appropriate personnel. Spouses, children, and even fellow students are not appropriate recipients of client information. The responsible student and nurse will understand that discussing a client's progress in a clinical post-conference has a validity that an after-class discussion at the local pizza parlor does not.

DUTY TO REPORT

Nurses must report situations that pose threats to client health or safety. Such situations may involve intentional torts, such as battery or breach of confidentiality, or unintentional torts, such as negligence resulting in a client fall. In making such a report, the nurse should first take care to document the situation clearly. Careful documentation will help determine whether the concern has merit or is merely a suspicion.

The nurse must then communicate the report to the proper personnel. In such circumstances, the nurse should follow the chain of authority and first notify the immediate supervisor of the individual identified in the report. Doing so gives the supervisor the opportunity to handle the situation.

If nothing happens, the nurse should contact supervisors at higher levels of authority.

LIABILITY

Liability may involve payment of legal costs, medical costs, lost wages, and compensation for physical or mental suffering. Those who commit wrongdoings bear the burden of liability. The bearer of such responsibility may be a nurse or an institution or both. For example, a nurse knows that a wheelchair has a faulty brake and works only intermittently. The matter has been reported several times to the maintenance department, which has not yet fixed the chair. Nevertheless, the nurse needs a wheelchair to discharge a client, and all other chairs on the floor are in use. Rather than wait for the next available wheelchair, the nurse decides to use the faulty chair one last time. The nurse wheels the client and belongings outside to the curb. Then, while the nurse is transferring belongings into the client's car, the brake fails and the client and wheelchair collide with the car, injuring the client's foot and denting the car door.

The client has several courses of redress. The client may be satisfied if the hospital administrator guarantees that the hospital will cover all costs for treating the foot and repairing the car. The client may, however, choose to pursue redress through the judicial process. If taken to court, the nurse may be found legally liable because of failure to exercise reasonable and prudent judgment in electing to use faulty equipment. The hospital may also be found liable for failing to repair or remove the faulty wheelchair.

THE JUDICIAL PROCESS

A client injury resulting from an unintentional tort involving negligence and perhaps malpractice would be covered by private, or civil, law rather than by criminal law. When private law is involved, the judicial process consists of several steps: filing a complaint, filing an answer, discovery activity, and trial.

Filing a Complaint. The injured client files a written document, called a complaint, that describes the injury and the persons responsible, called the defendants. The person filing the complaint is called the plaintiff.

Filing an Answer. The defendant is called upon to respond to the complaint in a written document called an answer. This describes the situation from the defendant's point of view. The defendant has about 20 days to respond to the complaint (McHugh and Haas, 1991).

Discovery Activity. After filing the complaint and answer, the plaintiff and defendant engage in discovery activity. During the discovery activity, the court investigates the circumstances surrounding the incident. Documents may be examined and individuals may be questioned under oath. Individuals under oath may also answer written questions called interrogatories. The court may ask the nurse for a deposition, or an oral description, of the events leading to the client's injury.

As information about the incident becomes known to both sides during the discovery activity, many parties decide to settle out of court. Doing so can save court costs, prevent unwanted publicity, and ease the emotional stress of legal proceedings for both the plaintiff and the defendant.

Trial. If the involved parties cannot reach a settlement, the case goes to trial, where the pertinent facts are presented to either a judge or a jury. A judge renders a decision whereas a jury renders a verdict; if either judgment leaves the plaintiff or defendant feeling that justice has not been accomplished, either party may file an appeal.

If an accused nurse's actions are deemed to have been the result of gross negligence, the nurse may be subject to criminal law rather than civil law. Under criminal law, the state seeks to punish the wrongdoer. Such cases are tried in different courts, and the burden of proof involves demonstrating guilt beyond a reasonable doubt.

SPECIFIC LEGAL PROCEEDINGS

The nurse should be knowledgeable about several types of legal proceedings including giving a deposition and serving as a witness.

DEPOSITIONS

A deposition represents an individual's responses under oath to questioning by attorneys for both the plaintiff and the defendant. The individual may give the deposition in an attorney's office or at a health care facility. Depositions are more formal than responding to written interrogatories; attorneys for both sides are present and a court reporter records all answers. This written transcript may be used during a trial.

SERVING AS A WITNESS

The court may call on a nurse to serve as a material witness or an expert witness. A material witness testifies about the facts in a particular matter. A nurse may be called as a material witness to give information in a client injury case about defective equipment. The nurse might testify if and when the equipment was broken and whether or not repairs were requested. An expert witness, unlike a material witness, does not have to know the particular facts of a given situation. An expert witness may be called to help lay persons in the jury understand complicated matters, such as hospital care standards or what a nurse is expected to know about certain equipment or drugs. Both material and expert witnesses can be subpoenaed if they are unwilling to appear in court. A subpoena commands that the person appear at a particular time and place to give information.

TESTIFYING IN COURT

- *Be prepared.*
- *Review all records.*
- *Practice with attorney.*
- *Answer concisely.*
- *Request clarification.*
- *Know standards and policies.*

MATERIAL WITNESS

McHugh and Haas (1991) offer six suggestions to ensure that the nurse serving as a material witness seems competent and consistent. Most important, information given in oral testimony should coincide with that given in response to interrogatories. In addition, McHugh and Haas advise the following:

1. Never testify unprepared.

2. Review all documents, including medical records and responses to interrogatories and previous depositions. Also review relevant standards, such as hospital policies and departmental procedure manuals.

3. Practice with the attorney. Practice sessions should not occur on the trial day but rather several days in advance. The added time allows for reflection on the experience and may help prevent the nervousness that naturally attends trials.

4. Answer questions without elaboration.

5. Request clarification before answering a question that is not understood.

6. Review client care standards that pertain to the particular nursing unit.

Grippando and Mitchell (1989) characterize the ideal witness as one who tells the truth, speaks audibly and with confidence, does not argue or become angry, and maintains a polite and professional appearance. Ideal witness also are clear about what they actually saw and heard and what things require conjecture. Grippando and Mitchell also stress the importance of taking time to reflect before replying to questions.

EXPERT WITNESS

To serve as expert witnesses, nurses generally need advanced education and extensive clinical expertise in the area in question. Pesto (1991) suggests that the most important credential is current and relevant clinical experience. Pesto also advises prospective expert witnesses to consider the merits of the case and to examine the medical records as well as interrogatory and deposition responses. Doing so can help nurses decide if they would feel comfortable serving as witnesses. Nurses should also consider the time required to research the case and provide information at a deposition or trial. They should evaluate how well they will be able to respond to questions by the opposing attorney and identify any existing conflicts of interest, such as having worked for the hospital or with the nurse involved. Finally, prospective expert witnesses should determine what compensation should be offered.

Serving as an expert witness involves providing information about care standards, about how well the nurse in question adhered to policies and procedures, and about whether the nurse's actions reflected those of a reasonable and prudent professional. In the past, physicians usually served as the experts on nursing practice. Now nurses are expected to provide expert testimony concerning nursing standards and performance. For this reason, the nurse should consider serving as an expert witness as a personal opportunity and a professional duty to the nursing profession.

AREAS OF LEGAL CONCERN

Nurses confront legal matters in many different situations. They deal with living wills and other advance directives under the new Patient Self-Determination Act of 1989 that took effect nationally on December 1, 1991. They also have specific legal responsibilities regarding orders not to resuscitate, informed consent, abortion, and client death.

LIVING WILLS

A living will deals specifically with client wishes concerning the manner of dying and usually specifies whether or not the client desires the use of artificial life support. Beginning with California in 1976, states have begun to recognize the individual's right to decline or discontinue mechanical or heroic measures to preserve life. Such natural death acts (NDAs) typically recognize the client's right to refuse such treatment while protecting the professionals who honor such client wishes. Following a client's wishes about artificial life support can pose a bioethical dilemma for family members or staff whose values incline them to preserve life at all costs. Such dilemmas are described in extensive detail in Chapter 7, Ethical implications for nursing practice.

Nurses should familiarize themselves with their state's right-to-die statutes. If an NDA exists, the nurse must follow specific procedures. Generally, once treatment has begun, discontinuing it is difficult. Although most statutes protect the individual's right to decline treatment initiation, they do not so clearly support the removal of life support already in place.

The nurse should also know that the law specifically forbids both active and passive euthanasia, the painless putting to death of a terminally ill client or one suffering without relief. Active euthanasia, such as administering a lethal drug dose, and passive euthanasia, such as withholding a drug, constitute murder. Any action that would result in client death, other than recognizing a client's voluntary refusal of treatment as authorized by NDAs, is illegal. Chapter 7 deals with the legal and ethical dilemma of administering large doses of medication which may hasten a client's death in order to obtain adequate pain relief.

Two well-known cases involving the right to die are those of Karen Ann Quinlan and Nancy Cruzan. In 1976, Karen Ann Quinlan was left in a persistent vegetative state after cardiopulmonary resuscitation failed to revive her from a coma; her parents sought permission to have her taken off the ventilator. After a New Jersey Supreme Court decision, ventilator support was withdrawn, but artificial nutrition and hydration were continued. Karen Ann Quinlan lived an additional nine years in this condition.

The case of Nancy Cruzan, who was left in a permanently vegetative state after an automobile accident in 1983, resembles the Quinlan case. Although Nancy Cruzan had left no written instructions to family or physician concerning her wishes about artificial life support, her family pursued legal recourse to discontinue all life-support measures, including fluids and nutrition. Lower courts agreed to the discontinuance, but Missouri's attorney general appealed the case to the state supreme court, which ruled that the feeding, being done by gastrostomy tube, must continue. In 1990, the U.S. Supreme Court affirmed the state supreme court's decision on the basis that clear and convincing evidence regarding the client's wishes had not been provided. When the case was eventually reopened, friends of Nancy Cruzan presented new evidence and testimony (Hassmiller, 1991). As a result, the feeding tube was removed. Eleven days later, the Nancy

Cruzan died. Since 1991, many such cases have been heard in U.S. courts; in the majority of these cases, the courts have allowed discontinuation of treatment (Fiesta, September 1990).

Nurses should be aware that most states have still not determined what constitutes clear and convincing evidence that the client desires discontinuance of life-support measures. As people become aware of the importance of specifying how they want to be treated in a similar instance, appropriate responses may become easier for the courts and for health care personnel.

ADVANCE DIRECTIVES

The Patient Self-Determination Act went into effect in December 1991. This national act provides clients the opportunity to formulate advance directives to caregivers. To ensure that the intent of the new legislation is carried out, the following provisions must be met:

1. Institutions must inform competent clients about their right to accept or refuse treatment and to decide about such care in the advent of competence loss (Greve, 1991). The institution should describe not only related state laws but also the institution's policy on advance directives and treatment refusal.

2. The caregiver must ask clients about living wills, durable powers of attorney regarding health care (statements authorizing individuals to make decisions for incapacitated clients who are unable to make such decisions), and other advance directive forms. This information becomes part of the client's medical record.

3. The institution must inform staff of state laws and institutional policy regarding advance directives and a client's right to self-determination.

4. Staff must avoid discriminatory care based on the presence or absence of advance directives.

Nurses must receive support in how to approach clients about advance directives and how to care for clients who refuse resuscitation efforts. Bosek and Fitzpatrick (1991) suggest that nurses may fear that discussing advance directives can sadden or depress terminally ill clients. They suggest that the nurse show sensitivity to client statements about powerlessness or lack of control, perhaps pointing out to clients that advance directives are expressions of autonomy and choice. Bosek and Fitzpatrick also suggest that the nurse present advance directives as a natural part of dealing with life change and transition. They conclude that rather than being resentful about advance directives, many clients are relieved at being able to articulate their wishes and to free their families of any related burden.

DO NOT RESUSCITATE ORDERS

A physician may write a Do Not Resuscitate (DNR) order or a no-code order for a terminally ill client or for a client whose death appears imminent and for whom no further treatment exists. The order should appear on the client's chart, should summarize the circumstances of the case and reasons for the order, and should summarize any discussions with the client's family. The order may restrict the type of resuscitative effort. For example, it might state that the nurse is not to initiate artificial ventilation. The nurse should recognize that a DNR order does not mean that other measures, if ordered, should not be carried out. Continued care for dying clients is just as important as it is for those who will recover. Institutions should have policies that govern nursing action when DNR orders are in place.

It is important for nurses to distinguish between a DNR order and a slow-code order. A slow-code order is not a formal order; it refers to the decision to undertake a resuscitative effort but without real effort. Slow-code orders can place the nurse and institution in legal jeopardy and result in a wrongful death charge. Nurses faced with such an order, whether verbal or written, should request clarification with the support of their administration.

INFORMED CONSENT

The client entering a health care facility gives a general treatment consent, which covers routine care such as bathing, feeding, and routine diagnostic tests. If the client requires more involved procedures, such as a cardiac catheterization or fracture repair, the person performing the procedures, usually the physician, must obtain additional consents.

To give an informed consent, the client must receive information about the procedure to be performed, the person who will perform it, risks associated with the procedure, harm or serious side effects, and available treatment alternatives (Sweeney, 1991). The client must also be given the opportunity to consent in writing. Although the physician is usually responsible for providing this information, the nurse has similar responsibilities when implementing procedures under standing orders or as part of advanced practice. A nurse can also obtain a client's signature on a consent form if she has reasonable belief that the client has been adequately informed. The institution's policy and procedure manual should define the nurse's responsibility in assisting with informed consents. Witnessing a consent involves three elements:

- Authenticity: the signature is that of the correct client
- Capacity: the client exhibits the capacity to understand the information about the procedure
- Voluntariness: the client willingly consents to the procedure without coercion (Sweeney, 1991).

If the nurse believes that any of these elements necessary for witnessing a consent has not been fulfilled or that the client has rescinded consent, the nurse must contact the physician immediately and postpone the procedure until resolution is reached.

The nurse may read the consent to a client who cannot read because of visual impairment. The client can designate another person to sign the consent if the client cannot sign because of a physical disability or illiteracy. Depending on hospital policy, the nurse may also act as witness for the client who cannot write but who can make a mark.

LEGAL RIGHTS TO ABORTION

The U.S. Supreme Court has ruled in the case of Roe vs. Wade that constitutional rights of privacy provide women the unrestricted right to abort a fetus during the first trimester, as long as a qualified physician performs the abortion. During the second trimester, reasonable restrictions protecting the mother's health and safety require that abortions be performed in a licensed facility. The law has held that the state can prohibit abortion in the third trimester, on the basis that the interests of the now viable fetus outweigh the mother's right to privacy.

Hospitals may decline to perform abortions, and health care workers, including nurses, can decline to participate. Certain employers may expect the nurse to assist in abortions and subsequent client care. Nurses should understand obligations as stated in the institution's policy prior to hire and, if necessary, make provisions to be excepted from providing such care except in emergency situations.

Legal rights concerning abortion currently are under review by the U.S. Supreme Court. Several states have passed laws that restrict abortion in some cases; however, early in 1993, President Clinton signed an executive order restoring the right to give abortion counseling to nurses and other nonphysician health care workers in clinics receiving federal funds. Nurses should keep up to date about legal rulings that affect abortion practice where they work.

ORGAN DONATION, AUTOPSY, AND DEATH CERTIFICATION

Legal issues that arise upon a client's death include organ donation, autopsy, and death certification. Any competent individual over age 18 can donate a part or all of the body under the provisions of the Uniform Anatomical Gift Act. These provisions allow for organ donation to any hospital, medical or dental school, physician, storage facility, or specific individual for purposes of transplantation (Annas et al., 1981). Some states have attachments to driver's licenses that indicate individual consent to organ donation under specific conditions. Organ donation may be specified in a will or consented to by the client's family. Hospitals should have established procedures to guide nurses in dealing with organ donation, including how to present the option sensitively to family members.

The client before death or surviving family members must also consent to autopsy. The law requires an autopsy if a client dies within 48 hours of hospital admission or in instances of sudden and unexpected death. When a client dies, the attending physician usually signs and issues a death certificate. Copies are given to the family and to appropriate state and local governmental bodies.

Nurses have a responsibility for seeing that legally regulated activities such as organ donation, autopsy, and death certification are appropriately carried out. Being familiar with the state legal requirements and institutional policies is the first requirement. Carefully documenting all activities can help the nurse demonstrate that the legal requirements of each situation have been met.

REDUCING LEGAL LIABILITY

As clients have become more aware of their rights, the number of suits filed against physicians, hospitals, and nurses has increased. Clark (1991) states that the average award in cases involving nurses is about $150,000. Nurses can do several things to reduce legal liability. They can adhere to accepted practice standards, use risk management and quality assurance strategies to identify areas of concern, and encourage all staff to treat clients with dignity and respect. Documentation, as discussed in Chapter 1, Communication and interpersonal relations, should indicate that proper care has been provided. Nurses should also realize that individual malpractice insurance is an important part of professional practice.

Safe, competent professional practice remains the best defense against legal liability. Nurses should recall that remaining competent is one of the legal obligations of the nurse practice act; this involves continually updating clinical skills and knowledge, continuing to learn and grow. Nurses should also monitor changing care standards in their practice areas and should adapt their practice as changes occur in hospital policies and procedures.

Risk management and quality assurance are also important. Fiesta (February 1991) points out that risk management and quality assurance are two strategies for dealing with the same concern. Risk management may require that the nurse analyze incident or situation reports, client statements regarding care satisfaction, or safety reports from maintenance and operations. The nurse can then address identified risks through a program of quality assurance, which seeks to maximize good client care. For example, if risk management information indicates a problem with nurses competently using a new I.V. controller, a quality assurance action involving in-service education and scheduled nurse assessments can alleviate the problem.

Fiesta (1991) points out that effective risk management requires nursing personnel support; it should never be used punitively. Clark (1991) describes how risk management data was used to analyze legal cases involving the nursing care of premature neonates, term neonates, and infants. Analyzing the incidents enabled researchers to recommend specific changes to ensure safer pediatric nursing practice.

The nurse can also safeguard against suits by developing and maintaining good client relationships. Even when accidents occur, a client who has otherwise received professional and compassionate treatment may choose not to file a suit. A nurse who demonstrates client concern, who communicates effectively, and who is pleasant and solicitous is much less likely to encounter a client in court than a nurse who antagonizes or is rude to a client. The entire nursing staff should work together to create a respectful and caring working atmosphere.

LEGAL LIABILITY IN THE HOME CARE SETTING

Nurses practicing in the home care setting have special need for vigilance and concern. Because they may be the only regular contact between the client and the health care system, they should especially assess the home care setting for safety.

Nurses should also determine that the family is economically and personally able to provide competent client care. For example, an elderly client attempting to care for his or her spouse may suffer from exhaustion and become unable to properly provide care. As a result, the client may suffer unintentional neglect. Careful attention to such circumstances forms an important part of the home health nurse's responsibilities.

The economic burden of caring for an ill family member can cause the family to ignore other household needs. As a result, the nurse should assess any unsafe structural deterioration, such as inadequate electrical wiring, deteriorating floor coverings, or inadequate temperature control, and determine the appropriateness of continued home care.

Finally, the nurse should evaluate the client's medication use. Observing for medication interactions, possible abuse, or lack of regimen compliance can enable the nurse to identify any threats to client safety or well-being.

MALPRACTICE INSURANCE

Most hospitals carry malpractice insurance policies that cover the institution and its employees, including nurses. Nurses should also have individual policies to protect them if, for example, a hospital chooses to countersue in a suit or if hospital coverage does not provide nurses with independent legal counsel.

Less than half the nurses giving direct client care have their own malpractice insurance (Clark, 1991). Some erroneously believe that they are protecting themselves against suits by not having insurance, thinking that they cannot be sued if they do not carry insurance. A suit, however, may result in a judgment levied against property. Furthermore, an uninsured nurse may be faced with expenses greatly in excess of any malpractice insurance costs.

Ellis and Hartley (1988) suggest that nurses consider the following when purchasing malpractice insurance: purchasing cost, situations covered and not covered, monetary limits, renewability, and recourse to independent counsel. Nurses should consider whether the policy covers instances brought during the period the policy was in force (called "claims occurred coverage") or covers incidents only as long as the individual remains insured (called "claims brought coverage"). Nurses can purchase insurance from insurance companies or through professional nursing associations.

SUMMARY

This chapter discusses the complex relations between nursing and law. It begins by describing the various types of law (common, statutory, and constitutional), distinguishing between private law and public law. The chapter then discusses the effects of law on nursing and credentialing, including licensure, certification, and accreditation.

The chapter describes the standards of professional nursing performance and the characteristics of negligence and malpractice. It covers the legal proceedings in which nurses are most commonly involved. These include giving depositions, responding to interrogatories, and serving as material and expert witnesses. The judicial process is also described.

The chapter also concentrates on the most common causes of legal action against nurses and suggests strategies to reduce legal vulnerability. Areas in which applicable legal standards are in flux are described; these include the natural death acts and the use of advance directives.

Many of the issues discussed in this chapter also have ethical and moral implications. For example, although the legal obligation to help a client place a living will in the medical record may be clear, the conflict this may cause for other family members or for the nurse must also be addressed. Similarly, although the duty to report an impaired colleague or an unsafe working condition may be legally explicit, loyalty to colleagues and employers must also be acknowledged. Chapter 7 deals with such conflicts and ethical dilemmas.

Application exercise

Identify an institution in which you would like to work. Using the following questions as a guide, research the appropriate institutional procedure that you would use if you suspected a colleague of drug or alcohol abuse.

1. What written policies and procedures for the agency in general are in place? What unit policies and procedures are available? As a new employee of the unit, to whom would you first report suspected substance abuse? What chain of responsibility would you follow?

2. What documentation do you need to provide? Are specific reporting forms available in your unit? How are employees who report colleague substance abuse supported? What institutional policies are in place to support the colleague identified as abusing drugs and alcohol? Is a diversion program available?

Review questions

1. How do statutory law and common law differ?

2. Explain the difference between public law and private law. Describe how public law affects nursing practice, giving examples of misdemeanors and felonies that nurses might commit. Describe how private law affects nursing practice, giving examples of intentional and unintentional torts that nurses might commit.

3. Compare and contrast tort law and contract law.

4. How does negligence differ from malpractice?

5. How does credentialing safeguard nursing?

6. How can nurses avoid malpractice? What role does quality assurance and risk management play?

References

Annas, G.J., et al. The Right of Doctors, Nurses, and Allied Health Professionals. New York: Avon Books, 1981.

Bosek, M.S., and Fitzpatrick, J. "Finding the Right Words," *RN* 54(11):66-67, November 1991.

Braun, K., et al. "Verbal Abuse of Nurses and Non-nurses," *Nursing Management* 22(3):72-76, March 1991.

Clark, M.D. "Toward Safer Nursing Practice," *Nursing Management* 22(3):88-93, March 1991.

Ellis, J.R., and Hartley, C.L., *Nursing in Today's World: Challenges, Issues and Trends*, 3rd ed. New York: J.B. Lippincott Co., 1988.

Fagin, C.M. "Nurses Rights," *American Journal of Nursing* 75:82-85, January 1975.

Fiesta, J. "QA and Risk Management: Reducing Liability Exposure," *Nursing Management* 22(2):14-15, February 1991.

Fiesta, J. "Safeguarding Your Nursing License," *Nursing Management* 21(8):20-21, August 1990.

Fiesta, J. "The Cruzan Case—No Right to Die," *Nursing Management* 21(9):22, September 1990.

Greve, P. "Advance Directives—What the New Law Means to You," *RN* 54(11):63-67, November 1991.

Grippando, G.M., and Mitchell, P.R. *Nursing Perspectives and Issues.* Albany, N.Y.: Delmar Publishers, 1989.

Hassmiller, S., "Bringing the Patient Self-Determination Act into Practice," *Nursing Management* 22(12):29-32, December 1991.

McHugh, M., and Haas, S.S. "The Nurse as a Witness," *Critical Care Nursing* 11(7):68-70, July/August 1991.

Pesto, M.M. "If You're Asked to Be an Expert Witness," *RN* 54(12):65-70, December 1991.

"Sixteen Thousand RNs Take Certification Exams," *The American Nurse* 12, November/December 1991.

Sweeney, M.L. "Your Role in Informed Consent," *RN* 54(8):55-60, August 1991.

RECOMMENDATIONS FOR FURTHER STUDY

Donovan, N.M. "Confidentiality vs. Duty to Warn: Whose Life Is It, Anyway?" *Nursing and Health Care* 12(8):432-436, 1991.

Fiesta, J. "Patient Falls—No Liability," *Nursing Management* 22(11):22-23, November 1991.

Haddad, A.M. "Where Do You Stand on Euthanasia?" RN 54(4):38-43, April 1991.

7

ETHICAL IMPLICATIONS FOR NURSING PRACTICE

OBJECTIVES

After studying this chapter, the reader should be able to:

1. Describe the relations between ethics and rights, morals, values, and duty.

2. Compare beneficence, nonmaleficence, autonomy, justice, and fidelity.

3. Contrast teleological, deontological, and pluralistic approaches to ethics.

4. Describe Rawls' theory of justice.

5. Identify and discuss social factors that influence ethical problems for today's nurses.

6. Describe how the American Nurses' Association (ANA) Code for Nurses affects the care of clients who refuse foods and fluids.

7. Identify the ethical issues surrounding euthanasia and acquired immunodeficiency syndrome (AIDS).

8. Apply an ethical decision-making model to a bioethical dilemma.

INTRODUCTION

Ethics comprises the study of values, morals, and the ideal human character. According to Fowler and Levine-Ariff (1987), the study of ethics as it applies to nursing focuses on specific dilemmas. Ethical dilemmas can occur on a nurse/client level, such as when nurses must decide whether or not to give pain medication in amounts that would alleviate client suffering but also perhaps hasten death. Nurses may face ethical dilemmas in other areas as well; for example, when they must decide whether or not to report a drug-dependent colleague. In such a dilemma, nurses must choose between colleague loyalty and responsibility for protecting clients.

Studying ethics enables nurses to develop an ethical framework that they can apply to specific dilemmas and to the nursing practice in general. This chapter begins by presenting the ANA Code for Nurses and discussing the connections between ethics and its associated concepts—rights, morals, values, and duty. It then describes other ethical concepts, including beneficence, nonmaleficence, autonomy, justice, and fidelity, and outlines teleological and deontological ethical theories as well as the theory of natural law. The chapter goes on to explain how societal factors affect ethical problems and reviews ethical issues related to withholding food and fluids, treating AIDS and human immunodeficiency virus (HIV) clients, client self-determination, substance abuse by nurses, and euthanasia. The chapter concludes by proposing several approaches to solving bioethical dilemmas.

ANA CODE FOR NURSES

The ANA Code for Nurses formally enumerates nursing's primary goals and values. Upon entering the profession, nurses "make a moral commitment to uphold the values and special moral obligations expressed in their code" (American Nurses' Association, 1985). In any given situation, nurses must consider not only their own ethical standards but also those of their profession as a whole. Principle among nurses' professional obligations is responsibility to support and enhance the client's ability to make health care decisions. "In this context, health is not necessarily an end in itself, but rather a means to a life that is meaningful from the client's perspective" (American Nurses' Association, 1985).

The ANA Code consists of eleven statements:

1. The nurse provides services with respect for human dignity and the uniqueness of the client, unrestricted by considerations of social or economic status, personal attributes, or the nature of the health problems.

2. The nurse safeguards the client's rights to privacy by judiciously protecting information of a confidential nature.

3. The nurse acts to safeguard the client and the public when health care and safety are affected by the incompetent, unethical, or illegal practice of any person.

4. The nurse assumes responsibility and accountability for individual nursing judgments and actions.

5. The nurse maintains competence in nursing.

6. The nurse exercises informed judgment and uses individual competence and qualifications as criteria in seeking consultation, accepting responsibilities, and delegating nursing activities to others.

7. The nurse participates in activities that contribute to the ongoing development of the profession's body of knowledge.

8. The nurse participates in the profession's efforts to implement and improve standards of nursing.

9. The nurse participates in the profession's efforts to establish and maintain conditions of employment conducive to high quality nursing care.

10. The nurse participates in the profession's effort to protect the public from misinformation and misrepresentation and to maintain the integrity of nursing.

11. The nurse collaborates with members of the health professions and other citizens in promoting community and national efforts to meet the health needs of the public.

ETHICS AND RIGHTS

A right is a just claim or privilege to which one is entitled. The Bill of Rights in the U.S. Constitution ensures certain general rights, such as freedom of religion, speech, and assembly. Other rights, such as the well-publicized "right to remain silent" when arrested, are more explicit. The National

League for Nursing Patient's Bill of Rights outlines the care to which clients are entitled (see Chapter 6, Legal implications for nursing practice). Sometimes these client rights conflict, resulting in ethical dilemmas for the nurse. For example, clients have the right to refuse treatment, but they also have the right to be protected against decisions made when they are not competent; furthermore, nurses may restrain suicidal clients and thereby avoid client self-injury at the expense of infringing on clients' basic right to make their own health care decisions.

Many rights are guaranteed by law; however, when one individual's rights conflict with another's, the law makes certain provisions. For example, individuals generally have the right to confidentiality of information. However, in the case of someone with venereal disease, the law provides that suitable disclosure can be made in an effort to protect those who may have been exposed to the disease. In such situations, the dilemma is an ethical one.

ETHICS AND MORALITY

Morality has historically been viewed as "the relationship of human actions to the norm or rule of what ought to be" (Glenn, 1947). Certainly to some degree, culture and the times determine moral conduct. For example, U.S. culture once considered the practice of premarital sex to be immoral. Those engaging in such sexual practices, particularly women, were severely censured. With the advent of birth control and effective treatment for sexually transmitted diseases, premarital sex between consenting adults has become more common and more accepted. Yet there are some people who believe premarital sex is intrinsically immoral and, therefore, wrong. Another act which is considered inherently immoral is killing. Can turning off a life-support system be considered killing? This complex debate involves how and when people should be maintained on a life-support systems, who should receive life support (for example, an unconscious or incompetent client), and who should make the decision to initiate or discontinue life support.

MORAL DEVELOPMENT

The educational theories of John Dewey (1851-1931) and the developmental theories of Jean Piaget (1896-1980) served as a basis for early theories of moral development. Dewey described three developmental stages: the premoral (or preconventional), the conventional, and the autonomous. In the premoral stage, individual actions result from biological as well as social needs and drives. At the conventional level, individuals' actions reflect the values of their society. At the autonomous level, critical thinking and independent judgment help determine actions. Piaget used similar terms—premoral, heterogenous, and autonomous—in his description of childhood development. Both theories maintained that although general developmental stages could be identified, individuals of the same age did not uniformly advance from stage to stage, and not all individuals reached the final stage.

Today's nurse may find several current models of moral development useful. One proposed by Kohlberg (1987) emphasizes the importance of rights and rules in determining fairness. Another developed by Gilligan (1982) contends that Kohlberg's conception does not accurately reflect the moral development or experience of women. Gilligan's model emphasizes the understanding of responsibilities and relationships as indications of moral development.

Kohlberg's (1987) model consists of three levels, each with two stages. The first level, called the Preconventional level, occurs during early childhood at a time when the individual must depend on others. During the initial stage of this level, moral behavior is that which avoids punishment. At the second stage of the Preconventional level, the child learns to respect the behavioral judgments of powerful others, such as parents.

The second level in Kohlberg's model is the Conventional. The first stage of the Conventional level begins as individuals develop the ability to weigh alternative courses of action. During this stage, the individual still depends on powerful others for defining moral action. The individual progresses to the second stage of the Conventional level when societal authority becomes the basis for judging behavior.

The third, or Postconventional, level also has two stages. During the first stage of the Postconventional level, the individual focuses on rights, obligations, and contracts between individuals. The second stage begins when the individual becomes able to see the merit of moral behavior even when not specifically prescribed by law. At this stage, morality does not merely reflect the individual's desire to avoid punishment, please powerful others, conform to societal expectations, or obey the law. Individuals can see themselves in relation to humanity as a whole. Like Dewey and Piaget before him, Kohlberg maintains that not all individuals develop in the same way at the same time, and that not every individual reaches the final stage.

As previously stated, Gilligan (1982) maintains that Kohlberg's model, particularly at the Postconventional level, does not accurately describe the moral development of women. Gilligan believes that although moral development in men can be linked to an understanding of rights and rules, such development in women also involves an understanding of individual responsibilities to others.

According to Gilligan, adult men emphasize the abstract nature of morality, whereas women emphasize the contextual application of moral principles within relationships and in relation to the individual's responsibilities to others. For example, in evaluating a client's potential candidacy for a study requiring experimental drug use, a male health care professional might focus his evaluation on the client's disease state, age, and other, similar considerations. His female counterpart might focus on relationships and responsibilities to a greater extent, evaluating the impact of the client's participation on family structure and functioning.

The suggestion that women and men may have different views of morality is important. Understanding the nature of the various parties involved in an ethical dilemma and considering the different issues each may emphasize during the decision-making process can help lead to an equitable and mutually satisfying resolution.

ETHICS AND VALUES

Values comprise the ideals and principles that influence our outlook on life and guide our behavior. They also influence our decisions about what is ethical and what is not. Values result from interaction with parents, society, and culture (see Chapter 5, Cultural implications for nursing practice). For many people, religion represents another important source of values. Professional values are learned during schooling and through socialization in the work setting; they are reflected in codes of behavior and professional standards.

Clarifying values can help the nurse to delineate personal and professional values and to identify causes of conflicts that can result when the two types are consistent. For example, a nurse's religious beliefs may lead the nurse to value life above all other considerations. Such a nurse might want to undertake all measures to preserve life. At the same time, the nurse's professional values would lead the nurse to support client autonomy in making choices about treatments and interventions, even if such a client choice involved refusing treatment that would prolong life. Being aware of inconsistencies between personal and professional values cannot remove all difficulty, but it can help the nurse to understand the conflict and to clarify situations in which professional values must be followed.

The nurse can also help the client identify values and, possibly, related conflicts. The client needs to inventory valued goals as well as the means of achieving these goals. For example, the client may identify as a valued goal a lifestyle that promotes health but realize through questioning by the nurse that goal has not been properly pursued because of the client's present interest in achieving academic success. The long hours of study required for this second goal may be interfering with the need for adequate exercise, proper diet, and rest required for a healthy lifestyle.

Understanding their own personal and professional values as well as the values of the cultural groups with whom they have the most contact can enable nurses to provide more appropriate care consistent with those values and principles.

ETHICS AND DUTY

Duty is that which an individual is bound to do by moral obligation. As it relates to nursing, duty might be associated with client rights: The client's right to competent care, for example, obliges the health care professional to provide such care. If a nurse fails to provide competent care because of lack of up-to-date knowledge, drug or alcohol abuse, or other reason, the nurse deprives the client of this right.

Duty can also be related to values and morals. A nurse may feel duty-bound to provide food for the poor, to assist with obtaining shelter for the homeless, or to spend part of each summer in Mexico providing medical and nursing care to underserved communities. Perceptions of duty, like those of rights, morals, and values, help to shape what the nurse considers ethical conduct.

ETHICAL PRINCIPLES

A competent grasp of ethics requires consideration of certain ethical principles, including beneficence, nonmaleficence, autonomy, justice, and fidelity. By considering these principles, the nurse will be better able to construct an ethical framework applicable to nursing practice.

Beneficence represents the obligation to do good. Knowing what is good, and therefore what the beneficent act should be, is not always self-evident. For example, is beneficence served by maintaining the life of a client in a persistent vegetative state? Is supporting a family unit beneficent when child abuse is suspected? Beneficence requires the nurse to examine an action or a problem from the standpoint of what good might result.

Nonmaleficence refers to the obligation to avoid doing harm. Although related to beneficence, this principle differs in ways that can lead to interesting consequences. For an illustration of these differences, consider the problem of a client who needs to be turned every 2 hours but who experiences extreme pain when this action is performed. Beneficence demands that the nurse "do good" by repositioning the client as ordered; at the same time, nonmaleficence demands that the nurse "avoid harm" by not causing pain. To follow both principles, the nurse could arrange for medication to relieve client discomfort caused by the turning. Explaining the need for repositioning to the client or family might also help to "avoid harm."

Autonomy is the principle of self-determination, or the right to make one's own decisions. Inherent in the exercise of autonomy is personal responsibility. Questions arise when considering the age at which one becomes autonomous and the circumstances under which autonomy is withheld. When autonomy is withheld, who makes decisions for the client? How is this person chosen? An ethical problem being examined by the courts concerns the rights of minors to have abortions and their autonomy in such matters. Many states grant minors the right to consent to their own medical care—excluding abortion. The minor desiring an abortion is not considered fully autonomous, and parental notification, if not consent, is required before the procedure can be performed.

Justice, also called fairness, involves the weighing of rights and responsibilities in an effort to achieve treatment equality. As with autonomy, deciding what constitutes justice can be problematic. Justice for one person may represent injustice for another. For example, in a community with limited resources, providing care for prenatal women may drain funds that otherwise would have been available for alcohol and substance abuse programs. A nurse must make a decision each shift how to apportion time among clients on an individual basis. For example, is it a priority to spend time talking with a new mother who is having difficulty breast-feeding or with another client who has previously miscarried and is now experiencing premature labor?

Fidelity calls upon individuals to honor commitments and agreements. The nurse, for example, is expected to honor written and unwritten contractual obligations to employers, clients, and colleagues. Problems arise when fidelity to one person produces a breach of contract with another. Consider the nurse who becomes aware that a colleague is stealing a client's prescribed injectable narcotic and substituting water.

**ETHICAL
PRINCIPLES**

- *Beneficence: the obligation to do good*
- *Nonmaleficence: the obligation to avoid harm*
- *Autonomy: the principle of self-determination*
- *Justice: the principle of fairness for all*
- *Fidelity: the principle of faithfulness.*

The nurse is bound by fidelity to honor a commitment to protect the client against the harmful actions of others. The nurse also has a responsibility to the employer to report unsafe situations and theft. Finally, the nurse has a responsibility to the colleague, who may lose be dismissed if the incident is reported. In this case, client fidelity takes priority, although fidelity to others may influence the course and manner of the nurse's action. The reporting nurse may seek information from the state nurses' association regarding drug diversion programs that assist addicted nurses and provide this information to the supervisor and hospital. By doing so, the nurse honors fidelity to the client and assists the addicted colleague, who may return to practice when rehabilitation is completed.

Although the principles of beneficence, nonmaleficence, autonomy, justice, and fidelity can help guide the ethical person's actions, they can also pose problems, especially when conflicts arise. Several theories of ethics can help the nurse make choices when conflicts involving ethical principles occur. These include teleological, deontological, and pluralistic theories.

THEORIES OF ETHICS

Teleological theory, also called consequentialism, examines the goodness or badness of action as it relates to the end results. Utilitarianism, conceived by Jeremy Bentham (1748-1832) and further developed by John Stuart Mill (1806-1873), is a teleological theory. Bentham and Stuart Mill believed that what was good could be determined by what benefited the greatest number of people. The problem with the utilitarian approach is its effect on minority populations. Suppose, for example, that health care funds are allocated primarily to provide extensive preventive care but only limited care for illnesses involving expensive technology. The larger, healthy population would benefit, but little money would be available for clients requiring heart-lung transplants for survival.

Deontological theory, also called nonconsequentialism, proposes that some actions are always good or bad, regardless of the consequences. To argue that abortion is always wrong under any circumstances is to argue deontologically. A person with this point of view would maintain that no reason, including rape, incest, or danger to the mother, could justify abortion. The weakness of deontological theory is that it does not allow for a consideration of individual circumstances.

A third ethical theory, pluralism, combines the teleological and deontological approaches. Pluralism recognizes the existence of inherently good and bad actions as well as actions that may be both. For example, a basically good action, such as pain alleviation, may also shorten a client's life. Using a pluralistic approach to solve an ethical dilemma requires the nurse to consider the potential consequences of an action. It also requires the nurse to consider intention. If the nurse administers a strong narcotic to alleviate pain, the action may be good. If, on the other hand, the nurse does so to shorten life, the action may be bad. Finally, the nurse using a pluralistic approach would consider whether an action's good effects outweigh its potential for harm. In the case of administering a narcotic that could shorten life, the nurse would have to weigh the benefits of pain relief against the potential life-threatening effects of the action.

The theory of justice developed by Rawls (1981) addresses the difficulties associated with teleological, deontological, and pluralistic theories. Rawls' theory proposes that two principles help determine what is good. First, all individuals must have the same opportunity and right to liberty provided for in the preamble to the U.S. Constitution. Second, social and economic inequities must be addressed in such a manner that the greatest benefits accrue to those most disadvantaged under a system of equal opportunity. The nurse using Rawls' theory to resolve an ethical dilemma would examine the client's rights and ensure that they are not limited by economic or social circumstances. For example, the decision about an expensive procedure, such as a heart-lung transplant, would not be influenced by the client's inability to pay. Rawls' theory is useful because it requires those making the decision to consider the decision's effects on individuals.

The nurse should realize that developing a personal approach to ethical decision-making may be fraught with difficulty and soul-searching, despite the aid of a specific, well-defined philosophy. Understanding ethical principles and theories, however, can help the nurse define ethical problems and consider them comprehensively.

SOCIAL FACTORS AFFECTING ETHICAL PROBLEMS

Many social factors complicate and contribute to ethical dilemmas. These include technological advances, increasing cultural diversity, economic inequities, the dissolution of the traditional family unit, and the lack of a national health care policy.

TECHNOLOGICAL ADVANCES

Technological advances complicate many health care decisions, even the most fundamental ones. The ability to maintain life in extraordinary circumstances complicates even our definition of death. Is a person existing on a respirator in a persistent vegetative state really alive? Should a life-extending procedure be performed simply because the technology exists?

One way to begin resolving such questions is to define "person." The most restrictive definition of "person" is "any human being, in whatever state." Thus defined, a person exists from conception until death, regardless of other considerations. Another definition that focuses on a being's functioning, or process, states that a "person" is a being that has abilities or power. Fletcher (1972) suggests that individuals become people as they develop. Accordingly, a not-yet-viable fetus and a person without cortical functioning are not "people." An individual without cortical functioning no longer has abilities and powers and has already experienced death. If Fletcher's definition is used, this same person has experienced death because there is no more development. Thus, the technological advances that have saved lives and kept bodies functioning require us to alter our definitions of and distinctions between life and death.

CULTURAL DIVERSITY

Cultural diversity in the United States can also complicate ethical considerations and lead to conflicts between people with different value systems. For this reason, nurses must have a strategy for dealing with situations in which their personal values and ethical beliefs conflict with those of clients or colleagues. As a first step, nurses should become familiar with the values and health care practices of the cultures with whom they most frequently come in contact (see Chapter 5, Cultural implications for nursing practice). Doing so enables nurses to approach problems involving ethical conflicts knowledgeably. Nurses must also analyze and understand their own values and beliefs (See "Ethics and Values" section). Finally, the nurse should use theories of ethics and decision-making strategies to help identify courses of action, recognize clients' rights, and act in a professional, ethical manner.

DISTRIBUTION OF RESOURCES

In the United States, economic resources are concentrated in a small upper class, with a large lower class possessing limited resources for meeting living and health care needs. Clients without insurance and those relying on Medicare and Medicaid do not have access to the same level of health care as do wealthier clients. Although nurses may work to expand benefits for all individuals, they must recognize that many health care decisions are influenced by the client's ability to pay. Acknowledging economic limitations enables the nurse to make more informed decisions.

DISSOLUTION OF TRADITIONAL FAMILY

The emergence of nontraditional families has complicated health care ethics. The nurse may frequently deal with single-parent families, blended families, extended families whose members are unrelated, and gay and lesbian families (see the "Families" section in Chapter 5, Cultural implications for nursing practice). Although it may be to determine who in a nontraditional family has legal custody and health care responsibility for a minor child, the nurse may still have to deal with queries from a parent who has no legal rights but who cares about the sick child's welfare.

Establishing legal responsibilities and honoring client wishes are important steps for the nurse to take in dealing with conflicts related to nontraditional families. If a nontraditional family structure conflicts with the nurse's moral or religious views, the nurse must take care not to impose actions that contradict the client's own desires and decisions. For example, a nurse who considers homosexuality abnormal or sinful should nevertheless recognize the client's right to choose a lifestyle and to have support from significant others. In such cases, nurses should assist the partner, providing information and support as they would for partners in a conventional family unit.

NATIONAL HEALTH CARE POLICY

The lack of a national health care policy in the United States contributes significantly to ethical dilemmas in health care. Resources and care vary from state to state and from locality to locality, resulting in ethically distressing inequities. A client in military service has access to health care that other citizens may not. Medicaid and Medicare clients have access to a level of services that working members of a lower economic class may lack. Care levels for psychiatric clients, prenatal clients, and other client types vary from state to state.

In the absence of a national health care policy, nurses can work to resolve each individual case as fairly and appropriately as possible, helping clients to understand and obtain the services and benefits for which they are eligible. On a broader scale, nurses can work with national nursing associations and other groups for passage of legislation that would provide more equitable access to health care.

Scott (1992) raises four questions that must be resolved in developing a national health care policy:

- *In times of limited resources, should public funds be used solely to finance care for poor clients?* This question suggests that many people who could provide for their own health care receive public funds. Scott contends that "today, much public financing for health care services goes for care of rich and middle-income senior citizens" and raises the issue of justice in the distribution of resources.

- *Should cost-effectiveness be an explicit criterion in approving new medical technologies?* This question suggests that the greatest benefit for the greatest number should govern the approval of new innovations. It also implies that introducing new treatments or technologies that benefit only a few clients and drain available funds, which in turn reduces the level of services for a greater number of clients, is ethically indefensible.

- *How responsible should individuals be for their own health status, and should the general public be asked to subsidize unhealthy lifestyles?* At issue here are clients who develop preventable illnesses from excessive drinking, smoking, engaging in unsafe sexual activities, or following dietary practices known to have a detrimental effect on health. Should public funds cover emergency department charges for injuries that result from drunk driving? Should the costs of lung cancer surgery be covered for a client who has smoked two packs of cigarettes daily for 30 years? Scott suggests that "we should tax alcohol and tobacco products sufficiently to cover the additional health care costs they engender" (Scott, 1992). In other words, people engaging in detrimental lifestyles would incur a behavior tax that would create health care funds. Doing so could avoid diverting other health care dollars from people who do not follow destructive lifestyles.

- *When should extreme or heroic measures to prolong life be stopped?* Scott contends that "all too often, emotionally charged decisions regarding life and death are made during a time of crisis at a loved-one's bedside, and the medical care being provided is futile" (Scott, 1992). The money spent on such care is then not available to others. Although advance directives, living wills, and other measures assist in determining care level, Scott contends that a national policy for dealing with "futile care" should be established.

MAJOR ETHICAL ISSUES IN NURSING

Many ethical issues confront contemporary nursing. Some of the more volatile and complex problems relate to withholding food and fluids, providing adequate pain relief when such relief may hasten or cause death, divulging client information concerning (AIDS) or HIV status, the care rights of AIDS clients, client rights of self-determination, and euthanasia.

WITHHOLDING OR WITHDRAWING FOOD AND FLUIDS

Wurzbach (1990) describes the dilemma of withholding or withdrawing nutrition from dying clients. Traditionally, food and fluid provision has been considered a way of maintaining not only life but also client comfort. Today, questions exist as to whether these measures contribute to client comfort or simply prolong the natural dying process. Abrams (1987) suggests that withholding food and fluids produces a semiconscious, azotemic state that may actually diminish pain perception. This suggests that the client may be more comfortable if artificially induced food and fluids are withheld.

Wurzbach (1990) points out the ethical conflicts accompanying this issue. Some people argue that withholding foods and fluids differs from withholding heroic or invasive treatments because foods and fluids are necessary for life, whereas heroic treatments are undertaken to forestall death. Considerable debate also exists as to whether foods and fluids constitute treatment or basic care. Some argue that the artificial administration of food and fluids should be considered a treatment, and as such can be refused by the client or another acting in his stead. Others point out that food and fluids differ from other treatments because withholding them always results in death. Underlying all these ethical conflicts are beliefs related to the right to die and to the sanctity of life. "For some, the right to life supersedes all other considerations; for others, dying with dignity is what is important" (Wurzbach, 1990).

Some people argue that if nurses and other health care providers relinquish their responsibility for preserving life at all costs, care will erode for clients deemed to be less deserving of life-sustaining measures. Such clients would include those in persistent vegetative states. People of this position also contend that the erosion of life-sustaining care will eventually lead to acceptance of euthanasia. This argument suggests that the only deterrent to such a progression is the unvarying support for life-sustaining treatments regardless of the client's condition or wishes.

The American Medical Association (AMA) and the ANA have taken positions on the issue of food and fluid withholding. The AMA's Council of Ethical and Judicial Affairs has stated that artificially administered food and fluids may be withheld when clients are in irreversible coma, even if death is not imminent. This extends the AMA's previous position allowing for food and fluid withdrawal in cases of imminent death.

The ANA's Committee on Ethics (1988) maintains that food and fluid withdrawal is morally impermissible except in specific circumstances, such as when food and fluid administration would more clearly harm than help the client or when a competent client refuses food and fluids. The nurse may also withhold or withdraw food and fluids when they severely burden the client or sustain life only long enough for the client to die of more painful causes (American Nurses' Association, 1988).

The dilemma associated with withholding food and fluid involves the ethical principles of beneficence and nonmaleficence. The ANA position values the importance of not doing harm over the importance of good. Wurzbach points out that the principle of justice is also involved because sustaining life may require scarce resources, which then become unavailable to another client. From a utilitarian point of view, the action that results in the greatest good should be followed. From a deontological perspective, if preserving life is always and intrinsically good, then any action that threatens preservation is bad, regardless of circumstances.

Regardless of the decision ultimately made regarding the provision of food and fluids for dying clients, the nurse must maintain client fidelity by providing supportive, respectful care. As Wurzbach describes, "[the] principle of fidelity means that the nurse protects the weak, vulnerable, and incompetent about whom the decision to remove foods and fluids is being made. A competent client may choose to refuse foods and fluids, or an incompetent client, once competent, may have written an Advance Directive refusing food and fluids. The client expects the nurse to cooperate with these directives and at the same time provide humane nursing care during the dying process" (Wurzbach, 1990).

U.S. and Australian nurses have displayed interestingly different expectations concerning the withholding of food and fluids from dying clients. Davis and Slater (1989) describe a study in which nurses from both countries were presented with a vignette in which an 83-year-old woman with advanced lung cancer and metastasis to the brain has repeatedly asked that nothing further be done for her. Most U.S. nurses thought that the client's wishes ought to be honored, allowing her to die; however, they also suspected that the client would receive treatment against her wishes. By contrast, most Australian nurses, who also thought that the client's wishes should be honored, expected that the client's wishes would be adhered to. Why did the expectations of the U.S. nurses differ from those of the Australian nurses? Australia's national health care service may be partly responsible. Under this system, "health professionals have seldom, if ever, had a malpractice suit lodged against them. This being the case, the looming shadow of the legal system does not tend to enter into the discussion of ethical dilemmas to the extent that it does in the United States" (Davis and Slater, 1989).

ADEQUATE PAIN RELIEF

Controversy exists over what constitutes an appropriate level of pain medication for terminally ill clients. Although most people agree that client suffering, particularly that which will end only in death, should be relieved, they do not agree that relief should be provided if doing so will hasten death. Other critics argue that pain medication should be withheld when the client is in danger of becoming addicted to the drug.

Cushing (1992) describes a successful suit involving the withholding of pain medication. The client was a 75-year-old man with stage III prostate adenocarcinoma and metastasis to the lumbar sacral spine and left femur. Having experienced a pathological hip fracture, the client was hospitalized for bone debridement. The extent of bone destruction prevented pinning. After discharge, his family briefly cared for him at home and then admitted him to a nursing home. The admitting physician described the client's prognosis as poor and indicated the short-term objective to be pain relief.

While in the hospital and at home, the client had been receiving Roxanol, a liquid form of morphine, 150 mg every 3 to 4 hours for pain. Despite the admitting physician's diagnosis and declared goal, the admitting nurse assessed that the client was addicted to morphine and decided to reduce the pain medication, substituting a tranquilizer that had also been ordered. The nursing director concurred with the admitting nurse, stating, "I have never heard of giving such high doses, at such frequent intervals. . . . I do not want the patient to hurt, but I have seen patients much sicker, in more pain, and on less medication. The staff and I did not think he needed that much morphine" (Cushing, 1992).

The nurses believed that the risks associated with addiction were more significant than the benefits of pain relief and that the client's interests would be better served by weaning him from the narcotic. During a 23-day period, the nurse did not medicate the client as ordered. During two 24-hour periods, the client received no Roxanol. The nurses did not communicate their plan or subsequent actions to the admitting physician.

UNRELIEVED PAIN

Of an estimated 26,000 clients who undergo surgery annually, about 40% receive inadequate pain medication (Gray, 1992).

The World Health Organization estimates that 80% of pain related to cancer is inadequately treated.

The North Carolina Department of Human Resources investigated the case and determined that the care rendered had endangered the client's health (Cushing, 1992). Recognizing that the client's rights had been violated, the North Carolina civil court awarded a multimillion dollar settlement for the nursing staff's failure to medicate and control the client's pain appropriately.

The ANA's position on pain relief for dying clients is clear. The ANA declares that "[nurses] should not hesitate to use full and effective doses of pain medication for the proper management of pain in the dying patient. The increasing titration of medication to achieve symptom control, even at the expense of life, thus hastening death secondarily, is ethically justified" (American Nurses' Association, 1992). The ANA places pain relief above maintaining life at any cost. The position statement also recognizes that tolerance to pain medications occurs frequently in clients requiring prolonged use. Acknowledging that doses may exceed those usually recommended, the ANA position states that nurses should identify the proper dose as "the dose that is sufficient to reduce pain and suffering." The ANA's stance values the client's right to death without pointless suffering.

Margo McCaffery (1992) points out that assessing pain is difficult. She notes that vital sign changes may not always accompany increasing pain. She also suggests that nurses may be unaware that some clients attempt to minimize their discomfort, stating that the pain is "not that bad." Nevertheless, McCaffery states that the single best indicator of client pain is the client and that client reports of pain should remain the primary means of diagnosis.

EUTHANASIA AND UNRELIEVED PAIN

Euthanasia is the practice of painlessly putting to death clients with incurable or untreatable, painful illness. Euthanasia can be passive (allowing the client to die by failing to take an action) or active (taking a specific action, such as administering a lethal injection). The difference between passive and active euthanasia is not always clear. For example, does administering a drug that controls a terminally ill client's pain but also hastens the client's death constitute active euthanasia? How does this differ from administering a massive overdose of the same drug with the intention of causing death? What if pain cannot be controlled by drugs? Are other measures to prevent suffering and end life ethically justified? According to the ANA ethics statement, the nurse caring for a dying client "may provide interventions to relieve symptoms in the dying client even when the interventions entail substantial risk of hastening death" (American Nurses' Association, 1985).

According to Virginia Shubert, president of the Hospice Nurses Association in California, the fear of intense, prolonged pain is the major reason clients request information on euthanasia and assisted suicide (Gray, 1992). Previous unpleasant experiences with pain and the difficulties in obtaining pain relief can lead clients, families, and even health care providers to make unwise choices when escape from unrelieved pain and suffering seem impossible. Clients may commit suicide or enlist the assistance of family members to accomplish an assisted suicide. Health care providers may take unapproved steps to provide additional pain medication to clients with unrelieved pain.

The case of the Hospice Six demonstrates the importance of providing client pain relief in an appropriate, reliable manner. The Hospice Six were nurses employed by a hospice facility in rural Montana. In the course of their duties, they had discovered that procuring pain medications for their clients during the middle of the night when physicians and pharmacies were unavailable was difficult and sometimes impossible. To avoid delays in administering medication that was ordered but not available, the nurses stockpiled narcotics from deceased clients and administered them, following the physician's orders, to clients who otherwise would have been forced to wait. When the nurses' actions were discovered, a zealous Montana prosecutor sought to punish the nurses to the full extent of the law despite the fact that no evidence existed that any client had received medication that had not been appropriately ordered. The nurses' fault, as Leah Curtin

ASSISTED SUICIDES

Janet Adkins was assisted in committing suicide in June of 1990 by Dr. Jack Kevorkian, a Michigan pathologist. Kevorkian remained with Adkins as she administered the medication that caused her death. A Michigan court ruled that the death was suicide rather than murder.

(1991) points out in her editorial "Free the Hospice 6," was not that they failed to administer medications correctly and according to the physician's orders. Curtain contends that no evidence exists that the Hospice 6 "did anything other than give the right [client] the right drug, in the right amount, by the right route, and (most certainly) at the right time" (Curtin, 1991). The prosecutor's case, however, focused on the nurses' methods of obtaining, storing, and dispensing controlled substances.

The Montana State Board of Nursing charged the nurses with misconduct for their stockpiling of controlled substances and ruled that they serve a 4- to 6-year probation, during which they were not to supervise any other staff. The nurses appealed the decision, which was then reviewed by the Montana State Supreme Court. Several years may pass before the case is resolved.

Regardless of the outcome, the nurses were clearly injudicious in their decisions to stockpile medications. However, if more appropriate avenues for obtaining pain medications had been available, the issue might not have arisen. The nurses had adopted a utilitarian approach in which a "minor" wrong achieved what they considered a "major" good—pain relief for the clients in their care. In this case, the negative result of the action fell heavily on the nurses. A beneficial byproduct of the court proceedings has been the wide exposure given to the problem of providing contingencies, such as longer pharmacy hours and better access to physicians, particularly in rural areas. Perhaps the case will spur reforms that can assure nurses and their clients that pain relief is consistently available.

Opponents of euthanasia fear that sanctioning the practice will enable health care personnel to extend the action to situations other than terminal illness. They argue that if euthanasia should become permissible to end pointless suffering for terminally ill clients, it may then become possible to hasten death for others, particularly those who cannot speak for themselves, such as the mentally ill or severely retarded. One reason for this concern is that some health care personnel have in the past abused their most basic trust and have actively caused client deaths. When such actions are exposed, they usually receive extensive publicity and cause public outcry about the dangers of caregivers too eager to release clients from pain and suffering, or from what the caregivers consider a meaningless existence.

The case of Richard Angelo, a night-shift supervisor in a Long Island Hospital in the state of New York, received extensive press coverage. Dubbed the "Angel of Death" by the press, Angelo was responsible for the deaths of several clients in his charge. Some of these deaths occurred even after nurses under Angelo's direct supervision had communicated their suspicions regarding his actions to his superiors. As Little (1991) points out, the unwillingness of coworkers and supervisors to pursue reports of concern is as distressing as actions that directly result in client death.

Euthanasia proponents argue that controlling terminal suffering with medications is not always possible and that the ability to decide when and how to die gives terminally ill clients a measure of control in their otherwise powerless position. In this teleological argument, circumstances outweigh the general good, the prolongation of life.

Despite the different ethical positions on active euthanasia, nurses should know the legal implications of their actions. Haddad (1991) describes a scenario in which a physician asks a nurse to prepare a lethal injection for a terminally ill client; the nurse questions the physician who indicates awareness that the injection is lethal and orders the nurse to proceed. Haddad points out that if the nurse follows the physician's order, the nurse may be charged as an accessory to murder, and suggests that the nurse refuse to comply and then report the incident to the nursing supervisor. Haddad also suggests that the problem be referred to the hospital's ethics committee to help the physician decide how best to handle the case. Haddad stresses that although several states are considering initiatives to allow euthanasia, such action is currently against the law.

ADVANCE DIRECTIVES

Advance directives legislation supports clients who would determine their care during a final illness. It affords them the opportunity to refuse treatments that would artificially prolong life and to decide about their care if they should become incompetent. The courts have affirmed the client and family right to have their wishes upheld by physicians and nurses, even when adhering to such wishes will result in the client's death (see Chapter 6, Legal implications for nursing practice).

Despite precautions, health care workers, family members, and individuals or agencies having no direct relationship to the client may find themselves in ethical conflicts related to advance directives. The conflicts usually reflect differences in teleological and deontological viewpoints; the client may value relief from suffering and the exercise of free choice; the family, health care worker, or agency may value life above individual circumstances. Such conflicts can occur when a client decides to terminate pregnancy in the first trimester or declines a life-saving blood transfusion because of religious convictions. To a person with a deontological point of view, these decisions would be ethically unacceptable because both would result in death.

Nurses can try to avoid such ethically difficult situations by understanding their own ethical beliefs and trying to work in situations that will not force them to confront ethically unacceptable activities. Because, however, such conflicts inevitably occur, nurses should remember that clients are legally guaranteed the right to make their own decisions regarding issues such as abortion, pain relief, and refusal of life-sustaining treatments. Adhering to these legal and ethical responsibilities can make dealing with ethically complex issues somewhat easier.

In dealing with family members whose ethics and values are different from the client's, the nurse may find the following actions helpful:

1. Explain the client's desires to the family. Doing so may involve having the client talk directly with the family or making the family aware of advance directives that the client filed before becoming incompetent.

2. Explain the client's legal rights to make treatment decisions as well as the institution's obligation to honor these decisions. Family members are often torn between wanting to honor a client's wishes and following their own conflicting ethical or religious principles. They may find comfort in knowing that the law dictates a course of action.

3. Encourage family members to voice feelings related to the conflict. Expressing guilt, helplessness, anger, or despair can help family members recognize that a conflict exists. Knowing that others are also in conflict can help everyone involved feel less isolated.

4. Inform clients and their families that support from biomedical ethics committees, knowledgeable staff, appropriate religious groups, or other sources is available. Having their decision to support the client's wishes validated can comfort family members.

NURSES AND SUBSTANCE ABUSE

Approximately 40,000 U.S. nurses are alcoholics, and one out of every three cases handled by the National Council of State Boards of Nursing is drug-related (Baywood, 1990). Nurses have both legal and ethical responsibilities in dealing with substance abuse. The ANA Committee on Ethics in Nursing places the responsibility for safeguarding clients directly on the registered nurse: "When nurses identify inappropriate or questionable practice in provision of health care, they should express concern to the person carrying out the practice. The nurse should clearly draw attention to the possible detrimental effect on the client's health and safety. At the same time, nurses must recognize that their first obligation is to protect the client. Nurses must intervene directly in any situation where the client's welfare is in immediate, serious jeopardy" (ANA, 1988).

In a discussion on dealing with substance abuse in the health care setting, Baywood (1990) suggests that nurses must address the following questions.

- *Why should we deal with the problem?* Dealing with substance abuse among health care professionals not only safeguards clients but helps the substance abuser. Many addicted nurses are described as the most responsible and dedicated members of their departments. Baywood further characterizes them as compulsive achievers who have usually performed well in their academic programs. Identifying occupational factors that place health care workers at substance abuse risk and creating a work environment that provides effective ways of relieving work-related stress can help prevent such abuses.
- *Who should deal with the problem?* Every nurse must deal with substance abuse when it occurs. Baywood suggests that the nurse must decide whether to confront a colleague directly or to report observations to a supervisor. The supervisor has an obligation to any involved clients, the agency, community, and impaired colleague.
- *How should we deal with the problem?* The first step is recognizing the problem's existence and accepting the fact that substance abuse is substantial among nurses, physicians, and other health care workers. In addition, the nurse should know that reporting such abuse and following up on the report are ethically and legally required. Finally, helping the impaired colleague get professional assistance, such as therapy and rehabilitation programs, can make dealing with the problem less difficult.

AIDS, CONFIDENTIALITY, AND THE DUTY TO PROVIDE CARE

An important ethical dilemma associated with the care of AIDS and HIV-positive clients involves the issue of confidentiality and the need to warn. Donovan (1991) describes a hypothetical case that graphically points out the conflicting obligations a nurse may confront. In this case, a Massachusetts man who is HIV positive charges that his right to confidentiality has been breached by a nurse who felt a responsibility to divulge the man's HIV status to his pregnant wife. The nurse is subsequently charged with unethical behavior (failing to maintain confidentiality) and causing the client grievous harm. (His wife deserts him and forbids him to contact his child after birth; because the man cannot meet his mortgage payments without his wife's income, he loses his home; and upon learning of his HIV status, the client's friends break off relations with him.)

The nurse's defense is ethically based. It maintains that in addition to having a duty to the husband, the nurse also had an obligation to prevent great harm coming to another. The defense argues that by warning the wife and thereby preventing harm to the unborn child, the nurse was fulfilling her ethical duty. The ANA Code for Nurses stipulates that "confidentiality is not absolute when innocent parties are in direct jeopardy" (American Nurses' Association 1985). In Massachusetts, however, where this hypothetical case is occurring, breaking confidentiality is legally defensible only when it relates to the contemplation or commission of a crime.

The hypothetical case presents a four-pronged unresolved dilemma:

- The client has the right of autonomy.
- The wife has a right to protection against foreseeable harm.
- The nurse has the right to practice within the limits of her conscience.
- Society has a right to health care that remains true to the principle of "do no harm."

The nurse in this case might have followed several courses of action before divulging the client's HIV status to his wife. First, the nurse should have been aware of state laws regarding disclosure and confidentiality. The nurse might also have contacted certain individuals or agencies, such as hospital bioethical committees, that are available to help and support staff in making decisions.

Other dilemmas arising during the care of AIDS and HIV-positive clients may be rooted more in ignorance than in ethics. When a nurse fears AIDS exposure, usually caused by lack of knowledge about its transmission, and also believes that AIDS clients are responsible for their condition either because of unsafe sexual practices or as retribution for their homosexuality, a pseudo-ethical dilemma ensues. Nurses may feel conflict about caring for clients who may endanger their own health and believe that they must choose between caring for themselves and caring for others. Nurses might also think that AIDS clients are less worthy of care than clients with other illnesses.

The first conflict, that related to caring for a client who might endanger the nurse, can usually be resolved by becoming better informed about AIDS transmission and transmission rates in health care workers. Acquiring such knowledge places the risk of contracting AIDS in perspective with others common to client care. Knowledgeable self-care, including the use of universal body fluid precautions, can also help relieve the nurse's conflict.

The issue of worthiness is more complex and frequently involves the nurse's personal ethics and possible prejudices. The nurse may think that an AIDS client's irresponsible lifestyle, including intravenous drug use and unsafe sexual practices, has led to the disease. The conflict can be further complicated if the AIDS client is homosexual and the nurse disapproves of homosexuality on ethical grounds. Regardless of the nurse's personal view of homosexuality, professional expectation dictates that the nurse care for all clients. The conflict, therefore, becomes one of personal versus professional ethical standards. The nurse either cares for the client, upholding professional ethical standards and sacrificing personal standards, or refuses to provide care, thereby upholding personal beliefs but sacrificing professional standards.

Many health care workers solve the dilemma a third way. They recognize that caring for a client does not imply that they approve of the client's lifestyle. From this point of view, individual beliefs regarding drug abuse, homosexuality, or promiscuity are not compromised by caring for a client whose illness may be related to these behaviors. Finally, nurses should realize that attacking the problems associated with drug abuse and unsafe sexual practices through preventive education and health care measures is much more likely to reduce the incidence of these diseases than refusing care.

Nurses whose personal beliefs would make caring for AIDS and HIV-positive clients difficult should follow the same course of action as nurses who, because of religious or other beliefs, cannot care for abortion clients. The nurse and employer should carefully work out care limitations so that the nurse does become involved in a situation in which such care is expected. A nurse who does not want to assist in abortions may choose to work in pediatrics rather than in obstetrics or the operating room, where care of abortion clients may be required. AIDS and HIV clients may be more difficult to avoid because most clients are unaware of their HIV status until hospital admission. A nurse who believes that caring for AIDS or HIV-positive clients will compromise personal ethics should consider other practice areas, such as school nursing, in which contact with such clients would be less likely.

Nurses should understand that in emergencies, when other nursing personnel are unavailable and when the four ANA criteria for client care at risk exist, they are expected to assist. Furthermore, if the nurse has accepted employment from an agency in which nursing staff are expected to care for AIDS and HIV-positive clients, the agency can reasonably expect the nurse to provide such services. Refusal to provide care may be grounds for dismissal.

ADDRESSING ETHICAL DILEMMAS

Several sources of assistance are available to nurses and other caregivers dealing with ethical dilemmas. Scanlon (1990) states that the number of hospital ethics committees and the nursing representation on these committees is steadily increasing. Currently, more than 60% of U.S. hospitals have some form of ethics committee. In surveying hospitals in metropolitan New York, Scanlon (1990) found that 58% had ethics committees to deal with problems such as Do Not Resuscitate orders, withholding or withdrawing treatment, AIDS, resource allocation, client's rights, death and dying issues, minor clients, professional practice issues, abortion, prison health, and institutional issues. An ethics committee can provide guidance in dealing with ethical problems and can provide a forum from which nurses can advocate for clients.

Scanlon (1990) identifies other formats for addressing ethical issues. These include nursing meetings, in-service education, hospital committees, interdisciplinary rounds, and individual discussion and consultation. For example, a nurse at a medical department staff meeting might bring up her concern that some staff are reluctant to provide care to AIDS clients. Another nurse might be concerned that all rooms do not have readily available gloves and disposal containers for used needles. The staff meeting might also be a forum for in-service education about AIDS and HIV transmission and universal precautions.

SOLVING ETHICAL DILEMMAS

Kozier et al. (1989) provide a five-step decision-making strategy for resolving ethical dilemmas in nursing:

- Establish a sound data base
- Identify conflicts presented by the situation
- Outline alternative actions and consider outcomes and consequences
- Determine who will make the decision and claim responsibility
- Define the nursing obligation.

As shown in the following example, the nurse can use this process to address ethical dilemmas involving complex problems with multiple, conflicting values.

> Mrs. Smith, an elderly client with metastatic cancer, enters the hospital for surgery. During the admission interview, the nurse discovers that although the client has signed the consent, she is unsure of whether she actually wants to have the surgery. She is unaware of her prognosis and the different treatment options open to her, and she has not discussed her wishes with her family. Her family have discussed treatment options with the physician, and they wish every medical effort be made to preserve her life. Mrs. Smith's prognosis, however, indicates that even with surgery, she is unlikely to live more than 6 additional months.

Establish a sound data base. The nurse should include in the data base the people involved, the proposed action, and the action's intent and consequences. The people involved include the client, physician, and family members. The proposed action is surgery, which Mrs. Smith is not sure she wants. The intent of the surgery is to comply with the requests of the family to prolong life. The surgery's consequences are more difficult to specify. Surgery may extend life slightly, but the client's prognosis offers no possibility of recovery. Other surgery outcomes include potential pain and suffering as well as monetary loss.

Identify conflicts presented by the situation. These conflicts include wanting to preserve Mrs. Smith's life, as desired by the family, versus wanting to allow her the option of making decisions about how her life will end. If Mrs. Smith chooses surgery, her life span may be slightly extended. If she elects not to have surgery, her life may be shorter, but she will not undergo the trauma of a surgery that cannot significantly affect the outcome of her disease process. The nurse's conflict is whether to go ahead with the surgery preparations or to help Mrs. Smith reexamine her decision.

Outline alternative actions and consider consequences and outcomes. In this step, the nurse considers other possible actions. The nurse could assist Mrs. Smith in raising questions about the proposed surgery and other treatment options. Consequences and outcomes might include choosing an alternate treatment or reaffirming the decision to undergo surgery. Outcomes the nurse might face include hostility from the family or physician. Conversely, the family may appreciate help in accepting Mrs. Smith's decisions.

Determine who will make the decision. Because Mrs. Smith is a competent adult, decisions regarding health care remain hers to make. Despite the fact that she is elderly and that her family do not want her to die, her wishes regarding treatment must be followed. Nevertheless, the nurse must acknowledge the values of the family and physician, especially if they differ from Mrs. Smith's.

Define the nursing obligation. Because Mrs. Smith is a competent adult and because she clearly has not given an informed consent, the nurse must alert the physician as soon as possible so that prognosis, proposed treatment outcomes, and alternative treatments can be discussed. Only then can the client's wishes be clearly identified. Two decisions are possible. Mrs. Smith, understanding the surgery's risks and relative benefits, may decide to have the operation. In this case, the nurse should support the client and prepare her for the procedure. If Mrs. Smith decides against the operation, the nurse's obligation remains the same; the nurse should support the client, perhaps assisting her to develop advance directives that precisely outline her decisions. The nurse may also help Mrs. Smith talk with her family and to gain their understanding and acceptance of her right to make such choices.

SUMMARY

Because nursing practice involves dealing with complex ethical problems, nurses must understand the relations between ethics and such concepts as rights, morals, values, and duty. They must also understand the different ways of approaching ethical dilemmas. Nurses must recognize the difference between personal and professional ethics and fully realize their obligation to uphold the client's legal right to self-determination. Confronting ethical dilemmas is made easier by better understanding one's personal values, learning about support sources such as professional organizations and hospital bioethics committees, and being able to apply an ethical problem-solving method.

APPLICATION EXERCISE

Identify a bioethical dilemma in a health care setting. With your instructor's assistance, compile the data you will need to apply the following decision-making strategy for resolving ethical dilemmas. Follow the strategy's five steps and determine how you would resolve the dilemma. If any fellow students examine the same dilemma, you might discuss your different interpretations at a seminar.

1. *Establish a sound data base.* Who is involved? What is the proposed action? What are the action's intents and consequences?

2. *Identify conflicts presented by the situation.* What issues are involved? What ethical concepts and theories are in conflict?

3. *Outline alternative actions and consider consequences and outcomes.* Identify available courses of action. What outcomes would each provide?

4. *Determine who will make the decision.* Is the client competent to make a decision? Do factors suggest that others should make the decision? Has the client left advance directives that apply in this situation? What decision should be made?

5. *Define the nursing obligation.* What is the nurse's responsibility in the situation? What would be the nurse's responsibility in possible alternative situations? What does the ANA Code for Nurses suggest for this situation?

ALTERNATE APPLICATION EXERCISE

With your instructor's assistance, identify an agency that has a committee or council to deal with bioethical problems. Request that the agency provide you information about committee membership and problems usually considered. If possible, arrange a visit to the committee and report on your observations.

REVIEW QUESTIONS

1. How do ethics differ from rights, morals, values, and duty? How do professional ethics differ from personal ethics?

2. Explain how teleological theory differs from deontological theory as each applies to ethical dilemmas.

3. Describe the impact of technology on ethical problems related to sustaining life at all costs.

4. What is the nurse's responsibility in caring for AIDS and HIV-positive clients? What is the nurse's responsibility in caring for competent, terminally ill clients who refuse food or fluids?

5. What should a nurse do when personal and professional ethics conflict?

References

Abrams, F.R. "Withholding Treatment When Death Is Not Imminent," *Geriatrics* 42(5):77-84, 1987.

American Nurses' Association. "ANA Statements Focus on Pain," *American Nurse* 7-8, February 1992.

American Nurses' Association. *Code for Nurses with Interpretive Statements.* Kansas City: American Nurses' Association, 1985.

American Nurses' Association. *Ethics in Nursing; Position Statements and Guidelines.* Kansas City: American Nurses Association, 1988.

Baywood, T. "Substance Abuse and Obligations to Colleagues," *Nursing Management* 21(8):40-41, August 1990.

Curtin, L.L. "Free the Hospice 6," *Nursing Management* 22(7):7-8, July 1991.

Cushing, M. "Pain Management on Trial," *American Journal of Nursing* 92(2):21-23, February 1992.

Davis, A.J., and Slater, P.V. "U.S. and Australian Nurses' Attitudes and Beliefs about the Good Death," *Image* 21(1):34-39, Spring 1989.

Donovan, N.M. "Confidentiality vs. Duty to Warn," *Nursing and Health Care* 12(8):432-436, October 1991.

Fletcher, J. "Indicator of Humanhood: a tentative profile of man," *Hastings Center Report* 2(2):3, November 1972.

Fowler, M.D.M., and Levine-Ariff, J. *Ethics at the Bedside; A Sourcebook for the Critical Care Nurse.* Philadelphia: J.B. Lippincott Co., 1987.

Gilligan, C. *In a Different Voice; Psychological Theory and Women's Development.* Cambridge, Mass.: Harvard University Press, 1982.

Gray, B. "An Update on the Hospice Six," *Nurseweek and California Nursing* 14(1):1,9, January/February 1992.

Gray, B.B. "Pain Management," *Nurseweek and California Nursing* 14(1):1,8, January/February 1992.

Haddad, A.M. "Where Do You Stand on Euthanasia?" *RN* 54(4):38-42, April 1991.

Kohlberg, L. *Child Psychology and Childhood Education; A Cognitive Developmental View.* New York: Longman, 1987.

Kozier, B., et al. *Introduction to Nursing,* Redwood City, Calif.: Addison-Wesley Publishing Co., 1989.

Little, C. "Nurses Who Kill," Nursing and Health Care 12(10):550, December 1991.

McCaffery, M. "RN's Assessment is Critical in Pain Control," American Nurse 24(2):4,12, February 1992.

Rawls, J.D. *A Theory of Justice.* Cambridge, Mass.: Harvard University Press, 1981.

Scanlon, C. "Confronting Ethical Issues: A Nursing Survey," *Nursing Management* 21(5):63-65, May 1990.

Scott, J.L. "Ethical Issues: A Washington Perspective," *Nursing Management* 23(1):52-56, January 1992.

Smith, S. "When Ethics and Orders Conflict," *RN* 54(9):61-68, September 1991.

Wurzbach, M.E. "The Dilemma of Withholding or Withdrawing Nutrition." *Image* 22(4):226-230, Winter 1990.

RECOMMENDATIONS FOR FURTHER STUDY

Certo-Guinan, M.J., and Waite, L.M. "The Director of Nursing and the Chemically Dependent Nurse," *Nursing Management* 22(4):52- 54, April 1991.

Edwards, B.S. "What the Nancy Cruzan Case Means for Nurses," *The Nursing Spectrum* 1(3):4, 1991.

Farber, D.A. "Constitutional Right to Die," *Trial* 26(1):23-26, 1990.

Griffin, S. "We Let This Patient Down," *RN* 55(3):49-51, March 1992.

Pinch, W.J. "Nursing Ethics: is Covering-up' ever Harmless'?" *Nursing Management* 21(9):60-62, September 1990.

Schwarz, J.K. "Living Wills and Health Care Proxies; Nurse Practice Implications," *Nursing and Health Care* 13(2):92-96, February 1992.

8

THE NURSE AS TEACHER

OBJECTIVES

After studying this chapter, the reader should be able to:

1. Describe the nurse's teaching responsibilities, based on the American Nurses' Association (ANA) clinical nursing practice standards.

2. Describe the three learning domains.

3. Compare the three major learning theories.

4. Identify barriers to learning and explain how to address them.

5. Identify facilitating factors.

6. Use the nursing process to develop a teaching plan.

7. Formulate behavioral objectives for the three learning domains.

8. Describe how using adult learning principles can facilitate staff teaching.

INTRODUCTION

Nurses have many types of teaching responsibilities. They teach clients and their families about impending surgeries, illnesses and treatments, and rights and responsibilities. They teach procedures to nursing assistants and other staff to whom they delegate responsibilities, and share their knowledge with their coworkers. To fulfill their role as teacher in these many circumstances, nurses are obliged to remain current in their field throughout their professional lives.

The ANA's Standards of Clinical Nursing Practice list eight professional performance standards; four (II, III, IV, and VII) have direct bearing on the teaching and learning process (American Nurses' Association, 1991):

- *Standard II. Performance Appraisal:* The nurse evaluates his/her own nursing practice in relation to professional practice standards and relevant statutes and regulations. This standard implies that the nurse should regularly engage in professional appraisal, evaluating strengths and weaknesses. It also implies that the nurse participates in peer reviews, seeks feedback from others, and takes action to achieve identified goals. Through such actions, the nurse can identify learning needs and devise a plan to meet them.
- *Standard III. Education:* The nurse acquires and maintains current knowledge in nursing practice. This standard requires the nurse to participate in educational activities to update clinical knowledge and professional skills as changes occur in the nurse's discipline and in the health care setting.
- *Standard IV. Collegiality:* The nurse contributes to the professional development of peers, colleagues, and others. This standard suggests that nurses share information with others and give constructive feedback to others regarding their performance.
- *Standard VII. Research:* The nurse uses research findings in practice. This standard suggests that nurses participate in research according to their individual educational level and practice environment and that they use research findings in practice.

Given these teaching and learning expectations, nurses must understand the teaching and learning process and acquire skills related to client, family, and colleague teaching. They must also acquire learning skills related to their own continuing education. This chapter discusses the three domains of learning and theories underlying the teaching and learning process. It next explores barriers to successful teaching and learning and describes factors that can facilitate learning. The chapter explains how to develop a teaching plan and reviews principles of adult education. Specific sections consider the problems of teaching staff, groups, and client families. The chapter concludes with a discussion of community health education.

LEARNING DOMAINS

The three learning domains are cognitive, psychomotor, and affective. Of the three, cognitive learning, the mastery of facts and figures, perhaps comes closest to what is popularly thought of as learning. When student nurses memorize the names of the bones in the hand or when clients learn to identify the parts of a syringe, they are engaged in cognitive learning.

Psychomotor learning occurs when a person acquires a physical skill. Nurses learn psychomotor skills ranging from the relatively simple task of taking an oral temperature to the complex process of performing a physical assessment. A client learning how to self-administer insulin is displaying psychomotor learning.

Affective learning requires changes in attitudes, values, and feelings. Such learning might be illustrated by the nurse whose feelings about caring for acquired immune deficiency (AIDS) clients shift from fear to responsibility and compassion. Learning about the actual risks of AIDS transmission and reexamining the professional ethics code governing client care practice might contribute to the nurse's change of attitude. A cardiovascular client who undergoes a cardiac rehabilitation program and subsequently adopts a more responsible attitude toward personal care also displays affective learning.

Client teaching frequently involves all three domains. For example, a diabetic client first masters information about the disease, dietary limitations, and treatment (cognitive). The client then learns to measure blood glucose and to self-administer insulin (psychomotor). Finally, the client develops a more positive attitude toward the disease and becomes more personally responsible for health behaviors (affective).

LEARNING DOMAINS

- *Cognitive domain: mastery of facts and figures*
- *Psychomotor domain: acquisition of physical skills*
- *Affective domain: changes in attitudes, values and feelings*

TEACHING AND LEARNING THEORIES

Behavioral, cognitive, and humanistic learning theories seek to explain how people learn. Each theory has its limitations, but together they offer a varied perspective on the learning process.

BEHAVIORAL LEARNING THEORY

Behavioral learning theory draws on the work of Ivan Pavlov (1849-1936) and John B. Watson (1878-1958). Pavlov, in exploring conditioned behavior, demonstrated the ability to "teach" a dog to salivate at the ringing of the bell by associating the presentation of food with the auditory stimulus produced by the bell. This form of psychomotor learning, called stimulus-response learning, involves linking an existing response to a new stimulus. In the case of Pavlov's dog, salivation (the existing response to food) became linked to a new stimulus (the ringing of the bell) when the bell alone became sufficient cause for the dog's salivation. The new response is called a conditioned response. Reinforcement, a reward for behavior that makes its repetition more likely to occur, is the driving force behind conditioning behavior. Reinforcement can be primary, such as food or drink, or secondary, such as money or grades. Primary reinforcements are directly usable, whereas secondary reinforcements provide the possibility of other rewards.

One of the more famous proponents of conditioning theory was B.F. Skinner, who pioneered operant conditioning. According to Skinner (1969), "[teaching] is the arrangement of contingencies of reinforcement which expedite learning." Teachers using operant conditioning break down desired responses into small elements, which are then taught sequentially, with the learner being immediately rewarded for each correct response.

Lamaze techniques for childbirth successfully use a form of operant conditioning, which is a form of behavioral learning. Clients learn to respond automatically to painful stimuli by breathing and relaxing, which distract the person feeling pain and thereby depress the pain sensation. In this case, the immediate primary reward is the relief from discomfort. Secondary reinforcement is provided by teacher approval.

The strengths of this approach include the careful identification of what is to be taught and the immediate identification of and reward for correct responses. This operant conditioning approach, however, is not easily applied in more complicated learning settings, where providing positive reinforcement is not always possible. Some people think that the process is too mechanical and that it devalues the learner's role in the teaching process.

Behavior modification is another outgrowth of behavioral learning theory. It has been used successfully to support clients' efforts to stop drinking or smoking or to learn to relax. Like other conditioning procedures, behavior modification relies on positive reinforcement for desired behavior.

COGNITIVE LEARNING THEORY

Developed by psychologists Kurt Lewin and Jean Piaget, among others, cognitive learning theory emphasizes the importance of an integrated learning experience. Learning within this context is not viewed as a conditioning process but rather as the development of understandings and appreciations that can help the individual function in a larger context. As a result, cognitive learning theory stresses the importance of social, emotional, and physical contexts in which learning occurs. Proponents argue that part of the teacher's role is to identify environmental factors that compromise learning. For example, a nurse might suggest that an overloud television program be turned off during a client teaching session.

The teacher-learner relationship is another factor important to cognitive learning theory. Accordingly, if the learner does not perceive the teacher positively and does not view what is being taught as important, little useful learning will ensue.

The strength of the cognitive learning theory is its holistic view of learning, which acknowledges the learner's motivations and environment. In addition, the theory encourages a teaching approach that is appropriate to each developmental level. The difficulty inherent in putting this theory into practice is that many of the environmental and motivational factors that influence a learning situation might be beyond the teacher's control.

HUMANISTIC LEARNING THEORY

Humanistic learning theory focuses on the feelings and attitudes of the student. This perspective emphasizes the importance of the individual in identifying learning needs and in taking responsibility for meeting them. The theory considers individuals to be generally interested in improvement and growth and suggests that with positive support and encouragement, individuals can become highly self-motivated learners.

A nurse using a humanistic approach would view the client as an individual who is self-motivated to learn. The client would identify current needs and desires, and these would serve as important guides for the nurse's teaching. Teaching would provide support and approval while emphasizing the client's role in working toward self-reliance and independence.

AN ECLECTIC APPROACH

Because teaching situations vary widely, nurses may choose to use an eclectic teaching approach, which draws on behavioral, cognitive, and humanistic theories. The following example illustrates how this might be accomplished.

> Jane is a 29-year old first-time mother who has just delivered and who wants to breast-feed her infant. So that Jane may succeed, the nurses must teach her psychomotor skills, such as how to attach the baby to the nipple and how to create breathing space for the infant during nursing. Jane also requires a cognitive learning approach to help her assimilate new information such as how long to nurse initially, how to interest the baby in the breast, and how to

prevent or treat sore nipples. Her nurses might also use an affective learning approach to help Jane address concerns she may have about being tied down by a nursing schedule because these feelings may influence her ability to learn.

Using concepts and principles from the three learning theories, Jane's nurses might:

- recognize that Jane is ultimately responsible for making decisions about her health and body, enlist her aid in identifying the information she requires on breast-feeding, and work with her to achieve her learning goals (humanistic)
- break down Jane's learning needs into discrete, manageable components, provide opportunities for her to practice, and give positive reinforcement each time she gets the baby to take the nipple properly and creates a breathing space by holding back the breast with the fingers (behavioral)
- make sure that Jane is comfortable and has uninterrupted time to focus on the instruction, form a positive teacher-learner relationship, and show her how her decision to breast-feed will have positive results for her and her baby (cognitive).

Nurses need to understand concepts from many theoretical sources and be able to apply them according to the demands of each situation. However, even when one theoretical approach seems appropriate, the nurse should consider the implications of other approaches. For example, the psychomotor skill breast-feeding might appear to be more easily taught with a behavioral learning approach. However, recent studies (Rentschler, 1991) have shown a significant correlation between breast-feeding knowledge and successful practice. Mothers with accurate information were significantly able to successfully breast-feed their infants. Conversely, many mothers who discontinued breast-feeding frequently cited as reasons a lack of milk and sore nipples, responses that suggest a lack of information about milk production and breast care. Apparently, information was, in this case, just as important as psychomotor skills to ensure successful learning.

LEARNING BARRIERS

Client learning barriers include a lack of learning motivation, a lack of developmental readiness, and cultural differences. Other barriers may be related to the learning environment or to the teacher. Anticipating barriers and taking steps to minimize them are important parts of successful teaching.

LACK OF LEARNING MOTIVATION

Various factors can cause a lack of motivation in the learner. Lack of motivation may result from ignorance, dissatisfaction with proposed treatment, or a quality-of-life decision that precludes compliance. For example, a client who has no intention of following the dietary plan a nurse is teaching is not likely to learn the numbers of calories, fat percentages, and other nutritional considerations related to food selection.

When a client lacks motivation because of ignorance, the nurse should identify what information needs to be communicated and in what form. The nurse should work with the client to determine learning goals. If the unmotivated client does not agree with treatment goals, solving the problem may be more difficult. The nurse should first explain the importance of following the prescribed treatment. If the client remains unconvinced, the nurse should explore the client's ideas about the treatment. Doing so may reveal that the client harbors unrealistic expectations, which the nurse may be able to address. A client in a state of denial regarding the consequences of a disease or treatment might also display a lack of motivation that will probably continue to block learning until the denial is overcome. If, however, the client has made a conscious and informed decision to decline treatment and related teaching, the nurse must respect this decision.

A client's preoccupation with other needs can also cause a lack of motivation. When basic needs are unmet, clients frequently cannot focus on other goals. For example, a client who is facing surgery and is concerned about the possibility of a mastectomy may be unable to concentrate on the preoperative instruction about coughing and deep breathing after surgery. Recognizing that basic safety and integrity needs are paramount, the nurse of such a client should first address the client's fears and concerns and then proceed with instruction in such a way that the client recognizes the immediate usefulness of learning.

LACK OF DEVELOPMENTAL READINESS

Developmental readiness is a consideration in teaching pediatric clients. The nurse should structure teaching according to the child's developmental level. For example, the nurse might best teach a preschool child about the anesthetic mask by placing the mask on the face of a doll or stuffed animal.

Frederick (1991) describes how to prepare a child for I.V. infusion, a procedure frequently traumatic for children. As Frederick points out, the nurse must prepare not only the child but also the parents: "Well-informed parents are more likely to stay calm, and their infant or toddler will pick up on that and be less apprehensive, too." Frederick suggests reviewing the procedure step by step, encouraging the child and parents to ask questions. For older children, the nurse can use story books and coloring books showing I.V. placement. For younger children, the nurse can use a stuffed animal or doll to show how the I.V. will be inserted. Acknowledging the child's emotional needs is important and can be accomplished through the use of finger puppets who express "fears" about the procedure and describe how they felt when it was actually done. The nurse should allow the child to voice any fears and concerns and help the child to understand that these fears are normal.

Although the nurse should deal sensitively with the child's apprehensions, the nurse should avoid offering the child a choice when none exists. For the child being prepared for I.V. infusion, Frederick (1991) cautions against asking, "It's time to start your I.V. now, O.K.?" because the procedure must be undertaken whether the child gives consent or not. The nurse should also realize that children may associate feelings about an experience with the environment in which it occurs. If the I.V. procedure is performed in a separate treatment room, the child's room will remain a place associated with secure feelings.

Nurses should allow parents to remain with the child throughout the procedure but not ask them to help restrain the child. After the procedure, the nurse should encourage the child and parents to express their feelings about it. At this time, too, the nurse should also teach the parents how to help protect the I.V. Learning motivation is usually high at this point.

The nurse should also consider developmental readiness with adult clients. For example, new mothers are not all equally ready to learn about their infants or about their own postpartum care. Furthermore, readiness to learn about diapering, feeding, bathing and infant handling is not necessarily age-related. Some adolescent new mothers may be more developmentally ready to learn about their infants than older new mothers who have focused on building careers and who might be torn between the conflicting demands of motherhood and career.

CULTURAL IMPEDIMENTS

Learning impediments related to culture include language barriers, differences in cultural expectations, and disagreement over learning goals. Language barriers are especially significant in the teaching and learning process. Non-English-speaking clients should be taught, if at all possible, by someone who speaks the client's language. If this is not possible, a translator should assist the teaching nurse. The nurse may ask family members to help in translating instructions, but this practice has certain drawbacks. The family member might have difficultly translating unfamiliar medical terms. The family member might also exercise independent judgment about what the client should or shouldn't know and thereby fail to communicate important information.

Cultural expectations can also make teaching difficult. For example, a new mother from a culture in which family members typically care for new mothers and infants may display little interest in learning to become independent. A nurse teaching prenatal classes should realize that some cultural groups value the participation of female family members but do not expect the husband to be present at delivery.

Disagreement over teaching goals can result from differing cultural expectations but might also result from differing nurse and client expectations. A nurse might independently decide that a post-cardiac bypass client should achieve a particular knowledge level by a certain time. If the client does not share this goal, teaching will be impeded and both parties will probably become frustrated. Understanding the client's goals and recognizing any cultural factors involved can enable the nurse to design a teaching plan that allows the client to proceed at a comfortable pace.

ENVIRONMENTAL BARRIERS

Various environmental factors can impede effective teaching. The physical environment of the teaching setting can detract from learning. If the room is too hot or too cold, the client might have difficulty concentrating. If the room is not well lit, the client might not be able to see materials clearly. If the room is noisy, the client may have difficulty hearing and concentrating.

The nurse should also consider client privacy. If post-mastectomy teaching involves exposure of the wound, the client may not be able to concentrate if others are in the same room, even if a screen is used. Nurses should be aware that visual privacy alone may not be sufficient for client ease. If teaching involves discussion of private information, such as sexual practices, the client may be too preoccupied with others overhearing to concentrate on the material being taught.

Conversely, the physical environment can be an effective teaching tool. A room might be designed to encourage clients' curiosity about topics they might otherwise be unwilling to bring up. Pearsey (1991) describes a teaching environment that encourages interested individuals to take the first step in getting information about (AIDS) transmission. Pearsey arranged for displays of posters and pamphlets that clients could read and review independently without having to interact with any staff members.

Nearly 1,000 pamphlets were taken in an 8-week period, and the number of AIDS-related questions increased substantially in the clinic, which until then had not had a single AIDS client. As clients acquired knowledge about the disease, they became more comfortable in approaching staff with questions. Pearsey's experience suggests that clients respond favorably to an informal and unobtrusive presentation of information and as a consequence become more inclined to seek learning opportunities.

The physical environment includes not only the client's room or other teaching area but also the larger environment of the hospital. Nurses functioning as teachers must balance that duty with their obligations to other clients. The nurse must consider this limitation when developing a teaching plan. If, for example, the nurse does not make specific arrangements for uninterrupted instruction, other responsibilities may intervene. The resulting interruption may lead the client to think that the teaching nurse lacks interest or commitment.

TEACHER-RELATED FACTORS

The nurse's approach to teaching can either facilitate or hinder learning. Teaching is most successful when nurses acknowledge clients' abilities and individual worth. It is impeded when it is coercive or when it devalues the learners. For example, if nurses view teaching alcoholic clients as "putting them straight," or teaching post–myocardial infarction clients as "telling them what they did wrong," the implicit message given to clients is that they are basically inept and unworthy. Using the humanistic learning theory as a guide, nurses should refrain from imposing judgments and instead should communicate a sense of positive regard, a more powerful motivational tool for helping clients to learn and develop healthier ways of coping with illness.

FACILITATING FACTORS

Facilitating factors to some degree represent ways of preventing the barriers discussed in the preceding section. They include assessing and stimulating motivation, acknowledging developmental level and readiness, considering cultural differences, and approaching the learner and the material to be taught positively. Other specific techniques facilitate learning, These include multiple teaching forms, generous reinforcement and positive feedback, the breaking down of complicated concepts into component elements, adherence to simplicity and clarity, and the exhibition of professional competence as a teacher.

USING MULTIPLE FORMS

Communicating the same information in multiple forms can help to ensure that learning occurs. An adult client might react well to printed information and to a videotaped presentation of preoperative instruction. A child learns better through role play and stories. A nurse teaching new mothers infant bathing might begin a teaching session by demonstrating the bath. The nurse might next have the new mothers practice the skill themselves, providing supervision and support as needed. Finally, the nurse might give the mothers printed materials designed to help them remember the main points.

The nurse should always use printed material cautiously and with a view of its appropriateness and to the client's reading ability. A pamphlet describing insulin injection and requiring a 12th-grade reading level would be inappropriate for a client with an 8th-grade reading level. Using the pamphlet in this case could even be hazardous if the client misunderstood the information. The nurse could try to have available printed materials written at several levels, especially if reading ability varies widely among clients.

Pictures, illustrations, and models can be effective teaching aids, but the nurse should consider client receptivity to graphic portrayals of body organs or parts. Material that violates the client's sense of propriety may impede learning.

FACTORS THAT FACILITATE LEARNING

- *Multiple forms of presentation*
- *Reinforcement and positive feedback*
- *Breaking down complex concepts or skills to component parts*
- *Simplicity and clarity*
- *Professional presentation*

The nurse should simply ask if the client would like to see a picture of what is being discussed. Pictures and models should also be appropriate to the learner's developmental stage.

REINFORCEMENT AND POSITIVE FEEDBACK

Behavioral theories of education indicate that learning is enhanced by reinforcement and positive feedback. Such reinforcement should follow the desired behavior as rapidly as possible. For example, upon observing a diabetic client's first independent injection, the nurse should immediately validate the success. The nurse should also reinforce client success before critiquing the performance. Even though the diabetic client's injection might have taken longer than desired, the nurse should commend the performance before explaining what the client might do differently in the future. Furthermore, the nurse should reinforce not only the psychomotor skills displayed but also any affective components, such as overcoming the natural reluctance felt at injecting oneself.

BREAKING DOWN CONCEPTS AND SKILLS INTO COMPONENTS

When presenting complex information, the nurse should first explain the overall concept and then teach each element step by step. When teaching self-injection, for example, the nurse would begin by giving an overall demonstration of the task: drawing up the medication, identifying and preparing the site, inserting the needle, and completing the injection. Then the nurse might go back and begin with drawing up medications, letting the client become familiar with the syringe and medication vial, and observing as the client practices correctly drawing up the prescribed medication. The nurse might teach another discrete step, inserting the needle, by allowing the client to practice on an injection model or orange. After all components have been covered, the learner should demonstrate the complete process to ensure that all components have been mastered and integrated.

Breaking down a complex skill or concept into its component parts also helps to structure teaching. The nurse should plan a logical sequence of presentations and practice

How To DETERMINE READING LEVELS

The providers of educational materials often specify required reading levels. When reading levels have not been provided, the nurse could seek assistance from a college or university education department or from a high school reading specialist.

sessions, being sure to give the client adequate time to practice skills and gain confidence. If the nurse does not have time to complete instruction and the client must leave the hospital, breaking down concepts or skills can enable the nurse to identify what instruction remains to be given after discharge.

SIMPLICITY AND CLARITY

Unfamiliar terminology and medical jargon can make learning unnecessarily difficult. Nursing and medical personnel sometimes forget that their clients may not have the advantage of a background comprising anatomy, physiology, microbiology, and chemistry. Health care personnel may also forget that clients might not be familiar with everyday medical vocabulary. Clients who are embarrassed or unwilling to indicate that they do not understand a term being used cannot adequately learn. They may also misunderstand instruction, which can be dangerous. Spees (1991) polled hospitalized clients' and their family members' knowledge of 50 common medical terms. Of the 50 terms, only 9 were correctly understood by all clients and family members. Commonly misunderstood terms included "emesis," "coronary care," "voided," and the abbreviation "NPO." Spees (1991) recommends that nurses "make a conscious effort to utilize common terms and explain all medical terms used in conversations with clients and families." In addition, the nurse should solicit the client's help in identifying unfamiliar terms; doing so can help the client feel comfortable enough to ask for clarification.

EXHIBITING PROFESSIONAL COMPETENCE

By projecting a professional image, the nurse can enhance the learner's confidence in the nurse's teaching abilities. The nurse who beings teaching without first becoming familiar with the equipment being used and making sure that all necessary materials are in place risks losing the client's confidence. Although accidents and unforeseen circumstances can and will occur, the professional nurse recognizes that teaching is a process requiring the same degree of preparation and planning as any other nursing intervention.

DEVELOPING AND IMPLEMENTING A TEACHING PLAN

Teaching, like any nursing intervention, should implement the five components of the nursing process: assessment, diagnosis, planning, implementation, and evaluation. Nurses need to assess the clients' learning needs, formulate a learning objective (or diagnosis), develop a teaching plan, implement the teaching plan, and evaluate the results of the teaching plan. When developing a teaching plan, the nurse can use behavioral objectives to help ensure that appropriate knowledge and skills are taught.

USING BEHAVIORAL OBJECTIVES

Behavioral objectives are learning goals stated as activities or behaviors. For example, a behavioral objective for a prenatal class client might be to list the stages of labor. Developing behavioral objectives can help the nurse structure the teaching; they also provide the teacher with a concrete way to determine if learning has occurred. The nurse and client should collaborate to develop behavioral objectives, which should reflect the client's background knowledge and motivation level as well as the material to be learned.

Bloom (1956) developed one of the first and still most widely used taxonomies, or systems, for classifying behavioral objectives for the cognitive, psychomotor, and affective domains. After diagnosing the client's educational needs within each domain, the nurse can use Bloom's taxonomy to develop specific objectives to address each need (see *Cognitive domain,* page 277). The ability to identify appropriate learning expectations is important to teaching plan development.

Suppose, for example, a nurse uses Bloom's taxonomy to identify cognitive domain behavioral objectives for an expectant first mother who wants to use Lamaze techniques during labor and delivery. An appropriate objective for mastering knowledge might be to list the stages and phases of labor. An objective for client comprehension might be to understand how these phases relate to comfort levels and to the internal processes taking place. An objective for the client's application of knowledge might be to demonstrate how the learned information applies at any particular phase of labor. A behavioral objective for the client's analysis capability might be to demonstrate the ability to analyze her situation at any particular stage or phase of labor and to identify the techniques that will help her through them. The nurse could also develop synthesis and evaluation objectives. Behavioral objectives for this learner might be written as follows:

- *Knowledge:* The client can state the three stages and phases of labor.
- *Comprehension:* The client can describe the physical changes occurring in the second stage of labor and what she can expect to experience subjectively.
- *Application:* The client can apply knowledge of the stages and phases of labor and techniques for each to a simulated labor and delivery process.
- *Analysis:* The client can analyze information regarding contraction frequency and intensity and other physical signs of the transition phase and can modify her breathing appropriately.
- *Synthesis:* The client can plan for her labor and delivery, including identifying breathing and relaxation techniques to be used at each stage as well as materials to be taken to the hospital and can demonstrate other evidences of planning (transportation, notification of family).
- *Evaluation:* The client can identify the usefulness of learned techniques and skills regarding labor and can evaluate whether additional support (medication or other intervention) may be helpful.

The nurse for the same situation can develop learning objectives for the designated levels of the psychomotor domain (see *Psychomotor domain,* page 278). Take, for example, the psychomotor skill of slow chest breathing. The learner becomes perceptually aware of slow chest breathing by experimenting with its components: the effleurage, or

COGNITIVE DOMAIN

As described by Bloom (1956), the cognitive domain includes six learning levels related to the mastery of facts and figures.
1.00 Knowledge: ability to remember of information
2.00 Comprehension: understanding the meaning of information
3.00 Application: ability to apply information to a specific situation
4.00 Analysis: ability to break down information into its component parts
5.00 Synthesis: ability to put elements together to form a whole
6.00 Evaluation: ability to make judgments about the value of information

fingertip massage of the abdomen; the conscious relaxation of the body; and the controlled breathing pattern—in through the mouth and out through the nose—at the specified rate. The mental, physical, and emotional set is achieved when the learner is willing and able to begin performing the skill. The learner can then perform the behavior with the nurse's support and feedback. The learner achieves the mechanism level when she automatically begins slow chest breathing in response to a simulated contraction. The mechanism level is then refined until a complex overt response to the simulated contraction results in a finely coordinated motor response. The adaptation level is achieved when the learner is able to vary the slow chest breathing performance, for example, performing the effleurage on the tops of her thighs rather than on an abdomen that has become sensitive. The client attains the origination level when she is able to tailor the new motor responses to her individual tastes. For example, the client might ensure relaxation during slow chest breathing by playing a favorite cassette tape and using a positive suggestion relaxation sequence.

The nurse could develop behavioral objectives for the affective domain when the client requires an attitudinal change toward health or illness (see *Affective domain*, page 279). For example, a staff nurse antagonistic toward AIDS clients and seeking to avoid working with them might benefit

PSYCHOMOTOR DOMAIN

The designated levels of the psychomotor domain include the following:
1.00 Perception: awareness of objects through perception: the seeing, feeling, smelling, handling, and manipulation of objects
2.00 Set: mental, physical, and emotional readiness for a particular psychomotor activity
3.00 Guided Response: ability to perform physical activity under teacher guidance
4.00 Mechanism: automatic performance of psychomotor skill
5.00 Complex Overt Response: performance of a complex psychomotor skill with ease and confidence
6.00 Adaptation: ability to adjust the psychomotor activity to new situations
7.00 Origination: development of new psychomotor skills.

from affective domain instruction from the supervising nurse. A responding objective might be to develop an interest in caring for AIDS clients. A valuing objective might be to develop a professional commitment to the care of AIDS clients. At the highest level, the newly acquired value becomes an essential part of the individual's approach to life. As with the other domains, the nurse should develop objectives that consider the client's capacity and motivation.

ASSESSING LEARNING NEEDS

In assessing appropriate learning goals with regard to learner, situation, and subject matter, the nurse should elicit the client's perceptions of learning needs. For example, the nurse may not have included in a new mother's original teaching plan an objective related to discrete nursing in public. If the new mother expresses this concern, the nurse should modify the plan to include such instruction.

Getting the client involved during teaching plan development can also enhance the client's learning commitment. By helping to identify learning needs and the time frame required

AFFECTIVE DOMAIN

The affective domain describes levels in the development of attitudes, feelings, and values.

1.00 Awareness: willingness to be made aware of information and receptiveness to information

2.00 Responding: active interest in information, for example, looking for additional information on a subject

3.00 Valuing: preference for a particular value and commitment to a particular point of view

4.00 Organization: incorporation of the value into a value system; reconciliation of the value with other competing and perhaps opposing values

5.00 Characterization by a value: integration of the value into a belief system that serves as a basis for action.

for learning, the client assumes more responsibility for success. Involving family members in the teaching plan development, especially if they are going to assist in the client's care, again stimulates learning and helps family members to understand more fully the client's condition.

DIAGNOSING LEARNING NEEDS

The assessment of learning needs should identify cognitive, psychomotor, and affective skills and knowledge which clients need. Then nurses can develop specific objectives for the teaching and learning process. Objectives stated in general terms may be difficult to address and even more difficult to evaluate. For example, if a written learning objective reads, "The client will understand the relation between diet and blood sugar," what exactly the nurse should teach and the evaluation criteria remain unclear. Measurable objectives, on the other hand, provide a concrete way of determining what needs to be taught and how to determine client success. A measurable objective about diet might read, "The client will choose an appropriate, balanced menu using a prepared list of food groups for the day."

FORMING THE TEACHING PLAN

Once the nurse has assessed and diagnosed client learning needs and formulated them into specific behavioral objectives, the nurse can begin to develop the actual teaching plan. The plan should identify subject matter, required materials and supplies, time frame for teaching and evaluation, and any specific client or environmental variables that need to be considered. For example, a client's need for rest intervals would prohibit long teaching sessions. The nurse should also consider the client's home situation after discharge. If follow-up care from a home health agency is required, the nurse can plan for continued evaluation. Equipment substitutions may be needed, depending on home resources.

The teaching time frame should include the length of the teaching session, the interval between teaching sessions, and the points at which evaluation will occur. The nurse should also remember that complex concepts and skills are easier to learn when they have been broken down into smaller units.

IMPLEMENTATION

During implementation, the nurse carries out the teaching plan. Young and White (1992) describe a teaching plan for clients receiving enteral tube feedings at home. The complex procedure is divided into manageable components:

- Explain the purpose of the tube feedings.
- Identify the type of feeding tube and tip location.
- Demonstrate formula preparation.
- Demonstrate an understanding of enteral administration.
- Demonstrate proper tube care.
- Demonstrate an understanding of equipment operation, cleaning, and storage.
- Describe how to monitor nutritional status.
- Describe how to prevent and treat complications.

These objectives are stated in terms of nursing interventions. To develop a teaching plan stated as behavioral objectives, the nurse could modify the original objectives to describe client goals in each of the three domains of learning: cognitive, psychomotor, and affective. The following are selected examples of such modifications applied to the teaching plan for a client receiving enteral tube feeding.

Cognitive domain objectives
- The learner will describe how the enteral feeding works. (1.00 Knowledge)
- The learner will use appropriate terminology to describe anatomy and physiology involved in normal digestion and in the enteral feeding process. (2.00 Comprehension)

Psychomotor domain objectives
- The learner will independently and accurately calculate daily intake and output. (4.00 Mechanism)
- The learner will adapt the performance of enteral tube feeding to the home environment, appropriately substituting equipment found in the home for that used in the hospital. (6.00 Adaptation)

Affective domain objectives
- The learner will feel comfortable with the feeding tube and enteral feeding process. (2.00 Responding)
- The learner will value self as an individual who is able to administer enteral feedings at home. (3.00 Valuing).

When developing behavioral objectives for the different learning domains, the nurse should check that each objective is adequately addressed in each domain. For example, the client taught in the cognitive domain about how to set up the electronic pump should have a related psychomotor domain objective to ensure that the activity has been learned.

The nurse must also determine that the appropriate level within each domain has been identified. If the nurse expects the client to understand how the enteral feeding works, a cognitive objective at the 1.00 Knowledge level is insufficient. An objective at a higher level, such as 2.00 Comprehension or 5.00 Synthesis, may be more appropriate. The client also may not have sufficient time before discharge to attain psychomotor objectives at the 4.00 and 5.00 levels. In such cases, the nurse should identify client support, such as a home care agency, to use after discharge.

EVALUATION

If the nurse has developed appropriate behavioral objectives for the teaching plan, evaluation is straightforward. Teaching has been successful if the client can perform the behaviors and display mastery of the necessary knowledge and skills. In addition to evaluating the client's learning, the nurse should evaluate the development and implementation of the teaching plan. For example, the nurse may determine that inadequate attention was paid to environment, which may have been noisy, humid, or lacking in privacy. The nurse should remember this evaluation for future teaching scheduled in that setting. The nurse should also evaluate other elements. Were client needs appropriately assessed? Was client input sufficient? Were objectives comprehensive enough? Were teaching sessions appropriately scheduled? Were ancillary materials effective? What suggestions did the client make about the experience? The nurse can use a chart form for organizing the teaching plan from the planning stage through evaluation.

TEACHING STAFF

In addition to client teaching responsibilities, nurses also have staff teaching responsibilities. Nurses often delegate tasks to subordinates whose knowledge levels must be evaluated and validated. Nurses are also expected to help colleagues maintain professional currency by developing new skills and knowledge as the practice setting requires. Teaching responsibility may be formal or informal and may involve individuals or groups. For example, a new graduate may ask an experienced staff nurse for help in using an infusion pump; an experienced colleague may ask another for help in presenting new charting forms to the emergency department staff.

Whether teaching an individual informally or planning a formal lesson for an entire department, the nurse can facilitate learning by recalling certain principles of adult education. Adults learn best when they are actively involved, when their experiences and understandings are brought into play, and when they themselves have a role in designing the teaching experience.

Conners (1990) describes a hospital in-service education program based upon adult learning principles. Staff in an intensive care unit (ICU) had requested more hands-on learning, as an alternative to the traditional lecture format. A committee of ICU staff members, drawing on suggestions from nursing staff, created a series of interactive sessions designed to teach such topics as tissue plasminogen activator therapy, organ procurement, monitoring mixed venous oxygen saturation (SvO_2), and plasmapheresis. In the SvO_2 session, for example, the equipment was first demonstrated and explained. Participants then had the opportunity to role-play caring for a surgical client on an SvO_2 monitor. During the organ procurement session, nurses role-played the part of a staff member who approaches a family member of a multiple-trauma victim to ask about organ donation.

Such programs succeed because staff are actively involved and perceive the information as having immediate benefit because staff have helped shape the curriculum and because previous experiences and knowledge are put to good use.

Manthey and Spirlet (1992) describe a similar approach, using clinicians as teachers. An annual program known as Nursing Kaleidoscope features a day-long series of 30- to 45-minute presentations from staff nurses on various topics in their areas of expertise. Both the staff attending the presentations and the clinicians teaching them learn from the process, becoming more confident and more expert teachers.

Staff teaching can take other forms. Adams-Ender (1991) describes a mentoring process in which an experienced nurse, the mentor, teaches, supports, and helps advance the career of a usually younger and less experienced colleague. The mentoring relationship can be formal or informal. Mentors can be role models, advocates, teachers, counselors, and friends. Adams-Ender suggests that the younger, less experienced colleague approach the potential mentor directly and ask for help, taking care to have a specific goal in mind. Such goals could range from help with a specific technique to assistance in long-range career planning. Both parties then develop a plan that best serves the younger colleague's needs within the limitations of the mentor's available time.

Finding available time is a major problem that nurses encounter when teaching staff. Because instruction is most likely to occur during the working shift, both teacher and learner must be free to engage in the process. One way of dealing with this problem is to use extemporaneous demonstration opportunities, whereby a nurse performs a specific technique, such as adjusting the position of a client in traction, in the presence of the learner. In other cases, teaching can take place on breaks, at the end of shifts, or during shifts if another staff member can cover during instruction.

Occasionally staff nurses resist learning new skills or techniques, even though they may be having trouble with techniques or procedures they currently use. For example, a nurse's aide may be using an ambulating method that makes the client feel insecure and that is hazardous to both the client and the aide. Rather than directly telling the aide that the ambulating method is wrong, the nurse might take a more indirect approach, saying, "It looks as if you're having difficulty ambulating Mr. Smith with all his equipment; I know a way that will be easier for you and will make Mr. Smith feel less frightened."

The same overall approach to learning applies to staff teaching. The teaching nurse must evaluate learning needs, formulate objectives, develop teaching plans according to adult learning principles and with personal and environmental variables in mind, and formally evaluate the results.

TEACHING GROUPS

Whether teaching clients and families or other staff, nurses have many occasions to teach groups. Group teaching offers several advantages. It communicates information much more rapidly than repeating the same instruction individually. Sometimes, too, the group evolves into a support system, with learners helping to stimulate and assist one another. Competition, if it is positive and constructive, encourages individuals to keep pace with class learning and to master skills.

Group teaching also presents some pitfalls. Sometimes the teaching nurse must deal with individuals who want to monopolize the group. Such clients or staff may constantly interrupt the teaching to interject their own views or report their own experiences; they may be unsupportive or even hostile to other views. The nurse must deal quickly with such individuals because they can undermine group effectiveness and disrupt learning. The nurse may discuss with such individuals the expectations for group member participation, stressing that everyone is to have an opportunity to contribute. The nurse might also enlist the individual's assistance to teach a specific skill, with the understanding that others are then to have the opportunity to comment or to ask questions. For example, a mother with several children who is attending a class on bathing an infant and who constantly interrupts to discuss her experience with her older children might be enlisted to discuss a specific aspect, such as how to ensure that the water temperature is at the right level or how to shampoo the hair without getting soap in the child's eyes. If the individual continues to dominate the group, the nurse may have to set specific limits on the type and amount of participation.

Another difficulty occurs when a group consists of individuals at different educational, ability, or experience levels. Identifying the types of individuals in the group is the teacher's first step. For example, when planning to teach a group of postpartum mothers, the nurse might begin by asking if any have had children before. If most have, the teaching style and material presented would differ from those used for a class consisting mainly of first-time mothers. If the disparity among members is too great, the nurse may choose to create two groups. The nurse may also ask more knowledgeable group members to help those who are less knowledgeable.

The nurse can apply the same format for developing an individual learning plan to group learning. Assessing and diagnosing learning needs, identifying objectives, developing the teaching plan, implementing the teaching plan, and evaluating are all important. The nurse should also identify learning barriers, including environmental factors. Finally, involving the group in the learning plan development can maximize the group's advantages and minimize its difficulties.

TEACHING FAMILIES

Family groups can be small (mother and father of a pediatric client) or large (an extended family who are cooperating to share the care of an elderly relative). Nurses frequently discover that families have decided to take on client care responsibilities without having a specific understanding of what is to be done, or who is to do what. Such a situation points out the importance of assessment and planning and of involving family members in the teaching plan development. For example, if an elderly client will require assistance with bathing, dressing, ambulation, eating, and medication administration, the family must decide who will have what responsibilities. Helping the family to identify each member's expectations and learning needs is an important benefit of assessment.

Nurses also frequently encounter the problem of family role changes. When an elderly client has been an autonomous father or brother, other family members may have difficulty seeing him as a dependent person needing direction and support. Family members may initially be unable to take charge of such things as deciding when to bathe the client or when to administer medications. The nurse can help family members to recognize those decisions that can remain within the client's control and those that need to be determined by the caregivers.

Some family members may feel that they are exclusively responsible for client care. A daughter, for example, may feel that she is solely responsible for caring for her elderly mother. Nurses can help clients understand that such exclusive care may not be feasible or desirable, depending on individual circumstances. Family members may also compete to provide care or to demonstrate concern for the client. Designing learning sessions during which family members can share their concerns and feelings about caring for the client can minimize unhealthy competition and enable the family to work together in supporting the client and one another. Finally, the nurse must assess family customs related to dealing with sickness, subsequently encouraging beneficial customs and educating the family about harmful ones.

COMMUNITY HEALTH EDUCATION

Nurses have a professional responsibility to promote health education in the community. They accomplish this in several ways. Nurses help to develop and present radio public service announcements on topics ranging from autologous blood transfusions to sibling-grandparent programs (Manthey and Spirlet, 1992). Nurses participate in public forums about community health issues, such as prenatal care and infant immunization. They participate in health fairs and education weeks designed to make the community aware of specific health problems, including cancer, heart disease, and AIDS. Nurses also volunteer to present health topics at public schools, day-care centers, and homeless shelters. National Nurses Week can be an effective forum for presenting health information to the community. Nurses in rural San Luis Obispo, California, each year sponsor a tabloid insert in their local newspaper in which nurses describe their specialties and teach readers about public health concerns particular to their farming community. Finally, nurses can become involved as political advocates on behalf of health care consumers by helping to publicize problems and legislation, either at the state or federal level.

SUMMARY

Teaching is a vital part of nursing practice. Whether teaching clients and their families, staff and colleagues, or the general public, nurses should follow a planned approach. Developing the teaching plan involves assessing and diagnosing learning needs, creating a teaching plan, implementing the plan, and evaluating learning outcomes. During this process, the nurse should identify learning barriers and facilitating factors. To identify and formulate specific learning needs, the nurse can use the behavioral objectives of the three learning domains: cognitive, psychomotor, and affective. Finally, the nurse must plan for ongoing personal education to remain current in the field and to provide competent client care.

APPLICATION EXERCISE

Identify a client teaching need for which learning objectives in the cognitive, psychomotor, and affective domains need to be developed. Create a limited teaching plan to address the specific learning need.

Assessment. What is the client's educational level? What does the client think is important to learn?

Diagnosis. What are the client's learning needs? Using some of these learning needs, develop specific objectives in the cognitive, psychomotor, and affective domains.

Planning. How should you structure the teaching? What materials are available? How much time is available? What barriers and facilitating factors can you identify? In what order should you teach concepts and skills?

Implementation. After your instructor has reviewed your assessment, objectives, and plan, implement the teaching.

Evaluation. Evaluate how successfully the client has learned the necessary skills and knowledge. Then evaluate your teaching plan. How accurate was your assessment and diagnosis? How effectively was your teaching plan implemented? What changes would you make?

REVIEW QUESTIONS

1. How does Standard III of the ANA *Standards of Clinical Nursing Practice* illustrate the expectation that all nurses have responsibility for teaching and learning?

2. How does affective learning differ from cognitive learning?

3. Describe the major components of behavioral, cognitive, and humanistic learning theories.

4. Identify cultural factors that can affect teaching.

REFERENCES

Adams-Ender, C.L. "Mentoring: Nurses Helping Nurses," *RN* 54(4):21-23, April 1991.

American Nurses Association. *Standards of Clinical Nursing Practice.* Kansas City, Mo.: American Nurses Association, 1991.

Bloom, B.S. *Taxonomy of Educational Objectives: The Classification of Educational Goals.* New York: David McKay Co., 1956.

Conners, C.D. "This Program Breathes New Life Into Inservices," *RN* 53(12):12-16, December 1990.

Frederick, V. "Pediatric IV Therapy: Soothing the Patient," *RN* 54(12):40-42, December 1991.

Knowles, M.S. *The Modern Practice of Adult Education*, rev. ed. Chicago: Associated Press, 1980.

Manthey, M., and Spirlet, L.E. "Nursing Kaleidoscope: Clinicians as Teachers," *Nursing Management* 23(6):14-16, June 1992.

Pearsey, T. "We Teach All Our Patients About AIDS," *RN* 54(11):17-18, November 1991.

Rentschler, D.D. "Correlates of Successful Breastfeeding," *Image* 23(3):151-154, Fall 1991.

Skinner, B.F. *Contingencies of Reinforcement.* New York: Appleton-Century-Crofts, 1969.

Spees, C.M. "Knowledge of Medical Terminology Among Clients and Families," *Image* 23(4):225-229, Winter 1991.

Young, C.K., and White, S. "Preparing Patients for Tube Feeding at Home," *American Journal of Nursing* 92(4):46-53, April 1992.

RECOMMENDATIONS FOR FURTHER STUDY

Stump, D., and Landstrom, G.L. "Developing a Continuing Education Hours Plan," *Nursing Management* 22(5), May 1991.

Tuazon, N.C. "Discharge Teaching: Use This Model," *RN* 55(4):19-22, April 1992.

9

THE NATURE OF LEADERSHIP

OBJECTIVES

After studying this chapter, the reader should be able to:

1. Compare and contrast the concepts of leadership, management, and professionalism.

2. Contrast theories of leadership based on personal traits and those based on situational components.

3. Describe the contingency theory of leadership.

4. Identify the four types of motivation described by the House in the path-goal leadership theory.

5. Compare and contrast the autocratic, democratic, laissez-faire, and multicratic styles of leadership.

6. Discuss the role of follower and characteristics of ineffective followers.

7. Explain how leaders influence followers.

8. Describe how new graduates can prepare to be good followers.

9. Discuss responsibilities associated with delegation.

10. Describe how shared governance is changing decision-making responsibilities in health care institutions.

11. Identify effective and ineffective leadership behaviors and begin to develop a personal leadership style.

INTRODUCTION

The nursing profession provides many opportunities for leadership. Nurses must serve as client advocates and protectors; they champion the cause of children, elderly clients, and other underprivileged groups with insufficient access to health care. They work to protect clients against the unsafe actions of others. They serve on hospital boards and ethics committees and in state legislatures and Congress. All these activities require significant leadership skills.

At the same time, many factors deter nurses from functioning as leaders. Historically, the profession has been viewed as a subservient one, with the nurse's principal responsibilities being to ensure that the physician's orders are followed and to implement the medical care plan. Being predominantly women, nurses were expected to be submissive and compliant; those who became assertive and powerful were considered misfits acting contrary to their nature. Until recently, leadership and management were not major components of nursing education because they were thought to be the province of physicians and hospital administrators.

Nevertheless, certain individuals have successfully challenged the traditional nursing role and have emerged as effective leaders. The deaconess Phoebe set up nursing establishments in southern Italy at the time of Christ. Florence Nightingale championed nurses and nursing reforms during the Crimean War. From these historical figures to the current American Nurses' Association (ANA) president Virginia Trotter Betts, female nurses have challenged what was considered appropriate for their gender and profession.

Despite the stereotypical view of nursing as a female profession, men have from the beginning played a crucial role in its evolution. Men as well as women cared for the sick and injured in the Roman hospitals of the pre-Christian era. During the centuries after Christ, the Catholic Church established male and female religious orders to care for the sick; an important duty of Benedictine monks was to care for their brothers as well as for pilgrims, wayfarers, and refugees. During the crusades of the Middle Ages, the military order

Knights Hospitallers was formed to bring the injured from the battlefield and to provide nursing care. During the 14th-century plague epidemics, the Alexian Brotherhood cared for the afflicted and buried the dead. These early male and female nurses established nursing and health care norms and values that continue to evolve today.

Several factors have contributed to the continued evolution of nursing leaders. During the mid-20th century, nursing education moved from the hospital to the college and university. This move enabled nursing students to acquire a scientific background on which to base nursing judgments and initiatives. As education for women and minorities became more available and as more women returned to colleges for retraining after bearing children, more and more nursing students were exposed to the rigor of scientific thought. The idea that nurses had an independent role to play in health care provision gradually took root.

The women's movement and the opening of other professions to women have had an interesting effect on nursing. Because women can now pursue professions previously closed to them, fewer are choosing nursing. This situation has led over the past several decades to a nursing shortage, which in turn has led to changes in nursing that enable it to compete with other professions and to attract high-quality applicants. The results have been increased salaries and independence for nurses.

The civil rights movement has helped to open up the nursing profession to all individuals; it has emphasized the importance of attracting and educating professionals from all cultural groups to provide care for the culturally diverse U.S. population. The movement has also worked to make the special health care needs of minority populations known. This in turn has helped nursing leaders focus their efforts on ensuring appropriate and adequate care for all populations.

Legislation establishing equal pay for equal work has forced the reassessment of predominantly female jobs to ensure appropriate compensation. Recognizing the registered nurse's responsibilities for practice in both dependent and independent roles has led to increased remuneration for nurses. As they make more money, nurses are expected to display higher levels of professional competence and leadership.

The development of sophisticated health care technology has also promoted nursing leadership. As nurses become increasingly responsible for monitoring equipment and modifying client care involving technology, the degree of initiative and independent judgment required increases.

LEADERSHIP, MANAGEMENT, AND PROFESSIONALISM

Some people view leadership as synonymous with management and professionalism. In fact, all three terms have different but related meanings. Leadership comprises guiding, directing, teaching, and motivating others in goal setting and goal achievement. A registered nurse who directs group care, overseeing a nurse's aid and a licensed practical nurse (LPN), and who interacts with laboratory, pharmacy, housekeeping, physical therapy, and dietary personnel, is a leader.

Management is a leadership component. It refers to resource coordination and integration through planning, organizing, directing, and controlling to accomplish specific goals (Sullivan and Decker, 1988). Managers usually have specific responsibilities by virtue of their position in a hierarchy. Some leaders, such as the supervisor of surgical nursing and the vice-president for nursing services, have managerial responsibilities.

Professionalism describes an approach to one's occupation that distinguishes it from being merely a job. A profession has a body of specialized knowledge that is constantly being enlarged on or updated. Professionals usually receive their training in colleges or universities and tend to concern themselves with the good of society. They themselves formulate statements that describe their responsibilities. Importantly, a profession focuses on the ideal of service and usually follows a written code of ethics; professionals view their work as a lifetime commitment.

This chapter discusses leadership theories, including the Great Man, charismatic, trait, contingency, and path-goal theories as well as theories emphasizing the interaction between trait and environment. It also describes management styles, including autocratic, democratic, bureaucratic, and multicratic styles. The chapter then explains the reciprocal relationship between leaders and followers and delineates the delegation process. The chapter concludes by describing the major functions of leadership and management. The application exercise focuses on identifying personal leadership skills and traits and developing a plan for professional growth.

LEADERSHIP THEORIES

The emphasis of leadership theories varies. Most early theories stressed the importance of individual traits. Some, however, explored situational components, such as the interaction between trait and environment. Later theories have combined these two approaches and examine how effective leadership must change to accommodate differences in followers as well as differences in the tasks to be performed and in the leader's authority.

GREAT MAN THEORIES

Early leadership theories focused on the traits of so-called Great Men who were acknowledged to be successful leaders. The theories sought to identify physical, emotional, and spiritual characteristics that would explain successful leadership. Theorists thought that such characteristics were innate and that leaders were born and not made. Aristotle believed that some men were born to lead and others to follow. He did not consider women's characteristics because women were not citizens in the societies of ancient Greece and could not hold leadership positions.

The study of great men did not satisfactorily explain many observed leadership phenomena. For example, not all great men were good leaders, and circumstances seemed to dictate in part the characteristics required for effective leadership. The characteristics of an effective wartime leader often varied from those of a peacetime leader. Although limited, the Great Man theories initiated the analysis of traits thought to constitute leadership.

CHARISMATIC THEORY

An offshoot of the Great Man approach, charismatic theory postulates that some individuals are able to lead others because of their personal magnetism. Many religious leaders are charismatic individuals who inspire loyalty and commitment among their followers. Charismatic leaders frequently emerge during stressful times, presenting approaches to problems that differ significantly from existing policies. Recent charismatic leaders include Martin Luther King, Jr., Cesar Chavez, and Candy Lightner of Mothers Against Drunk Driving.

One difficulty associated with the charismatic theory is that not everyone is similarly affected by a charismatic individual. Although many people may respond favorably to a particular charismatic leader, just as many may respond negatively. Also, a leader may project charisma when dealing with certain issues but fail to do so when confronting others.

LATER TRAIT THEORIES

Trait theories evolved significantly when researchers acknowledged the possibility that leadership traits might be learned rather than inherited. Theorists began to explore how identified leadership traits could be encouraged. Commonly identified leadership traits included intelligence, self-discipline, energy and enthusiasm, creativity, communication and interpersonal relations skills, assertiveness, and ambition. In 1945, the Ohio State Leadership Studies group investigated 1,800 examples of leadership and identified two basic dimensions, which they termed consideration behaviors and initiating structure behaviors. Consideration behaviors included such person-oriented actions as being friendly and supportive, listening to others, and showing individual concern. Initiating structure behaviors included task-oriented actions such as planning, scheduling, assigning tasks, and coordinating work. Successful leaders seemed to use a combination of consideration behaviors and initiating structure behaviors, and the combination could vary from one situation to another.

Although trait theories were helpful in identifying inborn and developed characteristics that contribute to successful leadership, they did not explain why leaders were sometimes effective in one situation and ineffective in another. Trait theories also focused almost exclusively on the leader, with little thought given to the group being led. In the 1940s and 1950s, the main focus of leadership theory shifted.

SITUATIONAL THEORY

Situational leadership theory, which emerged in the 1940s, suggests that the type of leader who will be effective in a given situation varies according to the situation. The term situation refers to both the followers and the circumstances in which they and the leader operate. In examining the circumstances that might influence leader effectiveness, researchers focused on the structure and atmosphere of the organization being led and on the roles of leaders and followers within it. This thinking helped to explain why leaders might be effective in one situation and ineffective in another. It did not acknowledge the fact that individuals can vary their leadership approaches and, as a result, should be able to adapt to changing circumstances.

CONTINGENCY THEORY

During the 1960s, Fred Fiedler developed contingency theory as an outgrowth of situational theory. Fiedler maintained that no one leadership style was universally effective and that determining an effective leadership approach for any situation required examination of three components:

- the nature of the leader/member relationship
- the structure of the task to be performed
- the position power held by the leader.

Fielder described each component as existing on a continuum: leader-member relationships could range from supportive and respectful to hostile; the structure of the task to be performed could range from the complex to the simple and could be either well defined or poorly defined; and leader power could range from considerable to negligible. The most favorable leadership situation exists when members have confidence in the leader, the task is structured, and the leader has considerable power based on broad support. An unfavorable leadership situation exists when members lack confidence in the leader, the task is unstructured, and the leader has no effective power.

Fiedler also developed contingency tables describing preferred leadership behavior in different circumstances. For example, when leader-member relations are good, the task is structured, and the leader's position power is strong, the preferred leadership behavior is control. Interestingly, when leader-member relations are poor, the task is ill-defined, and the leader's position power is weak, the preferred leadership behavior is also control. In the middle of the spectrum, where one or more of the variables are unfavorable, a permissive leadership behavior is preferred. In other words, Fiedler contended that task-oriented, controlling leaders are more successful in situations that are either highly favorable or highly unfavorable. In intermediately favorable situations, a permissive, relationship-oriented leader is more successful.

The following example represents an intermediately favorable nursing situation. A new nurse manager takes charge of an emergency department that has had significant conflict between management and staff over staffing levels and work schedules. Leader-member relationships have been mediocre to poor. The hospital administration hopes that the new manager can reduce conflict and help the department become more effective. The new nurse manager's position power is strong. In addition, the staff are experienced and know their jobs well, giving their activities some structure and continuity.

According to Fiedler's contingency theory, the most effective manager in this situation would be the one who adopts a permissive, relationship-oriented leadership style, working to involve and build strong relationships with members. A controlling manager who emphasizes the tasks at hand at the expense of building relationships and involving members would be less successful. On the other hand, once good leader-member relationships are established, the nurse manager could effectively use a more controlling approach.

Contingency theory helps to identify situational components that make one leadership style more effective than another, but it does not identify how leaders can motivate subordinates to follow their direction.

PATH-GOAL THEORY

Building on contingency theory, path-goal theory principally explores how the leader motivates subordinates. It operates from the premise that most workers are goal-directed and act to promote goal achievement. The leader's goal is to facilitate goal accomplishment by providing support, minimizing obstacles, and emphasizing personal benefits of goal achievement to workers. House (1971) identifies four types of motivating leadership behavior that could be used by nurse leaders: directive, achievement-oriented, supportive, and participative.

Directive leadership. The nurse leader clearly identifies goals to be achieved and the mechanisms and steps needed to attain each goal. The nurse might give to staff detailed instructions, including specific policies and rules, to facilitate goal achievement.

Achievement-oriented leadership. The nurse leader focuses on developing challenging goals to which staff can aspire. The nurse does not develop specific policies and rules and considers staff to be capable and intrinsically goal-directed.

Supportive leadership. The nurse leader focuses on supporting and encouraging subordinates to create an environment in which they can work productively in pursuit of goals.

Participative leadership. Workers assume an active role in working with the nurse leader. Workers and leader share responsibilities for identifying goals and goal achievement methods (House, 1971).

In all four leadership behavior forms, the leader is responsible for keeping institutional goals and personal goals in view and for providing support and structure that will enable workers to achieve both types of goals.

MANAGEMENT STYLES

Douglas (1992) identifies differences between leaders' and managers' roles. Managers, unlike leaders, have an officially designated position; they are supervisors, charge nurses, head nurses, nurse clinicians, or vice-presidents for client care services. Managers, unlike leaders, have the power and authority to implement decisions. Managers rely on predetermined rules and regulations; leaders attempt to influence others. Managers enforce order and structure; leaders take risks and look for new approaches. Managers interact with others according to official roles; leaders react to others as individuals. Managers succeed by accomplishing institutional goals; leaders experience success by achieving personal goals.

Regardless of the sometimes different manager and leader roles, management ability remains an important component of effective leadership. This chapter describes three traditional management styles of leadership. These include the autocratic, democratic, and laissez-faire management styles. In addition, an approach combining the best elements of these traditional styles, the multicratic approach, is described.

Factors affecting the choice of management style include individual values and goals, the organization's structure, and the subordinates' characteristics. The manager working in a basically bureaucratic organization may adopt an autocratic approach. If the organizational structure of the institution encourages broad-based participation in decision making, the manager may prefer a democratic approach. If the employees are highly skilled professionals, the manager may opt for a laissez-faire approach.

MANAGEMENT STYLES

- *Autocratic*
- *Democratic*
- *Laissez-faire*
- *Multicratic*

AUTOCRATIC MANAGEMENT STYLE

Autocratic leadership relies heavily on rules and regulations. Autocratic leaders see themselves as the individuals with the most comprehensive view of the task at hand and, consequently, as the people best able to make decisions. Autocratic leaders in a typical bureaucratic structure also have power and influence related to their position in the hierarchy. This allows them to reinforce decisions and to require subordinate compliance. Communication with subordinates includes giving directions, reinforcing rules and regulations, and providing feedback on subordinate performance in pursuit of identified institutional goals.

The autocratic management style can be either effective or inappropriate, depending on the situation. The following example illustrates an effective use of this style.

> John D. is the supervisor of a busy operating department. He manages five operating rooms and the recovery room. He assigns nurses and technicians to cases depending on their skills and interests and is directly responsible for his department's efficiency. One day, his schedule is abruptly disrupted by the arrival of four clients who have been involved in a bus accident. All four require emergency surgery, although two can wait for several hours. Once the priority for surgery has been established, John D. reassigns some staff who were preparing to work on a now canceled elective surgical case to the first surgery. He then calls in off-duty staff to help with the second emergency case. Then he adjusts the schedules and responsibilities of the remaining staff to accommodate the regularly scheduled cases.

In this situation, John D. uses an autocratic style because decisions must be made rapidly and by someone familiar with staff skills and experience. No time is available for a discussion of case preferences. Once the crisis has passed, John D. could discuss with his staff the situation and the departmental response. Such discussion would allow for a performance critique and for staff input concerning how a similar situation might be handled in the future. In this example, the manager acted autocratically when the situation required that he do so but resumed a more collaborative, thereby democratic, style after the emergency.

The autocratic management style of leadership has several advantages: decisions can be arrived at rapidly and the person responsible for making decisions is clearly identified. Disadvantages include the possible lack of subordinate support for the leader if subordinates perceive the leader as uncaring or lacking in knowledge about them. The autocratic leader may also have a more difficult time gaining subordinate support for institutional goals that they have not helped to formulate.

DEMOCRATIC MANAGEMENT STYLE

Using a democratic managing style, a leader provides information to subordinates, assists group members to examine possible courses of action, and helps them to make decisions that reflect the group's best combined judgment. A democratic leader functions most productively when subordinates have a vested interest in the decision outcome, are knowledgeable about their roles, and have the requisite knowledge and experience to contribute to decisions. A decentralized organizational structure facilitates a democratic approach; however, even in a highly centralized organization, the leader may still use a democratic management style and involve subordinates in the decision-making process (see Chapter 3, How organizations are structured).

Like the autocratic style, the democratic style can be effective or ineffective. The following example illustrates an effective use of the democratic management style.

> Mary K. is a staff nurse in the medical department of a large hospital. She works with an LPN and a nursing assistant and knows both of them well. When Mary receives the nursing report from staff on the preceding shift, she and her team members meet to plan how they will care for clients assigned to them. Although Mary retains responsibility for the overall care, she asks for input from her subordinates and uses the knowledge and experience they bring to the joint task.
>
> In this way, Mary K. can draw on her subordinates' experience and knowledge when structuring their tasks, and the subordinates, feeling part of a team effort, are motivated to accomplish their jointly defined task.

A democratic management style works well in this situation because the leader has confidence in the subordinates' ability to contribute productively to the decision-making process. She is familiar with their strengths and confident that the subordinates will function according to their responsibilities. Furthermore, adequate time exists for the collaborative process required in a democratic management style.

A democratic management style offers several benefits, including the greater likelihood that subordinates will abide by decisions to which they have contributed. Also, by using group experience, the leader has more information on which to base decisions.

One disadvantage of a democratic style is that using it requires more time to plan and reach decisions. Furthermore, if subordinates are not knowledgeable or able to participate appropriately, reaching good decisions may be difficult. This style also requires a leader with a high tolerance for ambiguity and uncertainty at points in the decision-making process; however, ambiguity and uncertainty may be more easily tolerated when the leader has confidence in the group's ability to reach a sound decision, when the group is committed to a common goal, and when adequate time for the collaborative process exists.

LAISSEZ-FAIRE MANAGEMENT STYLE

The laissez-faire leader gives maximum freedom to subordinates. This permissive leadership style works best with fellow professionals who have well-defined responsibilities and need only logistical and personal support for their relatively independent functioning. Laissez-faire management style is illustrated by the following.

> June T. is the department head of a busy well-baby clinic; she oversees a staff of experienced nurses who have relatively autonomous responsibilities caring for the families who come to them for well-baby checks, immunizations, and routine screenings. June sees her job largely as one of supporting her staff. She ensures that her staff have the necessary supports to perform their jobs well and calls group meetings as needed to discuss departmental matters. Staff members work independently with the physicians,

laboratory aides, and other personnel to care for the children and families who visit the clinic.

If used when subordinates cannot function independently, laissez-faire management style can result in productivity loss and failure to achieve goals. Subordinates in such a situation may think that the leader has failed to provide adequate management and leadership. In such a case, an informal leader may arise and manage without having a formally designated position. Problems occur when the designated leader or upper management does not support the informal leader's decisions. Such problems can paralyze group functioning.

MULTICRATIC MANAGEMENT STYLE

A multicratic style allows a nurse to vary management and leadership tactics depending on the conditions present. John D. appropriately used an autocratic style during the operating department emergency, but his overall approach, which involved his staff in goal planning and departmental planning, was democratic. In managing the well-baby clinic, June T. may effectively use a laissez-faire style in most circumstances, but she may find an autocratic style necessary when conflicts occur over responsibilities or departmental policies. A leader using a multicratic management style assesses each situation and determines whether to use an autocratic, a democratic, or a laissez-faire approach.

Some evidence indicates that leaders may be limited in their ability to vary management styles. Johnson and D'Argenio (1991) studied the effect of leadership-management development training designed to encourage managers to adapt their style to varying situations. They discovered that although obtaining short-term leadership behavior changes was possible, the nurse managers tended to impose more task structure and greater relationship orientation than the subordinates desired or needed, thereby failing to adapt management style to the subordinates' characteristics. Johnson and D'Argenio concluded that this high-structure, high-relationship approach was "not the best for fostering the growth and development of followers" and emphasized the importance of matching management styles with subordinates' characteristics and ability to function independently.

REDDIN'S 3D THEORY OF LEADERSHIP AND MANAGEMENT

Reddin (1970) suggests that leadership and management can be examined from two basic perspectives—task orientation and relationship orientation—both of which can exist to either a high degree or a low degree in each leadership situation. He identifies four leadership styles: integrated, related, dedicated, and separated. The integrated style emphasizes both task orientation and relationship orientation. The related style emphasizes relationship orientation but not task orientation. The dedicated style emphasizes task orientation but not relationship orientation. The separated style reflects low relationship and low task orientation. Reddin further theorizes that each basic style can have an effective and a corresponding ineffective application. The following descriptions illustrate the effective and ineffective application of the integrated, related, dedicated, and separated leadership styles identified by Reddin.

Integrated leadership style

Executive. This manager uses a high orientation to task and relationships when such behaviors are appropriate. The leader involves members in planning as well as implementation but can also make decisions independently when necessary. The leader works effectively with people and accomplishes tasks.

Compromiser. This manager uses task orientation and relationship orientation, but in an unproductive manner. The compromiser can be too easily swayed by individual interests, with the result that management veers from one crisis to another without any progress on long-term goals. The compromiser is ineffective and indecisive.

Related leadership style

Developer. This manager uses a high relationship but low task orientation. The developer considers subordinates productive and capable of structuring tasks and works to support and assist them.

Missionary. Like the developer, this manager also uses a high relationship but low task orientation; unlike the developer, the missionary does so ineffectively, usually in situations requiring more attention to tasks. The missionary is usually pleasant but overly concerned with everybody getting along rather than with making concrete progress.

Dedicated leadership style

Benevolent Autocrat. This manager successfully relies on high task orientation and low relationship orientation. The benevolent autocrat achieves subordinate compliance by providing precise direction.

Autocrat. This manager uses the same basic approach but usually in inappropriate situations. As a result, subordinates view the autocrat as dictatorial and uncaring or as caring only for the bottom line.

Separated leadership style

Bureaucrat. This manager effectively uses low relationship and low task orientation. With rules and regulations in place, the bureaucrat allows subordinates to exercise individual initiative, which makes them feel trusted and competent.

Deserter. This manager also uses low relationship and low task orientation but without success. Subordinates feel as if the leader has abandoned leadership obligations and as if no one is providing required guidance, structure, and support.

Goodroe and Beres (1991) suggest that the changing roles of nursing staff and leaders require a new participatory approach, which the authors call "network leadership." Network leaders are coordinators rather than commanders; they acknowledge staff abilities and expertise and work with group members as an equal rather than as a superior.

THE ROLE OF FOLLOWER

Just as leader traits can influence the leadership and management styles implemented, follower characteristics also have their influence. Douglas (1992) suggests that key follower characteristics include knowledge, competency and preparation level, and experience. If workers require close supervision because of low preparation levels and inexperience, the leader may appropriately use a more directive style. A nurse leader must assess each team member's qualifications before determining the proper management style and delegating responsibilities.

Follower attitudes and needs also influence the leadership style selected. A subordinate who works best when expectations are clearly spelled out and decisions are made by management may experience difficulty working under a laissez-faire leadership, which doesn't provide such structure. On the other hand, a subordinate who works best when allowed to participate in decision making may not respond well under a rigidly controlled, autocratic leadership. Because nursing requires a considerable degree of teamwork and mutual goal-setting along with adherence to timelines and sequences, a democratic leadership style may more often than not meet subordinate needs better than a style that grants subordinates virtually independent functioning.

Effective followers are able to see the relation between their personal needs and institutional goals in all situations. Such nurses maintain a commitment to the institution while deriving satisfaction from their work. Effective leaders point out the mutuality of personal and institutional goals and work with subordinates to facilitate the achievement of both.

INEFFECTIVE FOLLOWERS

Just as leaders can be ineffective, so, too, can followers. This section discusses several types of ineffective followers, including uncommitted, hostile, and impaired followers.

UNCOMMITTED FOLLOWERS

Although today's nurses continue to have family and personal commitments and activities, they also more often than not demonstrate a professional commitment that transcends an 8-hour or 12-hour day. They participate in professional practice committees, bioethics committees, community volunteer organizations, and continuing education programs. Nevertheless, uncommitted nurses do exist.

When working with an uncommitted follower, the leader must first recognize the individual's attitude toward nursing and then endeavor to work constructively with it. An uncommitted follower may not want to participate in activities other than direct client care; if the health setting permits, the leader should allow the nurse this option. The perceptive leader may also be able to instill a greater professional sense in an uncommitted nurse by encouraging the nurse to explore some personal interest. For example, the nurse may be interested in researching ways to deliver better client care within the facility or in working with a community group that assists clients after mastectomy.

HOSTILE FOLLOWERS

The long, arduous hours that most nurses work often cause stress; unrelieved stress can result in what is known as burnout. Nurses experiencing burnout may be chronically tired and passively hostile or overtly angry and actively negative. Such nurses feel exploited and misunderstood and may view any change as a ploy to get them to work even harder. Such hostile behavior can also negatively affect the group's general attitude and operation. Hostile nurses may reject new ideas as impractical, or they may prophesy failure for proposed innovations. Trapped in this cycle of stress and anger, hostile followers may be unable to see a way out. Frequently the only solution seems to be leaving the job or perhaps even the profession.

In dealing with hostile followers, the leader must first identify as many specific problems as possible. Perhaps the follower has worked in a particular area for many years and has seen more and more ill clients having to be cared for by the same number of staff. Perhaps the worker cannot adapt to an evolving delivery mode and continues to assume responsibility for total client care when doing so is not feasible. In the intensive care and coronary care units and in the operating department, the continuous exposure to highly charged situations can be debilitating.

Once problems have been identified, the leader can help the hostile follower to examine possible alternatives for improving the situation. The nurse might benefit from a transfer to another area. Additional education and training may enable the nurse to deal more effectively with stress. Perhaps another health care setting altogether would provide less stressful and more fulfilling employment. After the leader and hostile nurse have discussed all possible alternatives, the leader or appropriate supervisor should counsel the nurse, explaining the negative impact that the hostility is having and clarifying expectations for improvement.

IMPAIRED FOLLOWERS

Today's nurses acknowledge the fact that they are working in a highly stressful profession and that they, like other professionals in highly stressful jobs, run a high risk of drug or alcohol addiction. Chapter 6, Legal implications for nursing practice, and Chapter 7, Ethical implications for nursing practice, discuss the legal and ethical ramifications of this problem. However, the leader's responsibilities to an impaired follower are not always clear-cut.

Once a problem has been identified, usually by staff with whom the impaired nurse works, the manager as leader must initiate the organizational response to suspected impairment. The leader must know whether to call in the institution's substance abuse team or local law enforcement authorities. The leader should also know what resources are available from the institution, the state board of nursing, and other professional and private organizations.

Regardless of the organizational response, the leader can adopt a collegial role and assist the impaired nurse to see the personal damage as well as the hazard to clients and coworkers that results from substance abuse. The leader can treat the nurse as a professional who can potentially return after rehabilitation to make an important contribution. Nevertheless, because of the danger to clients and staff, the leader cannot allow an impaired follower to continue to practice. Removal from the client care setting until treatment can be undertaken is imperative.

INFLUENCING INEFFECTIVE FOLLOWERS

Yukl (1981) describes several ways in which a leader can influence ineffective followers.

1. The leader can serve as a role model. A staff nurse desiring greater responsibilities and leadership opportunities might be influenced to return to school by the example of a leader who has done so; identifying with the leader's example encourages the follower to attempt a similar career change.

2. The leader can use persuasion. After identifying the follower's needs and goals, the leader can point out that change is in the follower's best interests. For example, a leader might persuade a follower to consider requesting a move from the intensive care unit to the home health service, pointing out that the follower has been wanting an opportunity to work with client families.

3. The leader can appeal to the follower's values and ideals. For example, a follower caring for pediatric clients might have become calloused to parent concerns and fail to respond constructively to parents' requests for information and help. In such circumstances, the leader might recall the value of involving parents in their children's care and nurses' obligation to treat the family as a unit.

4. The leader can use a particular expertise to influence followers. If the leader of the hospital's transplant team claims that a workshop on how to approach families about organ donation will help the follower to perform this expected task, the follower may defer to the leader's expertise and decide to attend.

5. The leader can involve the follower in decision-making processes. The more direct input followers have in determining a course of action, the more likely they are to support the action.

6. The leader can make a legitimate request. As manager, a leader may request that a follower change some behavior. For example, the leader may ask a follower to refrain from interrupting other workers with negative comments at staff meetings and to wait until the entire proposal has been presented before offering a point of view. The follower defers because the leader has the legitimate authority to make such a request.

7. The leader can require instrumental compliance and show the follower the benefits of compliance. For example, a leader might propose a schedule adjustment to enable a follower to pursue additional schooling, while making clear the expectation that the follower become an active, effective member of the hospital bioethics committee.

8. The leader can influence the work situation. The leader may change staffing patterns in a particular unit, thereby requiring the follower to change if the follower wants to continue working in that unit.

9. The leader can use coercion. The leader who possesses coercive power can request that the follower make certain changes or suffer the negative consequences, from reassignment to dismissal. For example, if a hostile follower consistently arrives late for work and takes longer than the allotted time for breaks, the leader can request a behavior change, while assuring the follower that refusing to do so will result in disciplinary action.

RECIPROCAL ROLES OF LEADERS AND FOLLOWERS

The reciprocal nature of leader and follower roles frequently requires that nurses move back and forth between both roles; a leader in one situation may be a follower in another. For example, a team leader in a pediatrics department may be a follower in another nurses' group developing a pediatric symposium for the hospital. Being able to function comfortably and appropriately in both the leader role and the follower role is an important nursing skill. A nurse who is unable to follow may interfere with a group's function. For example, if an emergency department supervisor participating as a follower in a safety committee meeting attempts to control the discussion rather than support the identified leader, the group may be pulled between the actions of the competing leaders. Good leaders can be good followers by acknowledging the structure and goals set out by the leader and working to support them.

NEW GRADUATES AS FOLLOWERS

In most situations, new graduates are followers. Grant (1991) suggests several specific actions to help new graduates function effectively in the follower's role.

1. Invest yourself. Part of being a good follower is feeling committed to the institution's goals and objectives. Identifying an institution's goals and seeing that they are compatible with your own is important when choosing employment. If you strongly disapprove of health care as a profit-making enterprise, you may feel more comfortable working for a public agency or nonprofit organization than for a corporate-owned agency. If you want to continue your education while working, check to see if the institution will assist with tuition reimbursement or flexible scheduling. Once you have chosen a particular agency and work setting, you should actively work to meet both personal and institutional goals.

2. Identify your responsibilities as a follower. Clearly understanding what is expected and required of you is essential. You can obtain this information during orientations and internships and in policy manuals and job descriptions. You can also identify individuals whom you could question as issues arise. Familiarizing yourself with evaluation criteria for workers in your area can help you pinpoint essential responsibilities and expected performance levels. Clearly understanding your responsibilities will help you work more effectively and comfortably.

3. Identify your leader expectations. During your orientation or internship, you will become acquainted with the leaders under whom you will be working. Observe the leadership style used. Identifying an autocratic, democratic, or laissez-faire style can help you determine your role in relation to the leader and other group members. Furthermore, you should have realistic expectations of the leader; expecting the leader to continue providing the close supervision and direction that characterized orientation is probably not feasible or appropriate. On the other hand, if you have specific learning needs, such as obtaining more experience inserting nasogastric tubes, you could appropriately inform your leader of them.

4. Support the leader and the group. Nurses have colleague and institution obligations. One such obligation is to work effectively in collaborative care provision. This does not mean that problems should be left unaddressed; however, it does mean that an effective follower works to satisfy group and institution goals, as well as client and personal goals.

5. Challenge your leader and group. Effective followers question procedures and commonly accepted ways of doing things but should do so in a constructive way, using accepted procedures. Doing so can lead to task innovations. For example, a new nurse might wonder why charting a particular client action in three separate places is necessary and bring this to the supervising nurse's attention; the supervising nurse might report the observation to the nursing team examining the forms; a review of documentation might lead the institution to streamline forms and minimize charting duplication.

DELEGATION

Effective leaders must be able to delegate responsibilities to others. Hansten and Washburn (1992) suggest that nurses are traditionally unwilling to relinquish responsibilities or to accept help from others. Nurses frequently think that they can perform tasks better themselves or that explaining or teaching the task to another takes too much time. Some nurses believe that they are not properly performing their job if they delegate responsibilities to another. Other nurses prefer to work alone, thinking that they retain better control over client care. Despite these feelings, more and more nurses are serving as coordinators and managers at all levels, and these nurses must learn to delegate responsibilities comfortably and effectively. The National Council of State Boards of Nursing (1990) defines delegation as "transferring to a competent individual authority to perform a selected nursing task in a selected situation."

To delegate responsibilities effectively, the nurse must:

- assess subordinates' abilities and competencies. The leader or manager can accomplish this assessment by asking the subordinate direct questions, such as, "Have you worked with Mrs. Smith yet?" or "Do you know how to help her adjust her position with that type of traction set up?" The manager may also consult others about a subordinate's competency and experience or review certification or education information.

- provide support and education for subordinates. If a subordinate has had minimal experience with a particular task or skill that will probably be delegated to that subordinate, the manager can provide appropriate teaching. The leader can have the subordinate observe another nurse performing the task; support the subordinate as the subordinate attempts the task; and provide additional learning opportunities.

- clearly identify the task to be performed. An assignment should specify the task to be performed, the manner in which it is to be accomplished, when it is to be completed, and the type of reporting required. If the leader anticipates difficulties, the assignment should also specify the extent of the subordinate's responsibility and when the subordinate should seek help.

- confirm task completion and evaluation. The leader can delegate tasks but not the responsibility for seeing that they are properly completed. Toward this end, the leader must follow up to ensure appropriate task performance. The leader should also give prompt feedback, which will contribute to subordinate learning.

DELEGATION

- *Assessment of abilities and competencies of subordinates*
- *Provision of support and education to subordinates*
- *Clear identification of tasks to be performed*
- *Confirmation of task completion and evaluation of performance*

Hansten and Washburn (1992) point out that appropriate delegation enables nurses to provide more and higher quality care than would be possible without subordinate assistance and also gives nurses more time to conduct management activities, which are just as crucial to good client care as direct contact. Delegation also enables the leader and subordinates to develop a sense of teamwork and mutual support.

EVOLUTION OF THE ROLES OF MANAGERS AND FOLLOWERS

Health care managers and followers are developing new ways of working together. The new nursing care standards from the Joint Commission on Accreditation of Healthcare Organizations (JCAHO) underscore these new relationships. Nurses are no longer simply to make assessments that are "consistent with the medical plan of care" but must "collaborate, as appropriate, with physicians and other clinical disciplines in making decisions regarding each [client's] need for nursing care" (Joint Commission on Accreditation of Healthcare Organizations 1991). This new standard emphasizes the staff nurse's participatory and collegial role. Hurley (1991) believes that the new standards will mean a greater voice for nurses in client care planning and in determining how hospitals are run.

According to Hurley (1991), the new standards also address other important issues. A portion of initial assessments and evaluations may now be delegated to assisting staff, but the manager must have documented their training and competency before making such delegations. The standards clearly describe the responsibility of nurses for planning client care and developing nursing practice standards. In addition, nurses can now have a voice in the institutional body responsible for addressing ethical problems. Now, too, one chief executive nurse is to represent nursing in discussions with other hospital officials as together they develop the institution's "mission statement, nursing budget, strategic plan, and quality assurance and improvement policies." All these changes underscore increased nurse participation at all management levels.

SHARED GOVERNANCE

Institutions can support these changes by implementing shared governance strategies. Shared governance describes the collaborative decision-making process used jointly by nursing and hospital management. Bower (1991) points out that shared governance can be structurally complex, with leaders formally elected at prescribed intervals, or relatively simple, with just a few basic guidelines. Shared governance usually is accomplished by a system of governing councils, each with related committees and each specifically responsible for an area such as nursing practice standards, quality assurance, resource allocation, education, and the overall direction of nursing services.

The nursing standards council develops and approves nursing job descriptions. The quality assurance council addresses such things as staff credentialing and nursing performance. The resource allocation council establishes institutional resource priorities. An education council assesses continuing education needs and provides needed programs for new and established staff. A coordinating council comprising the chairpersons of all other councils is responsible for overall communication among the various councils, decision making, and strategic planning.

Several factors have influenced the general institutional shift toward shared governance. These include dissatisfaction with traditional centralized decision making, the desire to involve more frontline staff in problem solving and planning, the recruitment potential of a collaborative approach, and the mandates of professional and accrediting bodies, such as the JCAHO, that nurses become directly involved in leading and managing client care activities.

Evolution from the traditional hierarchical structure to shared governance requires considerable effort. Not all institutions successfully make the transition. O'Grady (1989) suggests that some institutions claiming to practice shared governance fail to provide sufficient autonomy and responsibility. Furthermore, nursing staff may be reluctant to assume traditional management responsibilities. Nor can shared governance guarantee improved client care or a professionally fulfilled nursing staff; however, nursing participation at all management levels potentially expands the leadership opportunities for all nurses.

O'Grady (1989) points out that "successful shared governance demands the commitment of every nurse in the organization." Staff nurses must be encouraged to participate on governing councils. Managers must relinquish control and decision-making responsibilities to the new councils. When true shared governance is in place, nursing staff elect peers to governing positions, specific policies or bylaws govern council functioning, and nursing staff have input into institution-wide concerns such as wages, budgets, and staffing. In other words, nurses control nursing practice.

BECOMING A LEADER

Whether heading a colleague team for group client care or chairing a shared governance council, all leaders change and develop in their role. The leader can facilitate development by self-evaluation, personal effort, and an understanding of the traits that characterize an effective leader. These traits include:

- the ability to set clear goals. In a traditional setting, the leader may develop goals based on knowledge of the situation, with varying degrees of subordinate input. In shared governance, the leader acts with colleagues to set goals. Effective goal setting may involve establishing behavioral objectives, which are easier to grasp, plan for, and evaluate (see Chapter 8, The nurse as teacher). Regardless of the goal-setting approach, the leader must articulate the goals so that the group understands them.
- the ability to communicate. A leader must be committed to sharing information with subordinates. Ineffective leaders are sometimes described as people who really know their field but cannot communicate their knowledge to

others. Effective communication requires knowing the abilities and characteristics of the subordinates receiving the communication, clearly articulating the message, and confirming that subordinates have understood the communication.

- an understanding of organizational structure. Leaders must adapt their style to the institution in which they work. If the institution retains a traditional hierarchical structure, the leader should exercise a more directive management style. Appropriate adjustments should be made for more collaborative structures. Furthermore, leaders can work toward changing a hierarchical structure to a collaborative one but should implement changes as part of an overall move to a new structure.

- an understanding of preferred leadership style. Although leaders should be able to adopt and use all leadership styles, they usually prefer one or two above the others. Being aware of preferences can help leaders identify and correct weaknesses in their handling of certain situations. For example, a leader who prefers an autocratic leadership style may initially have trouble leading in a collaborative situation that calls for a laissez-faire style. The aware leader would be better able to make the necessary adjustments.

- a willingness to develop new methods and approaches. Nursing leadership must continually adapt to the rapid changes in health care delivery. As a result, learning and adhering to a specific way of handling responsibilities (managing a budget, evaluating staff, or preparing departmental strategies) are no longer sufficient. An effective nurse leader must be willing to learn new management and leadership skills and to make collaborative decisions with subordinates, colleagues, clients, and other bodies, such as boards of trustees and regulatory agencies.

- a willingness to serve assertively as an advocate. Being an effective leader means taking risks, involving oneself at a significant level, and assuming responsibility for advancing client, staff, and social causes.

Assuming Formal Leadership

As nurses gain experience and knowledge, they encounter leadership opportunities. Tuazon (1991) discusses one way in which staff nurses typically gain their first leadership experience: as charge nurse in a relief role. Before assuming charge nurse responsibilities, the staff nurse undergoes a 2-day management training during which experienced managers discuss expectations, potential problems, and available resources. Subsequently, the new charge nurse may make assignments based on client acuity and staff qualifications and may make decisions about unit admissions, in addition to having patient care assignments. Tuazon suggests that a new leader use the following guidelines:

1. Understand your role and the extent of your responsibilities.

2. Be aware of your clinical and managerial strengths and weaknesses, and arrange for appropriate support.

3. When faced with a problem, consider all options. New leaders often want to resolve problems immediately. Take time to explore the problem, identify solutions, and select the appropriate option.

4. Delegate duties and responsibilities appropriately. Effective delegation gives you more time and flexibility to respond to staff needs.

5. Listen to your staff. They can provide important information about clients, their assignments, and other concerns. Being a leader does not mean making all decisions unilaterally; include staff feedback in decisions.

6. Acknowledge good work. Acknowledging staff contributions can help to build staff rapport and leadership support.

Summary

Today all nurses need leadership skills, whether they are directing colleague teams at the bedside or serving as elected leaders within the health care organization. Many factors, including the women's movement and the civil rights movement, have contributed to nursing's increased demand for effective leaders. Whether using a predominantly autocratic, democratic, or laissez-faire leadership style, effective nurse leaders must be able to adjust their style to particular situations. They must also be able to work within a traditional hierarchical structure and as a participant in shared governance. In delegating power, effective leaders must understand the demands of their role as well as the characteristics and roles of their subordinates.

APPLICATION EXERCISE

Arrange with your instructor to observe a nurse leader during the course of the leader's workday. Keeping in mind the four principle leadership styles (autocratic, democratic, laissez-faire, and multicratic), note how the nurse leader interacts with staff and others. Identify what basic approach is used, and when or if the leader modifies that approach. Use the following questions to analyze the leadership style you observed and to develop an effective personal approach to leadership.

1. What basic leadership style did the nurse use? Which characteristics of this approach did this leader use?

2. Did the leader vary the leadership style? If so, under what circumstances?

3. Was the leader effective? Why or why not?

4. If you were a leader in the same circumstances, how would your leadership style resemble or differ from that of the leader you observed? What personal traits would influence your decision?

REVIEW QUESTIONS

1. What are the differences and similarities between leadership and management? Between professionalism and leadership?

2. Describe the 'Great Man' theory of leadership, and contrast it with later trait theories.

3. What advantages did situational and contingency theory bring to the examination of leadership?

4. According to House, how can a leader motivate followers?

5. How does leadership differ under autocratic, democratic, laissez-faire and multicratic leaders?

6. How are the roles of leader and follower related? How can a leader also be a good follower?

7. What must a nurse do before delegating responsibilities to another?

8. What is shared governance, and how does it differ from a traditional bureaucratic approach to management?

REFERENCES

Bower. F.L. "Shared Governance, Part III: Structural Implementation," *California Nursing* 12(2):33-35, March/April 1991.

Douglas, L.M. *The Effective Nurse Leader and Manager*, 4th ed. St. Louis: Mosby YearBook, 1992.

Goodroe, J.H., and Beres, M.E. "Network Leadership and Today's Nurse," *Nursing Management* 22(6):56-62, June 1992.

Grant, A.B. "Developing a Management Style," in *Managing and Coordinating Nursing Care.* Edited by Ellis, J.R. and Hartley, C.L. Philadelphia: J.B. Lippincott Co., 1991.

Hansten, R., and Washburn, M. "Delegation: How to Deliver Care Through Others," *American Journal of Nursing* 92(3):87-90, March 1992.

House, R.J. "A Path-Goal Theory of Leadership Effectiveness," *Administrative Science Quarterly* 16:321-228, 1971.

Hurley, M.L. "What Do the New JCAHO Standards Mean for You?" *RN* 54(6):42-47, June 1991.

Johnson, R., and D'Argenio, C. "Management Training Effects on Nurse Manager Leadership Behavior," *Nursing Economics* 9(4):249-254, July/August 1991.

Joint Commission on Accreditation of Healthcare Organizations. *Accreditation Manual for Hospitals: Vol. A. Standards.* N.C. 1.3.2. Oakbrook Terrace, Ill.: Joint Commission on Accreditation of Healthcare Organizations.

National Council of State Boards of Nursing: Concept paper on delegation. Chicago: National Council of State Boards of Nursing, 1990.

O'Grady, T.P. "Shared Governance: Reality or Sham?" *American Journal of Nursing* 89(3):350-351, March 1989.

Reddin, W. *Managerial Effectiveness.* New York: McGraw-Hill, 1970.

Sullivan E.J., and Decker, P.J. *Effective Management in Nursing,* 2nd ed. Reading, Mass.: Addison-Wesley Publishing Co., 1988.

Tuazon, N.C. "When Your Supervisor Hands You the Reins," *RN* 54(12):21-23, December 1991.

Yukl, G.A. *Leadership in Organizations.* Englewood Cliffs, N.J.: Prentice-Hall, 1981.

RECOMMENDATIONS FOR FURTHER STUDY

American Organization of Nurse Executives. "Nursing Management and JCAHO," *Nursing Management* 23(5):26-27, May 1992.

Bennis, W. *Why Leaders Can't Lead.* San Francisco: Jossey-Bass Publishers, 1989.

Bethel, S.M. *Making a Difference: Twelve Qualities That Can Make You a Leader.* New York: G.P. Putnam's Sons, 1990.

Hansten, R., and Washburn, M. "What Do You Say When You Delegate Work to Others?" *American Journal of Nursing* 92(7):48-50, July 1992.

Lufkin, S.R., et al. "Job Satisfaction in the Head Nurse Role," *Nursing Management* 23(3):27-29, March 1992.

Manning, G. "Invest: A Plan for Developing New Managers," *Nursing Management* 22(12):26-28, December 1991.

Mark, B.A., et al. "Knowledge and Skills for Nurse Administrators," *Nursing and Health Care* 11(4):185-189, April 1990.

Puetz, B.E., and Thomas, D.O. "What Skills Do You Need for a Management Job?" *RN* 54(1):83-84, January 1992.

Schmeiding, N.J. "Do Head Nurses Include Staff Nurses in Problem Solving?" *Nursing Management* 21(3):58-60 March 1990.

Stengrevics, S.S., et al. "Nurse Manager Job Satisfaction; The Massachusetts Perspective," *Nursing Management* 22(4):60-64, April 1991.

Taylor, J.K. "Management Style and Unit Productivity." *Nursing Management,* 21(8):49-50, August 1990.

10

DECISION MAKING IN NURSING

OBJECTIVES

After studying this chapter, the reader should be able to:

1. Explain how critical thinking, problem solving, and decision making are related.

2. Define and illustrate stereotypical thinking.

3. Compare the nursing process and the problem-solving process.

4. Identify four learning styles and describe the advantages and disadvantages of each.

5. Compare and contrast Type I and Type II methods of inquiry.

6. Compare and contrast the four forms of knowledge.

7. List and describe the steps involved in problem solving.

8. Describe decision-making strategies for individual and group use.

INTRODUCTION

Decision making is the act of determining which of several possible outcomes is preferable in a given situation. Every day, nurses apply decision-making skills to client care, colleague relations, obligations to employers, and a host of other concerns on short-term and long-term bases. Despite this, the formal teaching of decision making and related critical thinking and problem-solving strategies sometimes takes second place to the teaching of skills such as medication administration and physical assessment. Some nursing educators even view decision making as merely an application of the nursing process or a secondary skill of research methodology, project planning, or financing. In fact, nursing students should carefully study the decision making process to learn how to implement it in different health care settings. The following example should illustrate how decision making can directly affect nursing and client care.

> Two weeks after concluding her orientation to the medical-surgical floor of a busy rural hospital, a recently hired registered nurse (RN) arrives for work. She is enjoying her new position, even though the hospital is short-staffed. In addition, many physical repairs are in progress, including resurfacing the small hospital parking lot. Because she has difficulty finding a parking space, the nurse arrives on her assigned floor several minutes late. The evening shift RN, who has been eager to leave, is annoyed at the nurse's tardiness and begins to file a report before the new nurse can record her clients' names on her worksheet. While the hostile report is being transmitted, a call bell sounds from one of the rooms for which the new nurse is responsible. The nurse knows that no one else is available to answer the light because budgetary constraints have forced the reduction of night shift staffing. Because she doesn't want to further antagonize the evening shift RN, the new nurse asks the ward clerk to inquire over the intercom what is wanted. The ward clerk, busy with a physician, fails to do this, and the nursing report proceeds until suddenly a code is called. An elderly client has fallen out of bed while attempting to get to the bathroom and is now lying unconscious on the floor.

Several decisions made at varying levels produced the situation just described. The new nurse made some; some were made by others. Some decisions had a direct bearing on client care. Others related to financial, ethical, and legal issues. Some were short-term; others were long-term. All directly affected the new nurse's situation. More important, all affected the client.

If the new RN had better understood the decision-making process, she might have addressed the choices before her more satisfactorily. She needed to consider questions related

---

THREE RELATED CONCEPTS

- *Decision-making: process of reasonably evaluating options to arrive at optimal choice among alternatives*
- *Problem-solving: a subset of decision-making that addresses an actual or potential problem*
- *Critical thinking: a way to examine assumptions, beliefs, propositions, and arguments during decision-making and problem-solving*

---

to several areas: What was her responsibility to her client? to her coworker? to the institution? What short-term solutions would have supported the long-term goal? Knowing that her shift was short-staffed and that parking was a problem, she might have planned to arrive early enough to park her car and reach her floor on time. She might have asked the evening shift RN to delay the report while she prepared her worksheet. When the call bell was heard, she might have asked the evening shift RN to respond while she finished her preliminary notations. She might simply have interrupted the nurse's report to check on the client herself.

This chapter presents a comprehensive look at decision making and explains how it relates to critical thinking and problem solving. The chapter begins by discussing critical thinking and its role in the decision-making process. Factors that help the nurse determine an approach to decision making are then covered. The chapter goes on to examine the problem-solving process, pointing out the similarities it shares with the nursing process and the research process. The chapter concludes with a discussion of the broader responsibility of decision making and offers some specific strategies for making effective decisions.

CRITICAL THINKING

Critical thinking is a way of analyzing problems or phenomena. It enables the nurse to examine the "assumptions, beliefs, propositions and the meaning and uses of words, statements and arguments" associated with a problem (Bandman and Bandman, 1988). Critical thinking also enables the nurse to eliminate preconceptions, biases, and traditional interpretations that might obscure other, more reasonable explanations. Critical thinking can lead the nurse to the possible reasonable solutions to a problem. The nurse can then choose from among these possible solutions in making a decision.

Evaluating and integrating information are essential steps in the critical-thinking process. The nurse must first decide if the information on hand is accurate. If so, does the information actually apply to the situation? If it is both accurate and applicable, does it dictate a particular decision, or does it suggest several possible solutions? For example, a small, rural hospital in the South is considering adopting a new charting method that has proved effective in a large city hospital. The staff of the smaller hospital must first collect all data related to the new charting method. Then they must examine the data in terms of their relevance to their situation. What effectiveness parameters did the city hospital use? Would these parameters be appropriate to the rural setting, or would smaller hospitals have different charting needs and priorities? How reliable are the findings? What other variables might have been involved in the city hospital's evaluation? What new elements might influence the charting method's effectiveness in a small, rural hospital?

Critical thinking also enables the nurse to recognize and consider claims or allegations that may be distorted by emotion. Suppose, for example, that during a labor dispute, a nurse claims that management cares only for the budget and has no concern for staff. This claim, if it were to gain acceptance, could undermine staff confidence in management and thereby hinder further attempts to reach a resolution. To deal properly with such a claim, the other nurses might request that the nurse making the claim substantiate the claim with evidence. If such evidence exists, it should then be examined so that an objective conclusion about the reliability of the claim and the person making it can be drawn. In doing so, the nurses should try to determine if other factors, such as budgetary constraints, might be hampering management's ability to grant the requested pay increase.

Critical thinking demands a comprehensive look at problems and thereby helps to eliminate stereotypical thinking, which is characterized by unconsidered beliefs about people, cultures, or events. The nurse who holds a stereotypical view of a particular ethnic or national group may misinterpret a client's behavior as being "just how those people are" and, as a consequence, provide inadequate or inappropriate care. For example, the nurse with such a view of Hispanic culture might expect a Hispanic client to be overly demonstrative during labor and childbirth. Such stereotyping could cause the nurse to downplay the client's protestations of pain and lead to inappropriate decisions about client care. A more critical approach might help the nurse in this situation overcome the bias and make a more reasoned decision.

APPROACHES TO DECISION MAKING

Several factors influence the approach a nurse takes toward decision making. The nurse's preferred learning style is one such factor. Another is the dominant method of inquiry the nurse chooses to use. Understanding the different forms of knowledge that everyone possesses can also influence the approach the nurse takes toward decision making.

LEARNING STYLES

How nurses usually learn and assimilate ideas and experiences can influence the way they make decisions. Kolb (1976) identifies four types of learner based on the way that each deals with ideas and daily experiences. The categories are determined in part by the degree to which they incorporate reflexive observation (watching), abstract conceptualization (thinking), active experimentation (doing), or concrete experience (feeling).

Analytic Learners. These people learn best by taking things apart and examining relations and concepts. Analytic learners usually are comfortable in traditional learning settings and when faced with a problem, they think through it. They also are more interested in concepts than in people.

Common Sense Learners. These learners seek a practical application of facts and learn best when they can see how to apply information to real situations. Common sense learners are intolerant of "fuzzy" thinking and learn by testing theories.

Dynamic Learners. These people enjoy learning by trial and error and self-discovery. They are comfortable with change, and their strengths lie in acting out and testing various experiences.

Innovative Learners. These learners are divergent thinkers, capable of viewing concrete situations from different perspectives. They focus on social interaction, and their strengths include innovation and imagination.

The differences among the four learner types can be illustrated by their decision-making approaches to the following situation: A medical-surgical unit is considering the use of a new type of I.V. controller. Staff are asked to examine the controller and to give recommendations about purchase.

The Analytic Learner would thoroughly read the accompanying brochure, identify pros and cons, and analyze the facts before deciding. The Common Sense learner would read enough of the instructions to see how the I.V. controller works, hook up the controller to an I.V. set, and see how well it functioned before making a recommendation. The Dynamic Learner would briefly examine the instructions and then test how well the controller dealt with occlusions, empty bags, air in the line, and loss of power. The Innovative Learner would contact staff in other hospitals who had used the controller and have them identify difficulties encountered. The Innovative Learner would compare the new controller with the old ones and might recommend that with slight modification, the controller in use would be more advantageous than the newer model.

No single learning style is appropriate for all situations. In some situations, an innovative or dynamic approach might require too much time; in such cases, the nurse might better use a commonsense approach. Other situations may call for an analytic approach. Being able to vary the decision-making approach based on the circumstances and nature of the decision to be made enhances the nurse's decision-making abilities.

LEARNING STYLES

- *Analytic learners: analyze, dissect*
- *Common-sense learners: apply information to real situations*
- *Dynamic learners: learn by trial & error*
- *Innovative learners: consider situations from different points of view*

DEGREE OF CERTAINTY

In evaluating facts and information, the nurse must also determine their degree of certainty. The fact that a scalpel

METHODS OF INQUIRY

Type I and Type II methods of inquiry emphasize different processes.
- *Type I (positivist-empiricist)*
  - *Analysis*
  - *Measurement*
  - *Experimentation*
- *Type II (subjectivist)*
  - *Feeling*
  - *Intuition*

will fall to the floor when dropped has a high degree of certainty that can easily be verified. Concluding that willful neglect was responsible for a nurse's failure to change a dressing cannot be determined so assuredly and is more difficult to verify.

When making a decision, the nurse should use facts that can be inferred only when other evidence reinforces them. For example, deciding that a nurse willfully failed to carry out an order might be more easily concluded if the nurse had repeatedly failed to carry out orders properly and had stated in a report the belief that certain procedures were not needed.

PARADIGMATIC APPROACHES TO KNOWLEDGE

Two major methods or paradigms of inquiry enable the nurse to consider information in different ways. In making health-related decisions, nurses most frequently use the Type I, or positivist-empiricist, method (Tinkle and Beaton, 1983). This method relies on objective observation and experimentation and is thought of as the scientific method.

The Type II method is described as the Intuitive-Subjectivist method. It emphasizes the uniqueness of individual experience and the interconnectedness of facts. Nurses using the Type II method study facts in their context (cultural and social setting) rather than in isolation.

Suppose a nursing staff is trying to decide how to improve client preparation for repeat cesarean section. Using the Type I method, the nursing staff would use empirical observation to identify the teaching plan that best provides objective information about cesarean sections. The staff might proceed as follows:

- A client care committee is established to improve client preparation for repeat cesarean section.
- The committee reviews all available teaching plans and on the basis of effectiveness reports described in other studies selects three alternative plans for closer examination.
- The committee randomly assigns client groups to test the relative effectiveness of the three alternative plans as well as the plan in use.

- Clients are asked to answer a pretest and post-test questionnaire that evaluates knowledge and emotional preparedness. The committee uses the results of these questionnaires to assess the effectiveness of the plans.

A Type II method to the same concern might produce the following actions:

- A client care committee concerned about the knowledge and emotional preparedness levels of their repeat cesarean section clients decides to learn more about the reasons some clients seem more knowledgeable and emotionally prepared than others.
- The committee decides to interview clients and their families to see what variables, including educational level, previous experience, emotional support, and others suggested by the clients themselves, might have bearing on the issues of knowledge and emotional preparedness.
- Based on the information they receive, the committee will construct a series of teaching plans that take into consideration client characteristics.

Both methods of inquiry would provide information on the clients' knowledge and emotional preparedness but would do so in different ways. The Type I method emphasizes objective measurement; the Type II method is more subjective. Both methods could provide an appropriate basis for a new preoperative teaching plan.

Patterns of Knowledge

People acquire empirical knowledge through objective observation. Using this means, a nurse would assess a client for observable signs and symptoms on which to base planning, intervention, and assessment. Empirical knowledge gained through objective observation is augmented by aesthetic, ethical, and personal knowledge.

Aesthetic knowledge represents a nurse's empathy and understanding of a client's feelings. To attain it, the nurse must understand not only the client's physiologic functioning but also as much as possible about the client as a person, including the client's fears, desires, and aspirations. To the degree that a nurse can gather and use aesthetic knowledge, the nurse's ability to care for a particular client improves.

Ethical knowledge represents the nurse's understanding of different value systems and beliefs and of the ways in which the nurse can address problems involving ethical decisions. Chapter 7, Ethical implications for nursing practice, provides problem-solving and decision-making strategies that specifically address these difficult areas. The following situation illustrates how a nurse might use ethical knowledge in decision making.

> A physician asks a new nurse to assist in a sterile dressing change on a postoperative cholecystectomy client. The physician has a reputation for being intolerant of delays and of new, inexperienced nurses. During the procedure, the nurse notices that the physician has inadvertently brushed his gloved hand against the client's bedsheet, contaminating his glove and the sterile dressing he subsequently picks up. The nurse knows that calling this to the physician's attention will require delay while the physician regloves and waits for a new dressing. If the nurse ignores the matter, no one else will know, even if the client should develop a wound infection. The nurse's awareness of her ethical responsibilities to the client requires that she alert the physician to the client hazard, despite his probable annoyance.

Personal knowledge is the nurse's awareness of the therapeutic value of the nurse-client relationship. Without this component, nursing would be reduced to technical, if skillful, manipulation. The following example shows how a nurse might use personal knowledge.

Many posthysterectomy clients, even those past childbearing age, believe that they have lost an essential part of their womanhood; this perceived loss often leads to diminished self-worth. Furthermore, many premenopausal clients equate the loss of menses with a loss of femininity and productivity, which lowers self-esteem still more. The nurse, knowing that she can influence the client's attitude, demonstrates caring and regard to bolster the client's feelings of self-worth.

The nurse should be aware of and use the different forms of knowledge simultaneously. In the following example, notice how the different forms illuminate a complex problem.

> An elderly, terminally ill client arrives by ambulance, and his distraught family arrives soon after. The client, under the long-term care of an oncologist, has already communicated both verbally and in writing that no heroic measures should be taken. The family, deeply distressed by the nearness of their relative's death, desires that everything possible be done.

The nurse, in determining the extent of intervention, must rely on empirical knowledge of the client's condition; aesthetic knowledge of the family's feelings and concerns; ethical knowledge of the client's right to choose or reject treatment; and personal knowledge of how her relationship with the family can facilitate their acceptance of the client's wishes. Obtaining and utilizing knowledge from as many sources as possible helps enlarge the nurse's understanding of the problem and its potential solutions.

PROBLEM SOLVING

As stated earlier, critical thinking can lead the nurse to a number of potential solutions to a problem. It can also help the nurse limit the number of solutions by enabling the nurse to identify stereotypical thinking and emotionally laden claims. Problem solving, the next step to be explored, represents the careful examination of the information arrived at through critical thinking.

The processes most closely related to (and to a certain degree involving) problem solving are the nursing process and the research process. The nursing process begins with client assessment. The nurse gathers data relevant to the client's condition and formulates a nursing diagnosis. The nurse uses the nursing diagnosis as the basis for a client care plan, which is developed, implemented, and evaluated.

The research process, described in greater detail in Chapter 13, begins with a statement of the problem, which the researcher may alter as information is gathered. This general statement of the problem precedes the assessment of the

PROCESSES RELATED TO PROBLEM SOLVING

- *Nursing Process*
  - *Assessment*
  - *Diagnosis*
  - *Planning*
  - *Intervention*
  - *Evaluation*
- *Research Process*
  - *Statement of problem*
  - *Review of literature*
  - *Hypothesis formation*
  - *Research design*
  - *Data collection*
  - *Data analysis*
  - *Conclusions*

STEPS IN THE PROBLEM-SOLVING PROCESS

- *Assessing and accumulating data*
- *Defining the problem*
- *Determining options*
- *Taking action*
- *Evaluating outcomes*

phenomenon in question. After reviewing what previous research has suggested, the researcher develops a refined hypotheses. In an experimental study, the hypothesis may state a suspected relation that will be explored by research. The research design selected depends on the nature of the phenomenon under investigation, including the type of data available for collection, the relation being examined, and the degree to which the researcher can control the situation in question. Once data are collected, the researcher analyzes it to see if it supports the hypothesis. Based on the findings, the researcher then makes conclusions and generalizations.

Like the nursing process and research process, the basic problem-solving process involves a series of discrete actions (Tappen, 1989). These include assessing the problem and accumulating data, defining the problem, determining options, taking action, and evaluating outcomes. The problem-solving process both resembles and differs from the nursing process and the research process. Some of these similarities and differences are described in the following explanation of the problem-solving process.

Assessing and Accumulating Data. The first step in the problem-solving process resembles the first step in the nursing process during which the nurse assesses the client, performing a physical examination; examining laboratory, dietary, radiologic, and other data; reading what other caregivers have communicated regarding the problem; and consulting reference works and hospital protocols. Similarly, assessing a problem related to a diabetic client's diet compliance might require the nurse to assess and accumulate data concerning the client's knowledge level concerning the disease and diet, the client's resources for purchasing appropriate foods, client and family strategies for recordkeeping, family pressures related to food preparation and eating, and client self-image.

This beginning step is important because it provides the information on which succeeding steps will be based. Although additional information can be added as the problem-solving process proceeds, the nurse should keep in mind that the more information obtained at the beginning, the more efficient and the more expeditiously the solution.

Defining the Problem. Although the nurse has an idea-perhaps even a well-defined idea-of what the problem is, waiting until information has been gathered before defining the problem can help to ensure accuracy. Similarly, the nurse gathering data during the nursing process also increases the likelihood of an accurate diagnosis by performing a comprehensive assessment performed. At this point, the problem-solving process also differs from the nursing process. During the latter, a nursing diagnosis becomes the basis for action; when applying the problem-solving process, the nurse does not take action after defining the problem but proceeds to the next step, determining options.

Determining Options. Having defined the problem, the nurse next uses critical thinking to determine and examine its potential solutions. During this step, the nurse may rely on the traditional options of authority, historical precedent, and trial and error. In some circumstances, these options may provide the best solution to a problem. They do not, however, always provide the most appropriate solution. Take, for example, the nurse who must decide whether or not to allow a visitor during nonvisiting hours. The nurse understands that hospitals establish formal visiting hours to provide rest and quiet for clients. These hours may vary according to the type of unit and clients' needs for rest. Formal visiting hours, however, may be difficult for family members to observe because of work or other conflicts. If the nurse relies solely on the unit policy that permits visitors only during certain hours, the nurse may overlook other solutions, such as allowing the client to visit with family members on an outdoor patio where other clients will not be disturbed.

In determining options related to client care situations, the nurse must first identify who has the right to make the decision. Certain legal or ethical problems may be the responsibility of the client or client's family. For example, an adult client is admitted for hemorrhage and because of religious beliefs refuses transfusion. The decision in this case is the client's and not the nurse's, the physician's, or the hospital's. By accurately determining who has responsibility for decision making, the nurse can help clarify the roles of client, family, health care team, institution, courts, or state and local government in ensuring proper client care. Chapter 6, Legal implications for nursing practice, and Chapter 7, Ethical implications for nursing practice, provide more information on the issue of responsibility, including treatment in emergency situations and decision-making related to incompetent clients.

Sometimes a problem is best dealt with by "benign neglect," or allowing those involved in a problem to work the problem out for themselves. This option might be used by a nurse manager trying to decide who should clean the staff lounge when institution policy leaves such cleaning to the nursing staff. Some staff may want the nurse manager to assign staff at the end of each shift to clean the sink and put away coffee supplies. Others may try to avoid the problem, stating that the cleaning up should be done by housekeeping. Still others may think that everyone should be responsible for their own coffee cups and personal items. The nurse manager, believing that problems concerning the staff lounge are best dealt with by the staff themselves, might decide to treat the problem with benign neglect. Doing so might encourage the staff to resolve the problem on their own by developing a rotation system whereby everyone would take a turn at general cleanup.

An advantage of allowing individuals affected by a problem to solve that problem themselves is that this oftentimes produces more commitment to following through on the solution. It is important when treating a problem by giving it time to solve itself that progress be monitored. If it appears that a solution is not forthcoming, then more direct ways of addressing the problem may need to be implemented. The nurse can also consider benign neglect for client-related problems.

Sometimes problems resolve themselves. For example, the nursing staff may be dissatisfied with current charting forms because they are time-consuming and hard to read;

however, the forms may have already been scheduled for replacement in a short period of time. If the situation does not pose a threat to client safety, the nurse manager may choose to ignore the problem, knowing that it will shortly disappear.

More commonly, a nurse must examine and select from several options. In considering potential options, the nurse should first assess the feasibility of each. To do so, the nurse might evaluate financial, staff, and legal or ethical constraints as well as constraints related to the institution's physical plant. The nurse should also consider the benefits and costs of each option.

For example, a problem might arise concerning the contamination of open bottles of saline solution used to clear nasopharyngeal suction catheters and tubing. The nursing staff might believe that the safest course, from the client's standpoint, would be to discard the 500 ml bottle after each use and open a new bottle each time saline solution is needed. On examining costs, however, the nurses might discover that the client or hospital would have to bear the financial burden for increased quantities of sterile saline. The nurses might also discover that the physical plant does not allow for the storage of large quantities of sterile saline on each ward but can resupply each ward only twice a week. In view of these constraints, the nursing staff might dismiss their first option and formulate a policy that calls for nurses to discard all open saline bottles after a 24-hour period. They might further institute in-service education on cleaning suction catheters and using open saline bottles.

Taking Action. Having determined possible options, the nurse develops and implements a plan of action. Formulating a plan is not always possible. In the case of fire or cardiac arrest, the nurse must take immediate action. For such situations, health care facilities usually have standard action plans that allow everyone to know in advance what actions will be necessary and who will be responsible for each action.

In most cases the nurse has time to identify the best way of taking action and initiating change so that facilitating factors are maximized and hindering factors are minimized.

The nurse should remember that, as a general procedure, having those affected by the action or change participate in the action encourages them to work toward successful change.

The nurse should first eliminate any policy or procedural impediments to change. For example, nurses on a pediatrics unit might believe that changing from 8- to 12-hour shifts would enhance client care on the unit. The shift change would reduce the number of caregivers, providing a sense of continuity for the family, and minimize the number of nursing reports, reducing chances for error. Because the shift adjustment represents a policy change, the nurses must attend to the policy changes before implementing the shift changes. Doing so would involve clarifying the length of the shift and when overtime pay would be earned.

The nurse must then choose the appropriate style of the action to be taken. The action may require group participation (a committee deliberation to allot weekend duty); it may best be accomplished by an individual. In the latter case, involving others could unnecessarily complicate the action or even compromise its effectiveness. For example, reorganizing the crash cart based on recommendations from the emergency services committee might best be accomplished by an individual. Changes could subsequently be checked by other staff. In this case, having all staff offer suggestions about how the crash cart should be arranged might be needlessly time-consuming. The action style can appropriately range from autocratic to democratic, from individual to group, depending on the problem and the action to be taken.

Evaluation. The final step in the problem-solving process resembles the evaluation step in the nursing process and the data analysis step in the research process. Selecting and implementing an intervention with care doesn't necessarily mean that the problem will be solved. If a complicated problem has been only partially identified, the proposed solution may not adequately address the root cause of the difficulty. In such cases, the nurse would not only evaluate the effects of the action but also reexamine the nature of the problem.

Consider the problem posed by a 3-year-old client who has difficulty going to sleep at night. The mother tries multiple strategies, including reading aloud until the child is sleepy, providing warm drinks and a snack, singing lullabies, and keeping a teddy bear in bed and a night-light on. All "solutions" are effective for only a short time because the real difficulty relates to an older sibling's story about monsters that come out from under the bed at night. Until the real problem is identified and confronted, solutions will continue to be ineffective.

In emergency situations, the nurse may have to solve immediate problems while recognizing that other important problems may have to be addressed at a later date. After handling the immediate crisis, the nurse should focus evaluation on identifying those problems that remain and on determining long-term measures to ensure that the problem doesn't recur.

In most cases, evaluation requires little more than a general assessment of the solution's effects and perhaps some fine tuning of newly implemented changes.

DECISION-MAKING STRATEGIES

Decision-making differs from problem solving in that it is not necessarily undertaken in response to an identified difficulty, either potential or actual. Decision making represents a broader responsibility that attempts to minimize problem development by taking into account as many of the problem-producing elements as possible (Sullivan and Decker, 1988).

As stated at the beginning of this chapter, nurses make various kinds of decisions related to management, colleagues, subordinate personnel, and clients. They may find themselves faced with legal, ethical, and financial decisions. How the nurse chooses to deal with a decision depends in large part on its context. A decision related to experimental research may best be addressed by using the traditional research process. A decision involving an ethical conflict may require the nurse to use the ethical decision-making process outlined in Chapter 7, Ethical implications for nursing practice. Nurses also have at their disposal several formal and informal decision-making strategies, including brainstorming, the Delphi technique, the nominal group technique, critical path methodology (CPM), a listing of strengths and weaknesses, decision trees, and decision grids.

BRAINSTORMING

Brainstorming is a way of considering options through creative, even radical thinking before practical concerns intervene to limit considerations. It can be used by either an individual or a group. Nurses might use brainstorming to approach problems for which they have been unable to generate solutions. For example, a nurse may be trying to figure out how to get staff to department meetings on time. Traditional solutions, such as posted announcements and reminder memos, have not worked. As a result, meetings are regularly delayed for 10 to 15 minutes while latecomers arrive or information has to be repeated.

In brainstorming for solutions, the nurse might begin by asking, "If I have no limits on what I might select or consider, how can I more effectively get staff members to attend meetings on time?" The answers to this question would generate several options:

- fire late employees on the spot
- double-pay employees who arrive on time
- post the names of latecomers
- pass out candy before the meeting
- make latecomers pay a symbolic fine
- discuss the most important issues first
- lock the door once the meeting has started
- don't hold meetings.

Some of these strategies, such as firing latecomers and abandoning meetings, are clearly not feasible. They might, however, suggest other strategies. A nurse manager might decide that meeting promptness is an appropriate expectation to add to annual evaluations. The manager might decide that the staff might more easily handle fewer meetings of slightly longer duration. The nurse manager might decide to serve coffee and donuts 15 minutes before the meeting begins and to discuss as the first order of business an item of considerable interest to all staff.

Brainstorming is more frequently associated with group decision making. During group brainstorming, certain ground rules are necessary. One such ground rule might state that all suggestions are to be initially accepted without criticism but that modification suggestions are permissible. The problem under consideration should be clearly explained and a time limit for brainstorming set. After generating a suggestion list, the brainstorming group or another designated group can examine the suggestions for feasibility.

Including people with different perspectives in the group can help to ensure that a number of different solutions will be proposed. Suppose the nurse manager working on the problem of staff tardiness at department meetings had chosen group brainstorming as a decision-making strategy. The manager might have elected to brainstorm with staff nurses from different shifts, including some who always come late and some who are always on time. The group approach, although more time-consuming than an individual approach, can result in suggestions that the individual working alone might overlook.

DELPHI TECHNIQUE

Brainstorming involves active, face-to-face discussion with others. Consequently, more assertive group members can inhibit others from contributing. The Delphi technique is a means of obtaining opinions, suggestions, or decisions from others that has the benefit of group input without the face-to-face element (Polit and Hungler, 1987). As such, the Delphi technique offers several advantages over brainstorming.

In using the Delphi technique, a nurse manager might ask a group of staff to make suggestions concerning a problem by responding to a questionnaire. The results of the first questionnaire are summarized and a new questionnaire based

THE DELPHI TECHNIQUE

- *Advantages*
  - *Group constructed without regard to physical location*
  - *More time for deliberation and response*
  - *Responses not influenced by more vocal or powerful group members*
- *Disadvantages*
  - *High costs of preparing and distributing information*
  - *Process time-consuming*

on the initial responses is formulated and distributed to group members, who reply again, refining their responses and working towards consensus. Three questionnaire/summary/response rounds usually are sufficient to refine suggestions to a useful form.

The Delphi technique might, for example, be used to identify common needs of nursing students throughout a certain state. The pool of respondents could include students, nursing counselors, and nursing directors. The first questionnaire might ask them to rank known needs and to suggest others. The resulting lists might include tuition support, personal counseling, financial assistance for books and supplies, academic tutoring, part-time employment, and child care.

This information would then be summarized and distributed to respondents for their opinion of the ranking of needs. The results from the second round might change the order of needs somewhat, listing tuition support at the top followed by part-time employment, academic tutoring, and personal counseling. A third-round questionnaire might validate this ranking, resulting in a group consensus regarding nursing students' needs. This information could then be used by schools, scholarship organizations, and other groups to attract and retain nursing students.

NOMINAL GROUPS AND SYNECTICS

In between the potential frenzy and immediacy of brainstorming and the distance and lengthiness of the Delphi technique are nominal groups and synectics. A nominal group can generate the same creative responses as brainstorming but in a quiet, non verbal manner. Each group member thinks about the problem or decision to be made and makes suggestions in writing. The group leader can then read the suggestions. Anonymity prevents less powerful members from being inhibited and encourages participation. The lack of verbal interaction prevents more vocal participants from overshadowing others. The group then generates a list of preferred options either by open discussion or by written ranking.

An emergency department supervisor might use a nominal group approach to address decisions about how to get better participation in voluntary in-services. Each member of the department could offer written suggestions, which the supervisor could then list anonymously. Staff could continue to offer suggestions until possibilities had been exhausted. The supervisor could then list the options, and staff would discuss the relative merits or difficulties of each. A list of preferred options could then be drawn up.

Synectics is a decision-making technique based on cooperation. Group members are chosen to include diverse personalities, specialization areas, and points of view. As in a nominal group, members offer their suggestions anonymously. The synectic approach then encourages group members to consider how each suggestion might be implemented, modified, clarified, or enlarged on. Immediately cutting off discussion of what initially seems like an outlandish suggestion is not permitted. Each person has a responsibility to help the new idea grow rather than to focus immediately on its impediments. Once the group develops a list of options, staff members think of ways to make options work, regardless of how impractical or difficult they might appear initially. Synectics encourages and supports creative thinking and the exploration of suggested options.

CRITICAL PATH METHODOLOGY

Although considered a planning and implementation tool, CPM can also be effectively used as a decision-making strategy. CPM enables the nurse to identify the individual sequential steps required in making a decision or in implementing a solution successfully (Grant, 1983). Using CPM, the nurse breaks down a decision or action into separate parts, which are then graphically portrayed on a chart. The chart also depicts the interrelations among elements and can help the nurse identify those decisions that should be made first and those decisions that are the most likely to succeed.

A nurse manager might use CPM to make decisions related to the introduction of new charting forms in a medical-surgical department. The nurse manager would first identify the target date for introducing the new forms and then determine the flexibility of this target date. The manager next identifies all the decisions and activities necessary in introducing the new forms, plots a sequence of events, and estimates the time each event will require. Once the graphic depiction has been completed the manager can use the information to make other decisions. For example, if the hospital administrator decides that the new forms should be in place before the next accreditation visit, the nurse manager might use the chart to decide whether to have a staff committee or a full-time consultant work on the project.

By breaking a decision into component parts, the nurse using CPM can make informed decisions regarding component pieces. CPM takes some time to complete, however, and may not adequately indicate cost estimates and time constraints related to a problem.

LISTS OF STRENGTHS AND WEAKNESSES

Listing the strengths and weaknesses related to a given problem can effectively help the nurse identify the various elements that need to be considered in making a decision. In deciding whether or not to seek a night shift position, a new nurse might list the following strengths and weaknesses:

Strengths
- more positions available
- pay differential offered
- pace less hectic

Weaknesses
- difficulty in sleeping days
- less support staff available
- fewer opportunities for learning
    Considering each element can help the nurse arrive at a more satisfactory decision.

DECISION TREES

Slightly more complex than listing strengths and weaknesses, decision trees are useful when a problem requires multiple decisions. Moir, Molson, and Levine (1988) describe a hospital's use of a decision tree in deciding when to hire a companion for confused, agitated, depressed, or suicidal clients who cannot be adequately kept under observation using staff. Because is a costly alternative, the decision tree assists staff to examine other alternatives.

Staff must first decide if the client in question is a risk to self or others. If they decide that the client is a risk, the process proceeds to the next level, where staff must determine if a family member is available to stay with the client. If a family member is not available, the process proceeds to the next step, at which the staff considers if the family can afford to pay for a companion. If the answer to this is no, the unit supervisor must determine if staff is available for assignment to the client on a one-to-one basis. If the answer to this final decision is no and if no other hospital resources are available, then the hospital should hire a companion to protect the client from possible injury and itself from legal action.

The different decisions are represented as forks in a branching tree, with each response leading to a new decision. By proceeding in this manner, nurses and administration can make a reasoned decision, with all important considerations included at appropriate points in the process.

DECISION GRIDS

A decision grid enables the nurse to compare alternatives from several perspectives. The nurse lists alternatives along one axis and the various factors to be considered along the other. The nurse can also indicate each factor's importance by assigning a numerical value to each.

Suppose the staff of a medical-surgical unit are asked to consider two commercially available videotapes for use with preoperative clients and at the same time to consider the possibility of developing a videotape specifically for their unit. The staff decides to use a decision grid.

One commercially available tape is more comprehensive than the other but is also considerably more expensive. The first tape may also be too long for use with clients who are admitted the morning of their surgeries. The length and cost of the second commercial tape is more appropriate, but it lacks information that staff believe to be important. The option of developing their own videotape is attractive to the staff, but doing so would require considerable time. The decision grid enables the staff to weigh the relative importance of each factor. Because staff identified comprehensiveness as the most important factor, it carried a higher numerical value than either cost or length. Based on the outcome, the staff decide to develop their own videotape.

EVALUATING DECISIONS

Bernhardt and Walsh (1981) describe two types of decisions, optimizing and satisficing. An optimizing decision is the best solution, according to objectives. It is made after all potential solutions have been identified and examined. A satisficing decision is the choice of any solution that meets the minimum requirements of the problem.

When evaluating a decision, the nurse must consider its type. The expectations for an optimizing decision are not the same as those for a satisficing decision. For example, staff on an obstetric unit concerned about insufficient support for client teaching on the postpartum floor might choose as an optimizing decision to increase nursing staff assigned to the area. However, on discovering that this decision is not economically feasible, the staff make an alternate satisficing decision to add an additional part-time ward clerk to the staffing mix. Although the satisficing decision will not increase the number of RNs teaching clients, it will relieve staff of other responsibilities, which could increase the amount of time available for client teaching. In evaluating the decision, the nurse should keep the limitations of the satisficing decision in mind.

When evaluating decisions, the nurse should measure quality and acceptability. Quality refers to how well a decision met the established objectives. Acceptability refers to how well the individuals affected supported or continue to support the decision. Bernhardt and Walsh (1981) maintain that including acceptability as a criterion for selecting among options may help to identify the decision that will produce the best result. An optimizing decision that is not supported by those who must carry it out might produce less effective results than a satisficing decision supported by everyone. Finally, evaluation allows the nurse to determine whether or not other decisions related to the problem remain to be made.

SUMMARY

Critical thinking, problem solving, and decision making are essential and interconnected skills used by nurses functioning at all levels. To make effective decisions, nurses must understand their own preferred learning style as well as the different kinds of knowledge and capabilities that others may bring to a situation. They must also be able to think critically about information related to a problem; doing so can help nurses to avoid stereotypical thinking and to discover more original solutions to problems.

Different methods of inquiry and decision-making strategies for specific situations are available for nurses use as they deem appropriate. These methods and strategies enable nurses to examine data and information, generate potential solutions, and choose the most appropriate, effective solution among the options. In evaluating decisions, nurses must consider how well the decisions have met established objectives and to what degree they have been accepted and supported by the individuals or institutions involved.

APPLICATION EXERCISE

Identify a problem you have observed in a clinical setting. Using the format below, gather data and evaluate options. Based on your work, identify one preferred solution.

Short description of problem. Where and how is the problem manifested?

Assessing and accumulating data. What are the facts related to the problem? Which individuals are involved? How frequently does the problem occur? What types of data and information, other than empirically observable facts, should you consider?

Defining the problem. Based on your information, reexamine the problem and restate it so that it reflects what you have learned. In your definition, try to list as many of the factors involved as possible. Who has responsibility for the decision?

Determining options. Brainstorm to generate as many possible choices of action as possible. You might enlist fellow students to help in this process, either in a brainstorming session or in a nominal group/synectic approach. Generate a list of options accompanied by advantages and disadvantages.

Taking action. If you had the authority to implement your preferred option, what would you need to consider? Whom would the action affect? What supporting and inhibiting factors would you need to consider? What strategies for monitoring implementation might be helpful?

Evaluating. How will you know if your decision has been successful? Based on your assessment of potential problems, what plans for modifying your approach might be considered if evaluation shows this to be necessary?

Evaluating your own performance. What type of approach to the problem did you use? Did you consider different kinds of knowledge? What other strategies might you have used when generating options? How might you ensure a more open, creative approach to problem solving in the future?

REVIEW QUESTIONS

1. Briefly define critical thinking, problem solving, and decision making.

2. Identify and briefly describe the four forms of knowledge.

3. What are the different learning styles? What are the characteristics of each?

4. What is the main difference between the Type I and Type II methods of inquiry?

5. List the steps involved in problem solving.

6. Explain how the nominal group approach might be used to make a decision on scheduling.

REFERENCES

Bandman, E.L., and Bandman, B. *Critical Thinking in Nursing.* Norwalk, Conn.: Appleton & Lange, 1988.

Bernhard, L.A. *Leadership: The Key to Professionalization of Nursing.* New York: McGraw-Hill Book Co., 1988.

Carper, B.A. "Fundamental Patterns of Knowing in Nursing," *Advances in Nursing Science* 1(1):13-23, 1978.

Grant, D.P. *PERT and CPM: Network Methods for Project Planning, Scheduling and Control.* San Luis Obispo, Calif.: Small-Scale Master Builder Press, 1983.

Kolb, D.A. *Learning Style Inventory.* Boston: McBer and Co., 1976.

Moir, E.J., et al. "Managing Costs Through Guided Decision Making," *Nursing Management* 19(10):50, 1988.

Polit, D.F., and Hungler, B.P. *Nursing Research: Principles and Methods,* 3rd ed. Philadelphia: J.B. Lippincott Co., 1987.

Sullivan, E.J. and Decker, P. *Effective Management in Nursing,* 2nd ed. Menlo Park, Calif.: Addison-Wesley Publishing Co., 1988.

Tappen, R. *Nursing Leadership and Management: Concepts and Practice,* 2nd ed. Philadelphia: F.A. Davis Co., 1989.

Tinkle, M. B., and Beaton, J. L. "Toward a New View of Science: Implications for Nursing Research," *Advances in Nursing Science* 5(2):27-36, 1983.

RECOMMENDATIONS FOR FURTHER STUDY

Hughes, K.K.E. and Young, W.B. "Clinical Decision Making: Stability of Clinical Decisions," *Nurse Educator* 17(3):8-11, 1992.

Jenny, J., and Logan, J. "Knowing the Patient: One Aspect of Clinical Practice," *Image* 24(4):254-258, Winter 1992.

Klassens, E. "Strategies to Enhance Problem Solving," *Nurse Educator* 17(3):28-31, 1992.

White, J.E., et al. "Content and Process in Clinical Decision-Making by Nurse Practitioners," *Image* 24(2):153-158, Summer 1992.

11

THE NURSE AS CHANGE AGENT

OBJECTIVES

After studying this chapter, the reader should be able to:

1. Describe spontaneous, developmental, and active change.

2. Discuss internal and external factors that influence change.

3. Compare and contrast the normative-reeducative, empirical-rational, paradoxical, and power-coercive models of change.

4. Discuss the change agent's role.

5. Describe the phases through which employees involved in organizational change progress.

6. Explain how nurses can assist clients dealing with life transitions.

7. Explain how nurses can prepare to deal with catastrophic changes.

INTRODUCTION

People view change from many perspectives. Some see it as threatening and disruptive; others think of it as a natural part of growth and development. Some think of change as an evolutionary process, a gradual response to natural variations; others think of it as revolutionary and sudden in occurrence. In truth, change can assume any of these characteristics, and in all of its forms, is always with us.

Whether on a personal, an institutional, a professional, or a societal level, things change. Beginning nursing students are not the same people when they graduate. Health care institutions responding to legislation such as the Americans with Disabilities Act will significantly change the way they interact with clients. The nursing profession itself continues to change, evolving to meet individual needs as well as larger societal needs related to ethnicity, age, education, and economic conditions.

This chapter covers change in its many permutations and explores the role nurses play in helping themselves and others deal with this sometimes disturbing concept.

TYPES OF CHANGE

Change can be classified as fundamentally cyclical or structural. Cyclical change involves a return to an earlier condition. The rotation of the seasons and the change from night to day and back again to night are examples of cyclical change. Structural change produces progress in a given direction and does not include return to a former state. Depleting ozone from the atmosphere or destroying huge tracts of rain forest result in structural, irreversible changes. Beyond these two basic divisions, other types of change exist.

SPONTANEOUS CHANGE

Change can occur spontaneously. Accidents, natural disasters (floods, fires, and earthquakes), and random genetic mutations, such as that which resulted in the acquired immune deficiency syndrome (AIDS) virus, are examples of spontaneous change. Although a spontaneous change usually cannot be anticipated and planned for, sometimes preparatory steps can be taken. For example, communities living close to nuclear power plants have contingency plans for emergencies such as a radioactive leak from containment structures. Such plans usually identify local hospitals and other institutions that will serve as decontamination and treatment facilities.

*TYPES OF
CHANGE*

• *Spontaneous*
• *Developmental*
• *Active*

The staff of these institutions participate in regularly scheduled drills simulating nuclear accidents and practice the techniques needed for dealing with radiation exposure. Necessary supplies are also regularly inventoried and rotated.

DEVELOPMENTAL CHANGE

Developmental change results form natural growth processes, such as the physical progression from infancy through childhood to maturity and old age. Institutions also undergo developmental change, restructuring their administrations as the institution expands and as tasks become more complex.

Most people view developmental change as generally good, primarily because it represents a response to some natural progression. Furthermore, people can with some certainty anticipate and plan for developmental change. A young family with a new baby can anticipate the child's growth and development and his or her need for immunizations and later, socialization and schooling. Theoretically, change under these circumstances should proceed with maximum support and minimum disruption. Being able to anticipate change does not necessarily make coping with it easy. The new family may encounter financial difficulties related to the child's school or may have trouble dealing with the child as a teenager.

ACTIVE CHANGE

Active change differs from spontaneous and developmental change in that individuals play an active part in determining what is to occur and how change is to be implemented. A middle-aged woman who wants to return to school to complete a baccalaureate degree in nursing can actively plan the educational changes required. The hospital switching from a traditional autocratic administration to one based on shared governance is also involved in active change.

People often engage in active change in response to other types of change. A community developing contingency plans in the event of a nuclear power plant accident is involved in active change to offset a spontaneous change. Parents saving for their child's education are acting in response to developmental changes.

FORCES INFLUENCING CHANGE

Internal as well as external forces can influence the type and rate of change. At the client level, internal forces might include the client's motivation to stop smoking or to lose weight, or the client's ability to understand the relation between exercise and fitness. External forces could include the development of new drugs and treatment related to the client's care. On an institutional level, internal forces can include the institution's resources and staffing patterns. External factors, such as the cyclical nursing shortage, could change the composition of the institution's work force.

Some external factors influence all levels of society. Demographic changes, including the increase in the number of new citizens with less education and fewer economic resources, may change health care priorities for the nation as a whole. Relatively new diseases such as AIDS, and changes in old diseases, such as tuberculosis, can profoundly effect individuals, institutions, nations, and even the world.

STRESS AND CHANGE

Change almost always produces stress to some degree. Researchers studying the relations between stress and the onset of stress-related diseases, such as coronary artery disease, have discovered that even positive changes, if numerous and large enough, can detrimentally affect individuals.

Holmes and Rahe (1967) investigated the influence of cumulative change, both positive and negative, on individuals. They developed a rating scale that uses a system of weighted events to calculate stress levels within a given period. Different weights are attached to different stressful occurrences. These weights range from 100 for the death of a spouse to 11 for minor legal infractions. The authors discovered an association between higher illness and higher stress levels, regardless of whether the stresses resulted from positive or negative changes. Their work suggests that even positive events, such as graduations and marriages, can have a negative impact on health. This is an important consideration for nurses dealing with clients coping with a physical illness: Even positive change can aggravate an already stressful situation.

THEORIES OF CHANGE

Several theoretical models can enable the nurse to view change from different perspectives. These models include the normative-reeducative models of Lewin (1951) and Lippitt (1973), the empirical-rational models of Rogers and Shoemaker (1971), the paradoxical model of Watzlawick, Weak, and Fisch (1974), and the power-coercive models of Alinsky (1972), Haley (1969), and Zaltman and Duncan (1972).

THE NORMATIVE-REEDUCATIVE MODEL

Kurt Lewin (1951) was one of the first change theorists to produce a comprehensive model that considers the leader's role in the change process as well as the stages through which change is accomplished (see *Theories of Change*). He also examines the stages in which change occurs, forces that drive and restrain change, and how such forces might be dealt with effectively. The first stage of Lewin's model analyzes the system to be changed and identifies driving and restraining forces. This is followed by the unfreezing of the system, which allows movement to accomplish change, and finally by a refreezing of the system to solidify the change.

Lewin suggests that simply identifying a good idea and communicating it to others cannot in itself always accomplish desirable change. The pressure of tradition and vested interests often prevents a good idea from becoming anything more than an idea. Similarly, a powerful leader attempting to enforce a change may not always succeed. Lewin maintains that a planned, carefully structured approach to change produces the best results.

THEORIES OF CHANGE

- *Normative-reeducative model: Emphasizes the importance of the change agent and the stages through which change progresses*
- *Empirical-rational model: Emphasizes the importance of rational thinking and communication in producing change*
- *Paradoxical model: Emphasizes expected changes that fail to occur and unexpected changes*
- *Power-coercive model: Emphasizes the need for power and control in producing change, especially when change is viewed by individuals affected as potentially negative*

EXAMINING THE SYSTEM

The first stage of Lewin's model examines the system to be changed. The reasons why people like or dislike the current system and the norms that govern its operation are identified. The first stage also provides for an analysis of driving forces (those supporting change) and restraining factors (those resisting or hindering change). The following example illustrates both forces.

> An operating department supervisor wants to introduce a new type of surgical drape that is more cost-effective, more water repellent, easier to handle, and available in more varieties. She knows that such changes have historically been unwelcome. Nurses and physicians used to the current drapes will probably not like the fact that the packages have to be opened and unwrapped in a slightly different manner and that the new drape has a slightly different shape. The physicians and nurses may not see any benefit to changing and may resent the time they might have to spend learning how to use the new drapes.
>
> The supervisor identifies the following driving forces and restraining forces:
>
> *Driving forces*
>
> - fiscal advantage: cost of providing drapes reduced
> - client care advantage: drapes are more water repellent and less likely to become contaminated
> - operator advantage: drapes are available in more sizes and shapes should be easier for surgeons and nurses to use.

Restraining forces

- tradition: staff is comfortable with current drapes
- need for retraining: staff time and effort are required for familiarity with the new drapes
- territoriality: staff at this point is not involved in drape selection; they may think that they should have been included in the discussion.

This stage of Lewin's model also enables the nurse to identify how to enhance driving factors and minimize restraining factors. To enhance driving factors, the operating room supervisor might work with the materials manager to identify exactly how much money might be saved yearly by switching to the new drape (the savings might allow the operating department to purchase another piece of needed equipment). The supervisor might talk with the infection control officer about the number of surgical wounds that are suspected to have become contaminated during surgeries and about the possibility of the new, more repellent drapes helping to reduce this number. The supervisor could organize her findings in chart form for presentation to the operating department staff. She could also demonstrate the new drape's versatility.

In dealing with the restraining factors, the supervisor might identify a target group of experienced surgical nurses and ask them to participate in a pilot study to use and evaluate the new drape. The group might consist of nurses who easily adapt to change and those who resist change. Including both nurse types has beneficial effects: It involves staff in the drape evaluation and, if the drapes are indeed superior, assures the support of those individuals who might otherwise have resisted the change.

UNFREEZING THE SITUATION

After evaluating the system to be changed and identifying the driving and restraining forces, the leader deliberately introduces an unstable situation, which initiates change. Lewin refers to this process as "unfreezing." According to normative-reeducative theory, individuals in the unfreezing stage respond to information and to appeals to norms and values.

If the operating department supervisor can show the nurses and physicians that the current drape is inferior to the new one and convince them that nursing norms and values related to client care can be better upheld by using the new drape, she might be able to successfully effect change.

There are several ways to provide information and appeal to norms and values. Tappen (1989) identifies three strategies: introducing disconfirmation, introducing guilt and anxiety, and providing psychologic safety.

Introducing Disconfirmation. Using this strategy, the leader (the operating department supervisor) provides evidence that refutes or challenges a commonly held belief. The nurses and physicians currently using the old drapes believe that the drapes do a good job of isolating and protecting the surgical field. They are confident in their handling of the drapes and believe that the drapes provide the size, shape, and opening aperture required. They may believe that the cost of the drapes is not excessive because the drapes have been in use for a long time. According to normative-reeducative theory, if the supervisor, by presenting cost and infection rate information, can challenge these beliefs, the nurses and physicians will reexamine their position. In addition, emphasizing that clients will be better protected by the more water-repellent drape and that the draping will be more secure and appropriate because of the increased variety available can further sway the staff to consider change.

Introducing Guilt and Anxiety. The leader of change can introduce guilt and anxiety by describing the consequences of not changing. The supervisor might suggest that because less expensive, more effective drapes are available, the departmental budget for these items will be reduced. If administrative support for the change exists, it should be pointed out. Doing so can create anxiety among staff who recognize that resisting change will bring administrative displeasure. The supervisor can also appeal to the physicians' and nurses' responsibility to do no harm and to take all reasonable measures to protect clients. The supervisor might also introduce guilt by suggesting that all personnel have an obligation to continue learning and to stay current in their fields and that unwillingness to adjust to necessary change represents a failure to do so. Introducing guilt and anxiety is more heavy-handed than introducing disconfirmation and may cause resentment; however, Lewin suggests that it can be useful in resistant situations.

Providing Psychological Safety. One barrier to change is the natural fear people face when trying something new. Even the most experienced, competent people usually have some fear of failure or embarrassment when confronted with the need for change. For example, the nurses of the operating department may worry about appearing clumsy when opening or handling the new drape. They may worry about the physician's reception of the new drapes. The supervisor can facilitate unfreezing by ensuring that all staff, including nurses and physicians, are provided adequate opportunity for learning about the new drapes. She can arrange for hands-on practice with the new drapes and answer any questions. Nurses can role-play situations involving new physicians who have not had exposure to the new drapes.

The supervisor might display models of the new drapes in an appropriate place, and the nurses who participated in the pilot program might be available as resources or troubleshooters. The supervisor might also explain that if a drape is inadvertently contaminated, another will be supplied without comment or question.

CHANGING
Once unfreezing has occurred, the actual change can be initiated. For example, after the pilot study of the new drape and after the staff education of the drape's use, the supervisor can establish a timeline for phasing in the new drapes. This might resemble the following:

- *Phase I:* Pilot nurses introduce the use of the new drapes in minor surgery cases. Reports of the drapes' use and any concerns or problems are shared with the entire staff at regular in service meetings.

- *Phase II:* Drapes are introduced in more complex orthopedic and neurosurgical cases. Again, reports of use and any problems or concerns with these more complex procedures are shared. Adjustments are made as staff become more familiar with the new drape.
- *Phase III:* The new drape is used for all surgical cases; old drapes are no longer available. Because successful use of the new drape for more complex procedures has been demonstrated in Phase II, physicians and nurses serving in other specialties will be less likely to resist the change.

The leader can help to reduce concern and nervousness as changes are implemented by being available, providing backup information (charts), supporting the experienced pilot nurses, and encouraging the staff in their efforts. The operating department supervisor can remind her staff of the reasons for the change, including increased client safety and increased savings.

The supervisor can also provide a means for staff to vent frustrations. If, for example, a nurse has worked with a physician who had difficulty with the new drapes and demanded the old ones, the supervisor should allow the nurse to talk about the incident and then work with the physician to ensure that the problem is dealt with before the drapes are used again. The supervisor can also keep records on staff experiences with the new drapes. Making these records available for staff perusal enables the nurses to see their increasing proficiency and success with the new drape.

REFREEZING

Once change has been accomplished and the new system is in place, steps must be taken to prevent the system from reverting to the old ways of doing things. In the example of the surgical drapes, a nurse, in an attempt to eliminate friction or discord, might succumb to a physician's request for the old-style drapes. Doing so might undermine the whole system or result in confusion wherein both types of drapes would be used indiscriminately.

The supervisor needs to set up systems to maintain the change. She may continue to monitor staff education and training related to the new drapes; she may provide continuing support for their use. She could share information on cost savings and wound contamination reduction. The supervisor can institutionalize the change by delegating responsibility for ensuring its continuation to others and by making staff education on use of the new drape part of the department orientation. Such institutionalization helps to ensure a successful refreezing.

THE EMPIRICAL-RATIONAL MODEL

The empirical-rational model stresses the rational nature of individuals and the power of communication to produce change (see *Theories of Change*, page 353). Rogers and Shoemaker (1971) and Dutton, Rogers, and Jun (1987) propose that if a new idea is properly communicated and if the individuals involved perceive the change as being in their own interests, the change will be adopted. The following represents an effective use of the empirical-rational model.

> A busy well-baby clinic that sees clients on a walk-in basis finds that use patterns during the day and throughout the week vary. The staff see few clients in the early mornings or late afternoons and a larger number of clients on Mondays than on Fridays. Wanting to minimize client waiting time, the staff decide to share this information with clients as they sit in the waiting room. The staff believe that doing so will influence more clients to visit the clinic at less busy times. The staff post in the waiting room a chart showing the average time a client must wait during the period from 10:00 a.m. to 12:00 noon on Monday compared with 8:00 to 10:00 a.m. on Monday or 3:00 to 5:00 p.m. on Friday. The staff also provide this information in written form. Recognizing that some clients will not be able to adjust their schedule because of family or other conflicts, the staff nonetheless assumes that as rational individuals, many clients will make use of the information to change their behavior.

Providing information does not always produce the expected change. Many smokers, despite efforts to educate them about the dangers of smoking, find quitting difficult;

individuals with coronary artery disease find dietary changes difficult, despite intensive education on the relation between diet and their disease and often despite angina, myocardial infarctions, and coronary bypass surgery.

In the case of the well-baby clinic, other reasons may interfere with the anticipated client response. Some clients may enjoy the wait because it provides them an opportunity to talk with other new mothers. For some the visit provides a respite from their other children and household duties. If the anticipated response to the information does not occur, the staff must analyze the reasons for the failure and perhaps try other strategies.

Rogers and Shoemaker (1971) suggest that using the empirical-rational model requires three steps. These include inventing the change, diffusing information about the change, and adopting (or rejecting) the change.

Inventing the Change. Inventing the change means conceiving the idea on which change will be based. In the case of the well-baby clinic, the staff had first to imagine offering information on waiting times to the clients and then to design the means of gathering and communicating this information effectively. To gather the information, the staff had to identify those hours during which clients had shorter waiting times.

Diffusing Information About the Change. After identifying the change and collecting information pertaining to it, the staff had to devise a way to diffuse, or communicate, their findings. The well-baby clinic chose to present the information in chart and written form in the clinic's waiting room. Other circumstances might have demanded other means. The more effectively and widely information is disseminated, the more effective the change will be. Mass media campaigns, such as the one for AIDS, can provide nationwide education. Using well-known and respected individuals as information communicators can help to attract listeners. This step can also pose problems. People tend to resist information that runs contrary to their beliefs and values. For example, some groups have been offended by the explicitness of the AIDS prevention advertisements urging safe sex.

EMPIRICAL-RATIONAL MODEL

- *Inventing the change*
- *Diffusing information about the change*
- *Accepting or rejecting change*

Accepting or Rejecting Change. The last step in Rogers' process occurs when the group accepts or rejects the defined change. Acceptance consists of three stages: trial, installation, and institutionalization.

USES FOR THE EMPIRICAL-RATIONAL MODEL

Nurses may use the empirical-rational model to provide information about a problem, to correct erroneous information about a problem, and to persuade by providing specific inducements. The goal of all three actions is change. For example, providing information about a clinic's Saturday morning free immunization program can produce change (increased immunization) simply by making people aware that the service is available. This use does not involve education or persuasion. Correcting erroneous information can also result in change. Public service announcements that describe high blood pressure as the "silent killer" or the "invisible disease" help to reeducate the people about hypertension and thereby induce them to have regular checkups. Finally, the empirical-rational model provides for persuasive strategies and specific inducements that go beyond providing information and reeducating. A well-baby clinic may give away free toys; a hypertension screening clinic may offer free diaries for keeping track of blood pressure. Less tangible, long-term rewards, such as the potential for better health and longer life, can serve as inducements for change.

In summary, the empirical-rational model depends on individuals responding rationally to information that will enable them to make beneficial changes. Empirical-rational strategies are not always effective because factors other than a lack of information can cause people to resist change, even when the change would be in their own best interest.

THE PARADOXICAL MODEL

The paradoxical model attempts to explain how expected changes fail to occur or how changes occur through unexpected means (see *Theories of Change*, page 353). Watzlawick, Weakland, and Fisch (1974) observed that in some circumstances, efforts that normally produced change failed to do so. For example, the empirical-rational model presumes that people will normally be motivated to change when such change is logical and when appropriate rational information has been effectively provided. Paradoxical theory attempts to explain why under these circumstances change sometimes does not occur or occurs through unexpected means. The following example illustrates this use.

The staff of a busy obstetric department are expected to record the mother's name, date and time of birth, neonate's sex, and Apgar scores at 1 and 5 minutes in the delivery log. They are finding that doing so in a correct and timely manner is often difficult. When things are particularly hectic, the log may not be completed until after the mother has been moved to the postpartum area; occasionally the second Apgar score is not recorded.

According to the paradoxical model, attempts at change, called first-order changes, will be made. First-order changes do not alter the existing situation but instead reinforce it. For example, the obstetric department supervisor might write memos reminding the delivery staff to record all information immediately. A statement of this responsibility might be added to the procedure manual. Because nothing in these first-order changes requires a change, old behaviors are likely to persist, even though the staff may agree that change is needed.

Second-order changes can alter existing circumstance in unexpected ways and produce otherwise unexpected changes. Making second-order changes requires looking at the situation in a new way and seeing alternatives that had not been previously identified. In the case of the obstetric department, the supervisor assumed that the delivery nurses had to record the information in the delivery log and devoted her first order changes to ensuring that this would occur. On closer examination, the supervisor might notice that nursery nurses often assisted with neonate care in the delivery room. As a second-order change, the supervisor might propose that rather than having delivery nurses record Apgar scores, the nursery nurses should do so.

GAINING NEW PERSPECTIVES

Watzlawick, Weakland, and Fisch (1974) propose that specific steps can free the thinker from old patterns. Reframing includes:
- *identifying the problem*
- *listing all attempted solutions*
- *defining realistic changes*
- *identifying and implementing a second-order change strategy.*

The supervisor's second-order changes could produce change by restructuring the situation. They might also produce unexpected changes. For example, as the new plan is put into practice, the supervisor might notice that the delivery nurses become more conscientious and reliable in recording the Apgar scores; paradoxically, as the need for the delivery nurses to record the scores is being removed, they are doing so more efficiently. Within a short time, the supervisor may return this responsibility to the delivery nurses.

The paradoxical model can be successfully applied to many situations in which people have resisted normal solutions. One example is its use in assisting assault and rape victims to recover from their trauma. Such victims may experience flashbacks and fears of future attacks. They become afraid of going out at night or of confronting people whom they perceive as threatening. In one instance, a rape survivor became unwilling to go out after nightfall; she was also uncomfortable with men who made any overtures to her. The paradoxical model provided a solution to her fears and inability to relate normally to men. In a controlled environment, she was exposed to verbal and physical assault and was taught how to defend herself from such attacks. She practiced forceful defense against a heavily padded "assailant." During the training, the woman shared her fears about being attacked with women in similar circumstances. The woman also learned ways of avoiding situations in which she was likely to be vulnerable. In this case, the combination of rational, unemotional instruction and direct physical conflict succeeded when more traditional methods of assisting had failed.

POWER-COERCIVE MODEL

The power-coercive model relies on the application of power to make change (see *Theories of Change*, page 353). Change usually occurs because those involved see either the possibility of reward for compliance, or avoidance of punishment. Nurses usually implement these strategies only when other methods have failed. Because power-coercive strategies frequently involve working with unwilling participants, they require continual monitoring and surveillance to remain effective. Furthermore, effects may be short term if no structural changes are made or if the changes are not supported by those affected (Haffer, 1986).

The use of power strategies, such as autocratic decisions, can often be appropriate and invaluable. For example, when a fire breaks out in an extended-care facility, power may be exerted immediately and forcibly to remove clients from the facility. In this case, the nurse may exert power by pressing staff into unusual duties not covered by their job descriptions and coercing unwilling clients into leaving behind valued personal belongings and mementos. Power strategies may also be used simply because they are more rapidly applied and do not require initial education, persuasion, or training. Using power strategies inappropriately, however, can ultimately result in wasted time and effort spent policing compliance, which might have been avoided by education and training.

Power strategies can be used by people in authority, such as administrators and managers, or by others not in such positions. Individual nurses and nursing groups seeking professional or economic change have traditionally been considered to lack authority. Tappen (1989) summarizes the steps required by those without authority to develop and exercise power. These include:

- defining the issue and identifying the opponent
- organizing a following
- building a power base
- beginning the action phase
- keeping the pressure on
- the final struggle.

DEFINING THE ISSUE AND IDENTIFYING THE OPPONENT

In initiating the power-coercive model, the problem and the individual or agency responsible must be identified and isolated. For example, nurses working with low-income prenatal clients in California may be concerned about proposed legislation that would minimize or eliminate access to low-cost or free prenatal care. Nurses and clients decide to work together to prevent passage of the legislation. The clients, however, have other problems and difficulties; they are concerned about post delivery care and other problems related to housing, schooling, and jobs. In this situation, the nurses identify the issue as preventing passage of legislation that would cut back on low-cost or free prenatal care. The clients' other concerns are not at issue; they represent another, separate situation. The identified opponents include the governor and, the state legislature. They may also include county officials responsible for allocating state and federal funds for low-cost prenatal care and the general public, whose support the nurses want to enlist. Limiting the problem and targeting opponents can help the group focus their actions.

ORGANIZING A FOLLOWING

The second step in the power-coercive model involves developing a constituency to press for the desired change. Existing groups can be used or new groups can be created. The nurses and their prenatal clients might identify and enlist the support of professional organizations such as the American Nurses' Association, the California Nurses' Association, the California Medical Association, nursing specialty groups, and consumer rights groups.

BUILDING A POWER BASE

The nurses and clients can now evaluate their own power sources, including the constituency they developed in the preceding step, and those of the opposition. Once this has been done, effective opposition strategies can be devised. Legislators running for reelection might be targeted to receive information on the detrimental effects of the proposed cutbacks. The nurses and clients could form a public relations group to educate the public and pressure legislators through radio and television advertisements or through a demonstration on the steps of the state capitol.

BEGINNING THE ACTION PHASE

During the action phase, the group implements its plans for confronting the problem. They provide the media with news releases detailing the likely effects of reduced prenatal care, and they begin a letter-writing campaign to legislators. During this phase, the group can expect conflict as opponents recognize the threat and begin to respond. The governor and legislators might point out that funding for all social and medical services as well as educational programs is being cut and that the nurses and their prenatal clients are asking for special consideration.

KEEPING THE PRESSURE ON

As the conflict continues, the nurses and their clients must step up pressure on the opponents by using increasingly confrontational and visible means. At this point, the proposed state capital demonstration should occur. During the demonstration, the group should make maximum use of nursing expertise, enlisting eloquent nurse speakers to describe the need for prenatal services and to enumerate the detrimental effects that will result from not providing such care.

THE FINAL STRUGGLE

During this phase, the group exerts maximum pressure on the opponents and uses every power source to coerce the opponents into changing their position. The nurses and prenatal clients might present graphic evidence of the human and economic waste that results from inadequate prenatal care. Evidence might include public statements from parents whose children have suffered injuries that might have been mitigated or prevented with proper prenatal care.

THE AFTERMATH

Because power-coercive change models involve people in such consuming and visceral ways, those involved should plan for dealing with the aftermath, whether the outcome is positive or negative. If the action is successful, the nurses and their clients have a model to apply to other health care issues, such as obtaining well-baby care for underinsured and indigent clients. In the event of failure, the group should provide support for those who expended such effort. Toward this end, even small gains can be identified. For example, even if the group fails to prevent the cutbacks, they may have helped to minimize them. In addition, they may have increased public and legislative awareness of their problem, which might make future pushes for change easier. The group should maintain communication with the organizations of its power base, and individual contributions to the struggle should be recognized. Group members should also realize that affecting change in health care is seldom easy. Working for long-term change can help to deal with the setbacks that will inevitably occur along the way.

PEOPLE INVOLVED IN CHANGE

Thus far, this chapter has dealt with change in terms of theoretical models that, for the most part, emphasize situational factors. Change can also be examined from the point of view of the participants: the change agent and the individuals, including staff and clients, affected by the change.

THE CHANGE AGENT

Building on the work of Lewin (1951), Havelock (1973) and Lippitt (1973) developed a model that focuses on the role of the change agent, emphasizing the need for communication and interpersonal skills. Lane (1992) describes how this model can be used to plan unit-based change in an acute care hospital setting. Six phases in the change process are identified.

PHASE I: BUILDING A RELATIONSHIP

During this phase, Lane (1992) states that the change agent must gain the unit's trust. To do so, the agent can adopt an open and responsive manner, respond to the unit's needs in a productive way, and demonstrate competence. The change agent should establish relationships with staff in all the unit areas to be involved in the change, including staff from all shifts and job categories.

The new emergency department manager knows that each year many clients needing organ transplants die because of a lack of donor organs. To increase the number of donors, the manager wants to provide more information to emergency department clients and to make the staff more aware of appropriate ways to approach families of fatally injured clients who may be potential organ donors.

Before attempting any changes in staff behaviors or unit procedures, the new manager as change agent must first establish trust within the department. To accomplish this, he might by way of introduction tell the staff about his previous experience, certification, and training at an early staff meeting. As the manager continues to establish trust between himself and staff, he might begin sharing information on the importance of organ donation.

PHASE II: DIAGNOSIS

During this phase, the change agent more fully identifies the actual desired change. Lane (1992) recommends establishing a planning committee consisting of representatives from all shifts and job categories in the unit and outlines a three-meeting format in which the project is described, goals are outlined, and a "diagnosis" of the desired change is made.

The emergency department manager would help to establish a planning committee with broad-based representation from nurses, physicians, technicians, ward clerks, and receptionists. The manager would encourage input from all members concerning:

- why approaching families about organ donation is important
- why doing so is a difficult process
- how other staff members can support those responsible for approaching families
- how unit members can support the family in making a difficult decision.

Thinking creatively and looking outside the committee's immediate experience can lead to additional ideas and discoveries. For example, the group might suggest that working with families who do not have a critically ill family member could also be useful. They might recommend having informative brochures about organ transplantation available in the waiting room as a means of making more people aware of the need for organ donation.

The change agent is also responsible for guiding the planning team to consensus. After allowing ample discussion of the various issues, the manager should encourage the group to diagnose the change to be made. The emergency department committee might state their diagnosis as: Members of the emergency department staff will receive training and support in learning how to approach client families regarding organ donation, with the long-range goal of increasing the number of appropriate requests made.

PHASE III: ACQUIRING RELEVANT RESOURCES

During this phase, the change agent helps the planning committee to identify what they need to do to accomplish the change. Lane (1992) emphasizes the importance of having one committee member research the nursing literature for information; doing so is another way of looking outside the immediate experience of the unit and its members for solutions and suggestions. Lane also suggests that planning committee members talk with staff at other institutions who have instituted similar changes. At this time, the committee needs to assess:

- what knowledge and skills will be required
- what motivation exists for making the change
- what economic resources are needed and which are available
- what investment in time and energy will be required.

The emergency department planning group might decide that staff need a series of workshops on the organ donation process. In addition, the group might want to bring in a consultant or speaker to help staff become more supportive and effective in dealing with families about donation. As a way of making organ donation information available to all emergency department clients, the group might recommend a client-teaching video that describes the importance of organ donation and features interviews with organ recipients and their families. The committee would evaluate the cost and utility of such a video during this phase.

Those instituting change should carefully evaluate resistance to the proposed change and identify ways of dealing with the resistance. The emergency department manager and the committee might encounter staff who think that approaching family members about organ donation during a time when they are dealing with the death of a loved one is unfeeling. Other staff members may have religious views that oppose organ donation and transplantation. The committee might recommend staff education to deal with the issue.

PHASE IV: CHOOSING THE SOLUTION

During this phase, the change agent helps the group to identify specific goals and various strategies for accomplishing them. The more specific the goals and the more detailed the planning, the greater the likelihood of successful change.

The emergency department manager and committee might establish as a specific goal that all emergency department staff will participate in organ donation workshops by a specific date. They might also stipulate that the evening shift be the first to try out the new techniques for approaching families about organ donation. This tryout could take the form of a simulated drill or an actual incident. After the experience, the staff involved would discuss their performance, describing members' feelings and identifying those techniques that worked well and those that need modification.

PHASE V: GAINING ACCEPTANCE

During this phase, Lane proposes that the change agent and planning group seek support for the change. This involves communicating the change and its proposed results to the unit and to the institution as a whole. An agency newsletter, for example, might describe the emergency department's efforts to improve organ donation. The newsletter could also recognize individuals involved in the planning committee and point out the importance of the new process to other clients.

PHASE VI: STABILIZING AND GENERATING SELF-RENEWAL

During the final phase, the committee's suggestions would be implemented and the other shifts would begin using the new techniques. Procedure and policy changes would emphasize the expectation that all staff be knowledgeable about organ donation and have the skills and abilities to approach or support families concerning organ donation. Refresher courses and regularly scheduled reviews of staff expectations could help consolidate and maintain the change. Lane (1992) suggests keeping the planning committee together during this phase to ensure that continued assessment and support are provided.

ASSISTING EMPLOYEES TO DEAL WITH CHANGE

According to Peck (1987), all change is "a kind of death, and all growth requires that we go through depression." Kubler-Ross developed a five-stage model dealing with the adjustment to death. Perlman and Takacs (1990) expanded on this model to describe the emotional response of employees affected by change. Understanding the phases that employees undergo when accepting change can help both staff and managers navigate the process more successfully.

Equilibrium. During this phase, employees invested in the status quo are in a state of emotional equilibrium. They are made aware of the need for change and the impact the change will have.

Denial. Employees refuse to recognize that the change will occur. They expend energy denying the need for and inevitability of change. While supporting the need for change, the change agent must allow employees to vent their feelings.

Anger. As the reality of change becomes more inevitable, employees angrily resist. During this phase, the change agent should identify the sources of anger and attempt to answer employee concerns.

Bargaining. Employees try to modify the change during this phase. As in the anger phase, the change agent should identify specific concerns and work toward their resolution.

Chaos. Perlman and Takacs (1990) maintain that the chaos phase, marked by lack of control and disorientation, is normal in the change process. Employees who have actively resisted change and who have not wanted to discuss how it will be accomplished are most prone to these feelings. Perlman and Takacs suggest that the change agent continue to listen to staff and help them to recognize that their chaotic feelings are normal during such periods.

Depression. As change occurs, employees may become depressed, remembering the past and talking about "the good old days." The change agent or manager should continue to listen to and validate employee feelings during this stage while continuing to provide information about the change.

Resignation. During this phase, employees begin to passively accept the change. The manager or change agent can expect and encourage more compliance with the change.

Openness. As employees accept the change, they demonstrate increased energy and willingness. At this point, the change agent should again present information on the change because many employees will not have understood it when it was presented earlier. Employees should not be made to feel negligent for initially having not understood the information.

Readiness. Employees discard the old order and focus on the changed environment. The manager can assume a more direct approach when helping staff to become involved in the new processes.

Reemergence. Staff returns to a state of equilibrium and the new order is established. New institutional values and goals may be developed.

The degree to which an employee experiences the phases described by Perlman and Takacs depends on several factors. Employees who were not involved in identifying change needed and developing strategies to achieve it may require a longer adjustment period. Those personally threatened by a change, by either job or status loss, may react more strongly than those for whom the change has less significant impact. Steele (1990) describes three ways by which the anger and turmoil generated during change can be minimized:

- active listening
- networking
- active involvement
- stress reduction.

Active listening involves seeking correct information about the change on the part of both staff and management. Dispelling rumors and providing accurate information about the proposed change help to minimize employee uncertainty.

Networking can enable employees to develop a support group for dealing with the change and its aftermath. Steele (1990) stresses that because working relationships may change during reorganization periods, individuals should establish new networks while maintaining those formed in the past.

Active involvement by staff and management consists of looking for ways to support others as they adjust to change. By offering to help others with new equipment or new procedures, individuals can help one another adjust to the new order.

Stress reduction requires that individuals develop appropriate physical, emotional, and social avenues of expression during times of change. Steele (1990) suggests that those involved in change ensure that physical fitness, friendships and family, and social and cultural interests be maintained during times of change.

ASSISTING CLIENTS WITH LIFE TRANSITIONS

Helping clients to deal with changes is an integral part of nursing. The changes may be relatively minor and temporary, such as a broken arm, or permanent and life-changing, such as childhood leukemia diagnosis. Selder (1989) describes the process that individuals undergo in adapting to life transitions, including permanent injury or death of a family member.

REALITY AND UNCERTAINTY

Selder asserts that each person has a relatively stable vision of reality that can be disrupted by a life-changing event, such as a spinal cord injury. The disrupted reality results in uncertainty, which the individual tries to resolve by seeking information. Nurses can assist clients by providing information about what has occurred and what can be expected. Clients in life-changing circumstances may not be able to process information in a normal way. For example, the client with a spinal cord injury may not understand what has happened, even when explanations are offered, because the new reality is too fraught with uncertainties and fears to be acceptable. The nurse may have to repeat the information several times or present it in different contexts.

INFORMATION SEEKING

Selder (1989) reports that clients undergoing life transitions recall "asking all the nurses, aids, [physicians], and ancillary staff about this injury" and that the clients further describe their questioning as "a compulsive activity in which somehow, the answers to their questions don't make sense." Nurses should be prepared to deal with such repetitive questioning from clients and understand that continually providing information can help clients adjust to the change. Becoming frustrated with or refusing to answer repeated questions can interfere with client adjustment. Family members who withhold information can also interfere with client adjustment. Both nurse and family should realize that information, no matter how initially upsetting, enables the client to see circumstances clearly.

IDENTITY CONSTANCY AND RESOLUTION OF UNCERTAINTY

Resolution of uncertainty occurs as the client restructures reality to reflect the changed circumstance and forms a new identity. Selder (1989) describes the sense of self as identity constancy. It may involve appearance and function, both of which may require modification. Being able to participate, to whatever degree, in activities that were important to them before the life-changing event can help clients adjust to their changed circumstances. Driving a car, dressing oneself, and dialing a telephone can represent activities that help individuals to define themselves according to their new abilities. In supporting such activities, nurses might allow clients extra time to button their own shirts or feed themselves. Impatience with a client's attempts at independence may delay positive adjustment to change.

TIME DISRUPTION

Clients adjusting to major life changes may experience a disruption in the way they interpret time. Rather than being able to note days and times in the normal manner, a client may relate days and times to specific events having to do with the life change. Selder (1989) describes a surviving spouse who marked time as it related to the day she gave away her deceased husband's suits. Others may interpret time as it relates to the day a wedding ring was removed, or pictures put away. Primarily, though, clients adjusting to a major life change are oriented to the present; they may become more interested in the future when current circumstances are sorted out.

TRIGGER EVENTS

Certain trigger events can reactivate a client's sense of loss or cause the client to become acutely aware of the irrevocable change that has occurred. For example, finding a tennis racket or baseball mit in the closet may reactivate a sense of loss for a spinal injury client who is no longer able to engage in athletic activities. The client may feel the same sadness and grief he felt before adjusting to the change. By the same token, on seeing another couple dancing to a favorite tune, a spinal injury client may suddenly become acutely aware that reality for the client and the client's spouse has changed forever. Trigger events can also cause sadness over missed opportunities. A woman who has lost a teenaged child may experience such sadness when attending the wedding of another young couple.

Nurses should understand that clients adjusting to major life changes will inevitably encounter trigger events. To further promote adjustment, nurses can inform clients about such events and encourage clients to discuss any feelings of regret or pain when they are encountered.

As clients accept their changed reality, normal behaviors return. They may want to begin wearing street clothes; women may ask for cosmetics. Information about the future and about how to maximize functioning will become more important as clients forge new identities related to their major life changes.

DEALING WITH CATASTROPHIC CHANGE

As nurses become more familiar with the change process and learn how to support themselves and others during transition periods, the changes themselves become less stressful. However, on occasion, the magnitude of change confronted is so great that existing coping skills are insufficient. This kind of breakdown of coping skills can occur during natural disasters (floods, hurricanes, or earthquakes). Although individuals and communities may make efforts to prepare for such events, some catastrophes are overwhelming. Lippman (1992) describes what happens when nursing staff and health care institutions confront natural disasters that defy advance planning.

Most hospitals have disaster plans and practice semiannual drills mandated by the Joint Commission on Accreditation of Healthcare Organizations. Nonetheless, when a natural disaster strikes, instant decision making, which can be stressful to staff, is required. For example, a fire at the New York Downtown Hospital resulted in electricity loss to the hospital and much of the city. The administration had assumed that in such a situation, the hospital's emergency generator system would allow things to proceed without much interruption; however, the emergency generator failed. As a result, nursing staff had to deal with ventilator clients who required manual ventilation as well as other client needs involving electrical power. Other nurses made continuous rounds with flashlights because callbells were not functioning. A disaster status was declared, and nursing staff remained on duty beyond their normal shifts, some for as long as 20 hours.

Similar disasters have further illustrated the importance of planning for unexpected changes that go beyond those envisioned in the standard emergency drill. Lippman (1992) suggests that nurses do the following to critique their unit's preparedness for natural disaster:

1. Determine if plans exist for both internal and external disasters. Such plans might relate to fires within the hospital or to a hurricane or an earthquake that affects an entire metropolitan area.

2. Identify the location of the individual unit's command post as well as an alternate site in case the main site is affected by the catastrophe.

3. Identify alternate communication means for use when normal channels are nonfunctioning. This may involve identify staff who can serve as message runners or who can use shortwave radios.

4. Assess the semiannual disaster drills to make them more helpful. Drills should include scenarios in which backup electricity, water, and communication systems are not functioning. They should also require staff to use alternate ways of handling the problems that such system malfunctions could cause.

5. Plan for notification of off-duty staff. Some hospitals in flood- or hurricane-prone areas have preestablished schedules for use during disaster. Other hospitals rely on conventional telephone networks with backup systems to ensure that all staff are notified. Maintaining a current roster of staff and their responsibilities is of obvious importance.

6. Determine if the hospital disaster committee has the necessary membership to plan for the eventuality of a natural disaster.

As a result of experiencing large-scale disasters, some hospitals have developed "script cards," which provide direction for staff attempting to cope with sudden, massive change. Such cards describe immediate actions, such as shutting off oxygen or gas lines, and electrical power. Others describe how nurses should evacuate clients from particular areas. Unit emergency kits, including such things as flashlights, batteries, radios, and extension cords, are also valuable preparation.

After experiencing a catastrophe such as a natural disaster, staff should have the opportunity to react to the events in a supportive environment. Miller (1992) describes a debriefing strategy conducted within 48 to 72 hours of the crisis. Staff members meet with a trained facilitator in groups of 10 to discuss what happened, how they felt and thought at the time, and how they currently feel. In this meeting, staff divulge grief, anger, or sadness at being unable to prevent client injury. As group members become aware of shared feelings and concerns, they begin to understand that such reactions to overwhelming change are normal. They learn that they may continue to experience sadness or depression and may be troubled with nightmares or flashbacks. The group leader and members then devise strategies to defuse the stress and help everyone recover from the experience. The experiences can be used to devise better disaster plans.

Summary

Change is an integral part of life. It can be cyclical or unidirectional, temporary or permanent, minor or life-changing. Various models (normative-reeducative, empirical-rational, paradoxical, and power-coercive) can help the nurse understand the different phases that compose the change process. Understanding the roles of the change agent and the other individuals involved in a change, including staff and clients, better enables the nurse to initiate and respond positively to change, whether it be personal, institutional, or client change. Catastrophic changes, such as floods and fires, can nevertheless sometimes overwhelm even the most prepared nurse. To the extent that such changes can be prepared for, nurses and institutions can take certain measures, such as establishing centralized command posts and participating in emergency drills.

APPLICATION EXERCISE

With the help of your instructor, identify a limited change that you would like to make in a work or personal setting. For example, if nonsterile gloves are not readily available for staff use in a particular clinical area, you might want to suggest a procedural change that would result in easier access. On a personal level, you might want a schedule that allows for regular exercise. Then analyze the problem according to the following:

1. Precisely what is the desired change? Describe how the situation you would propose would differ from the current practice.

2. Identify factors that inhibit making such a change. Be sure to include economic, political, and cultural factors.

3. Identify factors that might support such a change, including economic, political, cultural, and other factors.

4. How would you reduce or mitigate the inhibiting factors? How would you strengthen supporting factors?

5. What steps should you take to unfreeze the situation and allow change to begin?

6. Describe how the change might be implemented.

7. What steps would have to be taken to refreeze the situation and thereby maintain the change?

REVIEW QUESTIONS

1. Compare and contrast spontaneous, developmental, and active change.

2. What internal and external forces can affect change at the client care level?

3. Briefly describe the stages of the normative-reeducative model.

4. Briefly describe the stages of the empirical-reeducative model.

5. How does the paradoxical model help to explain why expected changes fail to occur or how unexpected changes result from unanticipated causes?

6. What are the steps involved in applying the power-coercive model?

7. What are the strengths and weaknesses of the four theoretical models in terms of working with professional nurses?

8. Describe the change agent's role in planning unit-based change.

9. What are the phases an employee might pass through when adjusting to organizational changes? Briefly describe each phase.

10. How can nurses assist clients undergoing life transitions, such as those caused by function loss or terminal illness diagnosis?

11. How can nurses determine if their unit is prepared for catastrophic changes such as might occur during a fire or natural disaster?

REFERENCES

Alinsky, S.D. *Rules for Radicals: A Practical Guide for Realistic Radicals.* New York: Vintage Books, 1972.

Dutton, W.H., et al. "Diffusion and Social Impacts of Personal Computers," *Communication Research* 12:219-250, 1987.

Haffer, A. "Facilitating Change: Choosing the Appropriate Strategy," *JONA* 16:18-22, April 1986.

Haley, J. *The Power Tactics of Jesus Christ and Other Essays.* New York: Avon Books, 1969.

Havelock, R.G. *The Change Agent's Guide to Innovation in Education.* Englewood Cliffs, N.J.: Educational Technology Publications, 1973.

Holmes, T.H., and Rahe, R. "The Social Readjustment Rating Scale," *Journal of Psychosomatic Research* 2(4):213, 1967.

Lane, A.J. "Using Havelock's Model to Plan Unit-Based Change," *Nursing Management* 23(9):58-60, September 1992.

Lewin, K. *Field Theory in Social Science: Selected Theoretical Papers.* New York: Harper & Row, 1951.

Lippitt, G.S. *Visualizing Change: Model Building and the Change Process.* LaJolla, Calif.: University Associates, 1973.

Lippman, H. "When the Disaster Drill Is for Real," *RN* 55(9):54-60, September 1992.

Miller, D.M., "Care for the Caregivers," *RN*, 55(9):58-59, September 1992.

Peck, M.S. *The Different Drum: Community Making and Peace.* New York: Simon and Schuster, 1987.

Perlman, D., and Takacs, G.J. "The Ten Stages of Change," *Nursing Management*, 21(4):33-38, April 1990.

Rogers, E.M., and Shoemaker, F.F. *Communication in Innovation*, 2nd ed. New York: The Free Press, 1971.

Saltman, G., and Duncan, R. *Strategies for Planned Change.* New York: Vintage Books, 1972.

Selder, F. "Life Transition Theory: The Resolution of Uncertainty," *Nursing and Health Care* 10(8)437-451, October 1989.

Steele, P. "Surviving Organizational Change," *Nursing Management*, 21(12):50, December 1990.

Tappen, R.M. *Nursing Leadership and Management: Concepts and Practice*, 2nd ed. Philadelphia: F.A. Davis Co., 1989.

Watzlawick, P., et al. *Change: Principles of Problem Formation and Problem Resolution.* New York:W.W. Norton & Co., 1974.

RECOMMENDATIONS FOR FURTHER STUDY

Buller, P.F. "For Successful Strategic Change: Blend OD Practices with Strategic Management," *Organ Dynamics* 16:42-55, Winter 1988.

Cashman, J. "Effecting Change through the Stream of Analysis Process," *JONA* 19:37-44, May 1989.

Mathey, M. "The Art of Breaking Set," *Nursing Management* 23(2):20-21, February 1992.

Meyer, C. "Emergency Nursing: Always Changing, Always Challenging," *American Journal of Nursing* 92(4):67-72, September 1992.

Spradley, B.W. "Managing Change Creatively," *JONA* 10:32-37, May 1990.

Strudthoff, M. "Orchestrating Change in Nursing Service," *Nursing Management* 22(7):96-98, July 1991.

12

USING POWER

OBJECTIVES

After studying this chapter, the reader should be able to:

1. List the sources of power available to clinical nurses.

2. Describe ways in which nurses can enhance their expert power.

3. Define economic power and explain the use of collective bargaining as a means of exerting power in the work setting.

4. Discuss legislation relating to collective bargaining, and describe the special constraints imposed on professions that substantially affect public welfare.

5. Describe the process by which a collective bargaining group forms and negotiates contracts for workers.

6. Describe recent changes in the worker-management relationship that have modified traditional roles and power structures.

7. Explain how nurses can become more skillful at developing and using political power.

8. Explain how a nurse's self-image can affect that nurse's referent power.

INTRODUCTION

Power is many things to many people. Some think of it as the ability to influence the allocation of scarce resources. Others consider power to be the ability to get people to do what they don't want to do or the ability to refuse to do what others want you to do. Whether viewed negatively or positively, power, when it is exercised, almost always arouses strong feelings.

How power is used and the ends toward which it is used determine whether it is positive or negative. This is an important concept, especially for nurses, who have often viewed power as something belonging to others rather than to themselves and who historically have had ambivalent feelings about those within the profession who have sought power.

Because women have historically lacked social and professional power and because nursing has been a predominantly female profession, nurses have often used indirect power sources to accomplish their aims. They have frequently relied on the power of other groups, such as physicians, to promote a nursing agenda rather than assert their own authority to accomplish tasks or goals.

Furthermore, a woman's deliberate quest for power has often been considered "unladylike" and equated with a desire for personal advancement or glorification. Unfortunately, among nurses, the sentiment "I just want to take care of clients" is still commonly heard, indicating a reluctance to become involved in decision making and governance activities, even though such activities clearly help determine client care. In part, this reluctance to use or even to be associated with power results from a shunning of responsibility. Nurses who display such reluctance may believe that if others decide what is best and if the nurse's responsibility is to follow orders, then nurses have no responsibility for judging initial decisions or ultimate outcomes. These nurses may consider a dependent position more comfortable because it carries less personal risk.

Nursing as a profession has moved substantially beyond the "handmaiden" image to establish its own body of knowledge, code of ethics, and concept of professional nursing. As part of that image, many nurses now understand and appropriately use all the power sources they can rightfully claim. This chapter describes the different forms of power and how nurses can exercise them. Beginning with different conceptions of nursing power, the chapter then describes traditional types of power: physical, expert, position, economic, political, and referent.

POWER IN CLINICAL NURSING PRACTICE

In her classic work on clinical nursing excellence and power, Benner (1984) points out that viewing power from the usual feminine or masculine perspectives is misleading; the belief that women must behave as men to gain and exercise power assumes that power can be effectively used in only one way. Furthermore, as Benner (1984) states, "the disparagement of feminine perspectives on power is based upon the misguided assumptions that feminine values have kept women and nursing subservient, rather than recognizing that society's devaluing of, and discrimination against, women are the sources of the problem."

Benner describes six types of power that nurses exhibit in dealing with clients: transformational, integrative, advocacy, healing, participative/affirmative, and problem-solving. According to Benner, power is more than an assemblage of physical or economic might; it can reside in one's ability to give of oneself to others. Caring is an essential part of nursing power; without it, nursing becomes a mechanical function that can have a severely deleterious rather than healing effect.

TRANSFORMATIONAL POWER

Transformational power represents the ability to assist clients to change their self-image or vision of reality. Benner describes nurses exercising transformational power in their care of clients with long and protracted illnesses. The nurses' persistent, unconditional caring help the clients transform their self-image from one of worthlessness to one of value. Giving compassionate care to clients who are incontinent or unable to speak or perform normal daily activities can have the same effect.

INTEGRATIVE POWER

Integrative power is the nurse's ability to help clients return to their normal lives in a manner that accounts for their disabilities while involving the clients as fully as possible in life. By doing so, the nurse can enhance the clients' reintegration into their family and community. Benner gives the example of a nurse assisting a young muscular dystrophy client's return to school and job.

ADVOCACY POWER

Advocacy power enables the nurse to remove obstacles, to encourage, and to make the system work for the client. For example, the nurse caring for elderly clients who are unfamiliar with health care benefits and agencies can help the clients understand the bureaucracies and procedures that must be dealt with to receive assistance. Caring is a necessary component of advocate power because without it, the nurse's initiative to risk and expend the effort to advocate will not be strong enough.

HEALING POWER

Healing power refers to the nurse's ability to create a healing climate and relationship with the client. Benner contends that an affirming and caring nurse-client relationship provides the best basis for healing. A client who feels supported and encouraged will deal with disease more successfully than one who receives the same physical care but without the supportive, caring dimension.

PARTICIPATIVE/AFFIRMATIVE POWER

Participative/affirmative power is the nurse's ability to draw strength from a caring interaction with the client. Benner disputes the commonly held belief that a nurse has only so much caring or emotional strength to draw on and suggests that such power is renewed by investing it in others. Even when the situation involves suffering or death, Benner contends that the process of involvement and caring allows the nurse to draw strength from the interaction, and to avoid disillusionment and burnout.

PROBLEM SOLVING

The nurse working in a caring manner possesses problem-solving powers that the less involved nurse lacks. Benner (1984) suggests that "a committed stance provides a sensitivity to cues that allows persons to search for solutions and makes it possible to recognize a solution when they are not directly looking for it." The nurse's commitment and caring enhances receptivity to solutions in part by allowing intuition and feeling to play a role in problem solving. This can lead the nurse to create nontraditional solutions.

TRADITIONAL TYPES OF POWER

In addition to understanding the types of nursing power, nurses must be aware of the more traditional power types. Being so can help nurses develop power-building strategies as individuals and as members of the nursing profession. Traditional types include physical, expert, position, economic, political, and referent power.

PHYSICAL POWER

Many groups have been dominated or not on the basis of physical power. In prehistoric eras, men were considered powerful because they had the physical strength to kill animals for food, build shelters, and protect and subdue women. Women were dependent because they were physically less strong and because they relied on men for food, shelter, and protection for themselves and their offspring. The importance of these factors in relation to the exercise of power has greatly diminished. In fact, most jobs that require considerable physical strength now rely principally on machines for that strength.

Many occupations once judged to be appropriate only for men because the jobs required great physical power are now open to women. Such jobs include maneuvering heavy machinery, working in construction, mining, and farming. As power becomes less associated with gender and personal physical strength, occupations can attract individuals on the basis of ability rather than on stereotypical views of gender suitability.

EXPERT POWER

Expert power results from the individual's demonstration of competency and knowledge. The knowledge might be clinical, political, ethical, or legal in nature. Nurses with expert power are able not only to influence the actions or decisions of others but also to act effectively in their own right.

Expert power is most effective when shared. The experienced nurse who hoards knowledge or who refuses to share information with others loses power to the degree that she is considered uncooperative or unprofessional. Rather than diluting expert power, sharing skills and information with others develops a sense of authority and strength in the expert nurse as well as the nurses receiving assistance.

Nurses can develop expert power by continuing to develop professionally and remaining current in their individual practice areas. Taking advantage of continuing education offerings, joining groups that review nursing research articles, attending conferences and seminars, and seeking additional formal education are all ways to expand knowledge and expert power.

Nursing research enhances the expert power of all nurses by expanding the understanding of disease processes and the effects of nursing intervention. In reviewing the literature and research on the human immunodeficiency virus (HIV), Larson et al. (1991) report that between May 1987 and June 1990 a total of 54 formal research studies dealing with HIV were published. An additional 677 articles, which were primarily descriptive or anecdotal, also contributed to nurses' ability to work expertly with HIV clients.

POSITION POWER

Position power stems from an individual's official standing or job title. For example, a nursing supervisor has certain powers that accompany job responsibilities. The supervisor has the power to assign staff to particular duties, to develop a staffing schedule, to produce a budget and a list of departmental priorities, and to evaluate and counsel staff. Position power frequently includes the ability to reward or to punish. A nursing supervisor may be able to grant a request for a particular weekend off or support an employee's request to attend a conference. On the other hand, a nursing supervisor may dock an employee's pay for arriving late for work or recommend termination of an unsatisfactory employee.

Position power is strongest when it is supported by other types of power. For example, a supervising nurse who is also seen as an expert has increased authority and respect from subordinates. Position power is weakest when it is exercised unfairly or arbitrarily. As shared governance structures have developed and problem solving and decision making are accomplished collaboratively by management and employees, position power which relies strictly on an individual title alone is likely to be relatively ineffective. For example, a nursing supervisor may have the position power to assign an employee to accept a particular assignment, but if such assignments are seen to be arbitrary or unfair, other shared governance mechanisms, such as grievance procedures or joint governance councils, may be used to reverse the assignment and to counsel or perhaps censure the supervising nurse.

ECONOMIC POWER

Economic power represents the ability of individuals or groups to influence others by providing or withholding resources. It is the ability to tell a nurse to conform to expectations or risk forfeiting a paycheck; economic power is also the ability of nurses in a collective bargaining unit to gain wage and working condition concessions by threatening a legal strike.

Economic power is also the nurses' ability, through involvement in budget development processes and governing boards, to make decisions about hospital finances. In the past, management has exercised economic power mainly by threatening job loss; organized workers, by threatening strikes. This adversarial stance is changing as shared governance is implemented in more and more health care institutions.

COLLECTIVE BARGAINING

Nurses have long had an ambivalent relationship with unions and collective bargaining. Because many nurses considered leaving clients to conduct a strike contrary to nursing's image and purposes, they likewise viewed unions and collective bargaining as antithetical to the profession. In addition, because health care was viewed as an essential public service and because collective bargaining was considered a means of jeopardizing the provision of that service, many employees were barred from such activities. However, as professional nursing associations assumed responsibility for nurses' wage and working conditions, nurses began to view collective bargaining as a way of gaining influence over the practice conditions, as a tool that can be used appropriately or inappropriately.

HISTORICAL DEVELOPMENT OF COLLECTIVE BARGAINING

Passed during the Great Depression, the National Industrial Relations Act set national standards for wages and working conditions. The act prohibited child labor, limited the work week to 35 to 40 hours, and set wages at 30 to 40 cents per hour. In 1935, the National Labor Relations Act (NLRA), or Wagner Act, was enacted. The Wagner Act provided federal protection to employees seeking to establish unions and created the National Labor Relations Board (NLRB) to oversee legislation governing union formation and collective bargaining.

As early as 1931, the American Nurses' Association (ANA) had recognized that to represent nurses effectively, it had to represent nurses' concerns for wages and working conditions as well as their concern for client care issues. Most members believed that divided representation, with a professional association addressing professional issues and a separate nurses' union addressing economic concerns, would prove less effective in advocating for both issues. A study of employment conditions resulted in the ANA Economic Security Program, which urged ANA state affiliates to serve as professional collective bargaining units for nurses. Mirroring the societal perception of health care as a critical industry, the ANA maintained a no-strike policy until 1968.

The Wagner Act was amended in 1947 by the Taft-Hartley Act, which specifically excluded nonprofit hospitals from the collective bargaining process (despite this, many hospitals voluntarily entered into contracts with nursing unions during this period). The 1959 Ladrum-Griffin Act further controlled unions by providing them with specific election and financial accounting procedures.

Finally, in 1974, with the passage of the Nonprofit Health Care Amendments to the Taft-Hartley Act (Public Law 93-360), the rights and responsibilities of nurses working in nonprofit organizations, including hospitals, clinics, nursing homes, and other health care facilities, were acknowledged. Nurses in these work areas could now engage in collective bargaining. The amendments also provided safeguards for the public's welfare by requiring that any strike be preceded by a 10-day written notice and further defined the worker's right to join or not to join a collective bargaining unit.

The amendments also require a 60-day notification by the employer or bargaining unit of any intent to modify or terminate a collectively bargained agreement. Notification of such intent must be made to the Federal Mediation and Conciliation Service (FMCS), and both collective bargaining groups and employers are required to participate in mediation activities. Under the 1974 amendments, any action that threatens a substantial disruption of health care is subject to review by a board of inquiry. An employee strike or a management lockout of workers can be referred to the board of inquiry. With these safeguards in place, nurses could collectively bargain with management over wages, benefits, working conditions, and professional and client care concerns.

Various collective bargaining groups throughout the country now represent nurses. Professional representation of nursing staff through the state affiliate is referred to as the collective action division. In California, for example, the collective action division of the California Nurses' Association (CNA) is governed by the Economic and General Welfare Congress, which reports to the CNA House of Delegates ("CNA Directory," 1992). Congress members are elected by the collective bargaining units of facilities represented in agreements negotiated by the CNA.

PROCESS OF COLLECTIVE BARGAINING

When nurses determine that they want to be represented in negotiations with management by a collective bargaining agent, they must follow a specific process to establish the union or professional organization as the legally recognized representative. This process involves several stages, including organization of nurses, supervised election, contract negotiation, and contract administration (see *Collective Bargaining*, page 393).

Organization of Nurses. Nurses can work together to press for changes in working conditions, for a greater say in client care issues, or for salary or benefits adjustments. Electing to bargain collectively for such issues does not necessarily mean that a health care organization has been unresponsive to the nurses' needs; it does suggest that nurses see value in working together to advance such concerns and that they view collective bargaining as an appropriate means of expressing and using power.

The nurses who have the initial interest in forming a collective bargaining group contact their professional organization or unions that may be interested in representing them. The organization or union provides information to all the nurses employed at the agency and ascertains the level of interest in forming a union. This must be done according to legal requirements, which include using nonwork time for discussions in settings outside the work environment. If a majority of nurses are interested in being represented by a collective bargaining unit, the union or professional association provides authorization cards. At least 30% of the agency's nurses must sign the authorization cards for the selected union to begin acting on their behalf. At this point, some health care agencies voluntarily recognize the selected union and begin negotiations. In other cases, an election is held to determine the nurses' level of interest. If interest is sufficient, the NLRB certifies the union as the bargaining agent for the nurses in that facility.

Supervised Election. NLRB, which administers the NLRA, has two main functions: it conducts elections by secret ballot to determine whether a group of workers wants to be represented by a collective bargaining unit and it deals with unfair labor practices on the part of either employees or employers. The NLRB becomes involved when the employees first identify that the majority of them want to be represented by the collective bargaining agent. If the hospital or other agency does not voluntarily recognize a prospective collective bargaining group, the employees can request that the bargaining group send to the management a letter stating that the employees are organizing and that this activity is protected by law. When the employees have gathered the required number of votes, a petition is filed with the NLRB. The NLRB regional director then holds a formal hearing to establish the eligibility of the employees voting to form the union and sets the date, time, and place for the actual election.

The election is held during working hours at the agency, and all employees who worked during a specific recent payroll period are eligible to vote. This last requirement prevents management from hiring large numbers of new employees who will vote against representation by the collective bargaining group. Management, supervising employees, and temporary employees are not eligible to vote. Determining just what a supervising employee is can be difficult. In some agencies, charge nurses who have principally managerial responsibilities are considered management. In other settings, they may function principally as staff nurses, in which case they are classified as members of the bargaining unit. Generally, supervisors represent management if they are involved in activities such as hiring, assigning, or disciplining employees.

COLLECTIVE BARGAINING

Collective bargaining includes the following important steps:
- *organization of nurses: Nurses identify a need for representation by a collective bargaining group.*
- *supervised elections: Nurses employed at the agency vote to determine whether a majority want to be represented by the collective bargaining group.*
- *contract negotiations: Nurses and management negotiate agreements on wages, working conditions, grievance policies, and other issues.*
- *contract ratification: After negotiators reach an agreement, the collective bargaining group votes to ratify it.*

If agreement cannot be reached, the nurses may implement mediation, arbitration, or work stoppage to resolve differences.

The separation of "workers" and "supervisors" in the collective bargaining system has created special problems for nurses. Frequently in the past, supervisors and managers have worked for improved salaries and working conditions and for nursing involvement in client care. Because statutes prohibit supervisors from belonging to collective bargaining groups, many nursing leaders are unable to participate directly in the collective bargaining group. As a result, many state nursing associations now provide for distinct membership levels, in which managerial and supervisorial members can belong and pay dues to the professional organization but cannot belong or pay dues to the organization's economic and general welfare branch. This enables all nurses to be represented by one organization for all components of professional practice.

Once the election has occurred, the regional NLRB office counts the ballots and forwards the results to the NLRB General Council in Washington, D.C. Election results are then announced. If the vote does not support union formation, a year must pass before the nurses can make another attempt.

If the vote for union representation is successful, contract negotiations are begun.

Both employees and employer are subject to laws protecting against unfair labor practices. These include the employer's interference with or discrimination against employees attempting to form a collective bargaining group. Similarly, employees cannot attempt to coerce other employees into joining the collective bargaining group. Both groups are expected to bargain in good faith, put forth reasonable proposals, discuss issues, and attempt to reach agreement.

Contract Negotiations. The initial contract between health care workers and management describes the working relationships and responsibilities of each party. It usually begins with a statement of each group's objectives and includes agreements to work toward joint purposes and to formally recognize the union or professional group acting as the official bargaining agent. Specific articles then follow that govern wages and working conditions, fringe benefits such as insurance and retirement, and policies covering promotion, transfer, and layoff. The time period to be covered by the contract is identified, as is a policy for dealing with grievances related to contractual agreement violations and policies to handle individual disciplinary situations. The contract may require employees to join the union or to pay a fixed amount equivalent to the agency welfare fund. This last requirement prevents employees from benefiting from the collective bargaining process without having to make a financial contribution.

In addition, nurses may press for agreements that stipulate shared decision making and individual professional accountability. (See Chapter 9, The nature of leadership, page 315, for a discussion on collaborative decision-making councils.) Professional accountability may be advanced through interdisciplinary committees, professional standards committees, and the inclusion of nurses on committees dealing with concerns such as bioethical dilemmas.

In the past, contract negotiations have been adversarial, with union and management taking hard-line positions and using aggressive tactics to force the other side to make concessions. This traditional procedure, which frequently resulted in staff polarization into hostile camps, was an important reason why nurses were reluctant to become involved in collective bargaining and the union movement. Many health care agencies and unions representing nurses have moved away from this adversarial model to a more collaborative model (Porter-O'Grady, 1992).

Dealing with existing contracts. Benton (1992) describes contract negotiations in a long-term care setting. First, either the union or management makes proposals regarding wages, working conditions and benefits, union memberships, and dues. Benton suggests that proposals be made available before the first negotiating session. Both management and the union then choose negotiating teams and a spokesperson. Each side reviews the issues and attaches some degree of priority to each. Then both sides examine each issue and either agree or disagree about it. As Benton states, bartering is part of this stage, and both sides will take offensive or defensive positions. Negotiations usually start with the more easily negotiated issues and work up to the more difficult articles, which generally involve economic and union membership issues.

Contract negotiations can be protracted. Benton (1992) suggests that using time-outs and caucuses for discussion can reduce conflict. Including nurse managers in the bargaining can present advantages and disadvantages. If negotiations are positive and constructive, the presence of managers may provide a helpful nursing management perspective and may enhance later relations between management and employees. If, however, negotiations are acrimonious and antagonistic, keeping nursing management separate from the process can help to preserve positive relationships that exist between employees and managers.

Finally, the parties either agree on and ratify a new contract or reach a point where neither is willing to compromise further. If a stalemate results, the FMCS must be notified. Several courses of action can then be undertaken, including mediation, fact finding and recommendation, binding arbitration, or work stoppage.

Mediation. A mediator is "a professionally trained, unbiased person skilled at helping individuals resolve conflict" (Benton, 1992). Appointed by the FMCS, the mediator can talk to both parties in a more neutral context and move between the two parties to present options and choices. Mediators can suggest solutions, but neither party in the negotiations is bound to accept them. The mediator can help both parties to understand the positions and priorities of each and to develop acceptable compromises.

Fact Finding. The FMCS might appoint a fact-finding body to assess the situation and make public the body's conclusions, which sometimes helps the disputing parties move closer to agreement. The fact-finding approach is effective because it removes the issues from the closed bargaining context and subjects them to public scrutiny; an intransigent stance by either employees or employer becomes harder to maintain when seen as unreasonable in the eyes of those observing the discussions. The fact-finding approach can also validate or invalidate claims made by either party, thereby further objectifying the process.

Binding Arbitration. An arbitrator, like a mediator, is a trained, neutral party who investigates the dispute and makes recommendations. An arbitrator may be requested from the American Arbitration Association, from the FMCS, or from state mediation and conciliation services. In accepting binding arbitration, which may be part of an existing contract, each party presents and justifies its proposals and agrees to hold to the arbitrator's recommendations. If the negotiations involve an existing contract, the FMCS is notified 90 days before a contract is to be modified or terminated and 60 days before the expiration of the contract on which a new agreement has not been reached.

Work Stoppage. Work stoppages can result from a nurses' slowdown or strike or a management lockout. If a bargaining unit decides by a majority vote to initiate a strike, it must give

10 days notice to the institution involved. This allows the institution to transfer less critical clients to other facilities, cancel elective surgeries, and alert the public to the situation. Management will typically try to reassign supervisory personnel to provide client care. The bargaining unit prepares for the strike by establishing a strike headquarters and a means of communicating information to all workers (hot line, telephone tree, or newsletter) and organizes strike logistics, such as setting up picketing teams and identifying individuals to provide information to the public. Both sides will attempt to influence public perception of the strike, sometimes by discrediting or defaming the opposing sides.

Nurses frequently have difficulty deciding whether or not to strike. Many nurses believe that reducing or refusing to care for clients in need violates professional principles. Some collective bargaining groups avoid this dilemma by stipulating that they will continue to care for critically ill clients during a strike. Negotiating a binding arbitration agreement into the contract also helps nurses avoid the need for strike.

Other nurses believe that without the ability to strike, they are unable to affect significant changes in areas related to client care. They argue that nurses can no longer allow hospital management to dictate working conditions that are detrimental to client health and safety and that a strike is justified to achieve beneficial changes in these areas. All efforts to avert a strike usually are made, and the pressure of an impending strike may produce movements that forestall such action.

If a strike is called, bargaining should be continued or resumed as soon as possible. Efforts to reach an acceptable compromise should continue until a tentative agreement is reached between the opposing parties. The union members then review this agreement. If accepted, the agreement becomes the new contract under which employees and management will function for the agreed-on period.

CONTRACT ADMINISTRATION

Once they have signed the contract, both parties are expected to honor its provisions. If one party fails to do so, the other can file a grievance. Although either management or an employee can file a grievance, most grievances are brought by employees. This may occur because many firstline supervisors are not familiar with the contract's provisions and may violate an agreement due to lack of knowledge.

The process for dealing with a work conflict begins with discussion between the employee and the supervisor, who should make all reasonable efforts to resolve the conflict. Communicating directly and using joint problem-solving skills can help to prevent conflicts from escalating into the more formal grievance. If, however, an employee and a supervisor are unable to resolve a contractually governed issue, the employee begins an official grievance by making a complaint to the collective bargaining representative, called a steward. Then, within a specified time period, the steward and supervisor talk and try to reach a decision. If the grievance is not resolved at this level, it proceeds through further steps as specified in the contract, perhaps going to a joint employee-management committee or to the president of the collective bargaining group and the hospital administrator. The grievance can also be submitted to an arbitrator for final decision if so provided in the contract.

The employee and employer cooperating with good intentions can rapidly resolve many grievances. If an employer fails to grant a pay raise when one is due or produces a work schedule that violates one agreed on in the contract, the collective bargaining representative usually has only to confirm that the issue is covered by the contract. Management wants to avoid grievances because they are time-consuming and divisive.

Managing nurses should be as knowledgeable about collective bargaining matters, particularly contracts, as they are about any other agency operations. They should also orient new employees to the contract's requirements and protections. New employees should review and become familiar with their institution's contract and its provisions for wages, working conditions, and the grievance process. The new nurse should also note such things as clinical ladders or other scheduled advancements. If such information is not conveyed during the institution's orientation, the new employee should request such information from the personnel office.

DECERTIFICATION

If employees decide that they no longer want to be represented by their collective bargaining group, they may begin a decertification process. (Employers may also initiate decertification if they believe that the collective bargaining group no longer has the support of the majority of employees.) To initiate decertification, the employees sign a petition indicating their desire to discontinue representation. At least 30% of employees must sign (50% if decertification has been initiated by the employer) before the petition is filed with the NLRB. Petitions are usually filed 120 days before expiration of the current contract, although they can be filed on the expiration date.

The NLRB then officially notifies the employees, the employer, and the collective bargaining group about the decertification petition. The NLRB may hold hearings to explore issues, after which an election date is set to decide the issue. Actual campaigning for and against decertification is limited to the 24 hours before the election to ensure that the vote reflects the employees' current feeling regarding the representation. If the decertification is approved, the collective bargaining group no longer represents the employees. If it is not approved, contract negotiations resume.

RECENT CHANGES

Porter-O'Grady (1992) points out that radical changes are occurring in the workplace and between employers and employees. He believes that the interaction between collective bargaining groups and management must begin to reflect the workplace's new requirements or face obsolescence. Porter-O'Grady maintains that collective bargaining groups must understand the changing workplace, the nurse's changing role, and effective collaborative management structures, including shared governance.

The changing workplace

One of the most important changes in the workplace has been the development of a highly decentralized work environment. Unions have been effective in helping to define the job responsibilities of some workers. In an assembly-line environment, for example, a union contract describes precisely what the worker is expected to do and not do. In health care today, what a nurse does depends on a variety of factors, many of which cannot be precisely defined.

The nurse's changing role

Nurses are increasingly seeing the need for interdisciplinary practice and shared roles. As a result, traditional contractual language cannot always be used to codify role functions and job responsibilities. Nurses are also developing new ways to interact with the health care agency. Another important nursing development is the establishment of new work relationships and rewards. According to Porter-O'Grady, "gain sharing, shared ownership, bonusing, pay for performance, outcome pay, per diem contracting, case load payment structures and benefits smorgasbords are all signs of more creative and individual economic and services approaches" (1992).

Collaborative decision-making and shared governance

Shared governance management practically demands a change in how collective bargaining groups and employers interact. Nurses and employers who enter antagonistically into negotiations do not facilitate the process. As Porter-O'Grady (1992) suggests, "from mutually establishing goals and service targets to setting work policy affecting outcomes, management must permit local union leadership to. . .participate in diagramming and planning for the future." Such involvement of collective bargaining leadership in the management process would allow for collaborative problem solving and decision making but require a radical change in the way management has viewed such groups. Rather than seeing the union as an adversary, managers should include collective bargaining leaders in shared governance councils, planning teams, and policy development teams.

Although contracts would still describe agreements for wages and working conditions, they could be negotiated with the recent changes in the workplace and in the nurse's role in mind. In addition, contracts could address how goals are set, how job descriptions are created, how changes in the health care setting are introduced, and how problems are to be approached. Such a collaborative approach would reinforce the shared decision-making structures developing in many health care institutions.

POLITICAL POWER

Today's nurses are aware of the importance of gaining and exercising political power. Nurses are involved in politics at all levels, from county and city government to the U.S. Congress, and an increasing number are becoming successful politicians. As with other forms of power, nurses struggle against the stereotypical idea that the nurturing, caring, supportive image of the nurse is incompatible with the role of an active politician. However, Terry Agir, government relations commissioner for the CNA, suggests that nurses who think that they can focus on client care without understanding the political arena are naive (Gray, 1992). She contends that by actively providing information to political bodies about health care needs, nurses can affect the nature of health care legislation.

Nursing, a profession with over more than 1.9 million registered nurses and more than 1.5 million licensed practical nurses, holds considerable political clout. Nurses can endorse candidates, can be candidates, can contribute as individuals to campaigns, or can donate to a political action committee (PAC), such as the ANAPAC, which has supported candidates whose positions on health care issues were congruent with those of nursing. The ANA endorsed Bill Clinton in the 1992 presidential campaign. According to ANA president

Virginia Trotter Betts, among the ANA's top priorities is the election to Congress of nurses and others who support the nursing agenda for health care reform and who will work for the direct reimbursement of nursing services. Another politically important organization is the Tricouncil for Nursing, which is composed of our national nursing groups, the American Nurses Association (ANA), the National League for Nursing (NLN), the American Association of Colleges of Nursing (AACN) and the Association for Nurse Executives. The joint collaboration of these major organizations serves to enhance the political power of nursing.

Successful nursing involvement in politics is not new. Florence Nightingale was a consummate politician, able to work within a rigid system to obtain the ends she sought by bargaining, demanding, negotiating, and bringing pressure to bear from other powerful individuals and groups. Meyer (1992) identifies nurses who have more recently braved the political front with success (see *The Nurse's Political Power*, page 404). Marilyn Goldwater, who served in the Maryland legislature from 1975 to 1987 and who is now executive assistant for health issues for Maryland's governor, was instrumental in obtaining passage of bills mandating reimbursement by private insurance for both nurse practitioners and nurse midwives in Maryland.

Nurses can use political power outside the system as well. Meyer (1992) describes a successful political action by Colorado state-employed nurses who resigned en masse to protest a proposed salary cut, the result of a flawed state study that purportedly showed that nurses were overpaid by 5%. The nurses first conducted their own survey, which showed that nurses were actually underpaid by as much as 6.5%. To bring the issue to the attention of the public, the legislature, and the governor, the nurses developed fact sheets on the nursing shortage and the impact of a wage decrease. They also hired a lobbyist to represent their interests, recruited other nurses working in state service, and established telephone trees to coordinate and communicate information about the proposed action.

Despite meetings with the governor and the state budget committee, little progress was achieved. As the legislative session wound down and after a final, futile meeting with the governor, the nurses converged on the Colorado capital where they publicly tendered their resignations. (Colorado law prevents public employees from striking, but no law prevents public employees from resigning.) More than 250 nurses from the University of Colorado Health Sciences Center and 56 from Fort Logan submitted resignations. The numbers included many supervisors. This action inspired the governor to call two legislative committees back into session. He then assumed emergency powers, which he then used to grant a 7.5% raise to registered nurses and to identify other needed reforms, including merit pay and tuition assistance.

BECOMING POLITICALLY ACTIVE

Becoming politically active means becoming aware of the issues confronting nursing and health care and making a commitment to work for change. Nurses can become politically active by working for the passage of specific legislation, by supporting candidates who understand health care issues, and by running for local, state, or national office. In 1992, four nurses ran for Congress: critical care nurse Judy Jarvis of California; Cheryl Davis Knapp, a neonatal nurse manager from Florida; Virginia Collins, who has served six terms in the Alaska state legislature; and Eddie Bernice Johnson, who similarly served successful terms in the Texas house and senate.

Nursing students and newly graduated nurses can become politically active in a number of ways. Mason (1990) suggests that nurses can establish and develop political power not only in the workplace but also in government, professional nursing organizations, and the community. Regardless of the setting, developing political power requires that nurses become aware of the health care needs of the area in which they live and work, and that they understand political processes and the people involved.

THE NURSE'S POLITICAL POWER

Nurses can exert political power in the workplace, in the community, in nursing organizations, and in government.
- *Workplace: Nurses can develop personal power types, including expert power and positional power, by negotiating the presence of nurse-members on standing committees and boards of trustees. They can develop economic power through collective bargaining.*
- *Community: Nurse can develop expert power by serving as advocates for client groups, such as prenatal or AIDS clients. They can work with community organizations such as the American Cancer Society and the American Heart Association.*
- *Nursing organizations: Nurses can become politically active within regional, state, and national organizations; by serving as delegates to conventions or members of commissions, and by supporting the Nursing Agenda for Health Care Reform.*
- *Government: Nurses can act as legislative liaisons and information sources for state and national representatives. They can actively participate in the campaigns of politicians supportive of nursing and health care and run themselves for office.*

BECOMING KNOWLEDGEABLE

The nurse can become knowledgeable about local health care needs and issues by becoming active in volunteer organizations, such as the local chapter of the American Heart Association or the American Cancer Society, or with other groups, such as the American Association of Retired People, that have an agenda for health care reform. The nurse should understand the positions taken by the professional nursing associations, such as the Agenda for Health Care Reform proposed by the ANA and the National League for Nursing (see Chapter 3, How organizations are structured, and Chapter 4, Health care delivery).

Nurses should also understand the political process. They should identify representatives to local boards of supervisors, city councils, and state legislatures and know each representative's position on health care issues. Legislators at all levels usually have local offices and staff who can provide information or forward questions to the representatives. Contacting a representative's office can serve as the first step in becoming familiar with a particular politician. Having gained a basic understanding of health care needs and the existing political structure, nurses can begin to work for change. They can identify a specific issue or concern and develop a plan for political action.

DEVELOPING AND EXECUTING A PLAN

A new nurse or student nurse might choose to address health care issues at a local or state level. The nurse should develop a plan, based on change theories, that identifies the inhibiting and facilitating factors, the strengths and weaknesses of each factor, and the power sources available to the nurse (see Chapter 11, The nurse as change agent).

An example of political power exerted at the state level is the 1992 action of California nurses to defeat Proposition 166, the "Basic Health Care" proposition advanced by the California Medical Association. California nurses had been actively involved in seeking reform of the health care system, but on examining Proposition 166, they found that it did not address many health care concerns. In addition, it imposed an unfair burden on small businesses, which were to bear the financial brunt of the reforms. An estimated 375,000 jobs would have been lost as a result of employers cutting back on employees, quitting business, or moving out of state. In addition, the proposition did not describe how the new legislation would affect existing state insurance.

Nurses who opposed Proposition 166 used many strategies to inform voters of the proposal's deficiencies. They prepared and distributed printed press kits and held statewide scheduled news conferences. A broad representation of more than 60 organizations gathered under the umbrella organization "Health '92 Coalition," which included diverse groups such as the California Chambers of Commerce, the California chapter of the National Organization of Women, the American Association of Retired Persons, the California Farm Bureau, the California Manufacturers Association, and the American Federation of Labor. As a result of this political action, Proposition 166 was defeated.

REFERENT POWER

Referent power resides in the individual and reflects that person's strengths, energies, and talents. (Referent power is sometimes referred to as charismatic power. See Chapter 9, The nature of leadership). Referent power comprises all the other power types an individual may possess, each of which can be cultivated and developed. Nurses can enhance their expert power by developing skills and broadening knowledge; their political power by becoming politically aware and active; and their economic power by joining shared governance counsels or participating in collective bargaining activities. Components of referent power include commitment and action, and image.

Commitment and Action. Many theories attempt to describe nursing practice (see Chapter 2, A conceptual base for nursing practice). The most effective describe not only the components of the nursing role but also nurses' responsibility to act. A nurse's understanding of ethical or legal matters is insufficient if it fails to produce a corresponding action at the necessary time. Referent power depends on nurses acting in accordance with their commitments. Such actions may include serving as client advocates, functioning as change agents, or working to develop nursing's professional agenda.

Image. Image is the picture, or view, that others have of an individual. It is a composite of many things and can be positive or negative. Both the image of nursing as a profession and that of the nurse as an individual are important when assessing an individual's referent power.

Nursing's popular image has changed over the years. Female nurses have been seen as wise women, witches, servants, incompetents, handmaidens, and religious zealots whose goal is self-sacrifice in the service of others. In recent years, some television shows have even portrayed nurses as shallow, self-seeking, but seductive caregivers only peripherally interested in nursing the sick. The male nurse's image has also gone through several transmutations ranging from wizard to soldier to a man somehow less masculine than his counterparts in other professions.

The popular image of nursing has improved as nurses' education and preparation have become more equivalent to of other professions. Professional nursing organizations have also done much to correct the popular image of the nurse. The 1981 National League of Nurses (NLN) recruitment videotape, "Nursing: A Career for All Reasons," portrays nursing in a realistic light as a career that allows men and women to make meaningful, professional contributions. The NLN and other nursing organizations have formed task forces to educate the public further about the nurse's role. Articles describing nursing's contribution during the 1991 Gulf War helped the public to better understand the nature of nursing. Donley and Flaherty (1990) suggest that nurses themselves can improve and correct their popular image by exerting the powers available to them. They also suggest that changing nurses' self-image will correct the public's idea of nursing.

Each individual's self-image depends on many variables, including personal values, goals, and expectations. For example, nurses who achieve licensure as registered nurses and who work competently and caringly on a medical floor of an acute-care hospital may rightly feel that they are making an important contribution and meeting personal and professional goals. Such nurses, reinforced by institutional respect and recognition, have a positive outlook on their jobs, which in turn affects the way they interact with others and the way others perceive them. On the other hand, nurses who feel trapped in a profession that fails to provide the autonomy, status, or compensation desired will have a less positive self-image. Nurses dissatisfaction can cause them to feel powerless, angry, and resentful. They may view their profession as "only a job." When this happens, nurses will develop a negative self-image and professional image. Having a clear idea of personal values and goals can help nurses act in accord with their beliefs. Doing so enhances self-image and helps nurses to avoid compromising situations that can have deleterious effects on self-image.

In the past, the starched, military-styled nursing uniforms suggested to the public a commitment and dedication to order and discipline. Although nurses need no longer resort to the styles of the past, they can enhance their public image by other means that communicate the same commitment to order, discipline, and caring. For example, when communicating with clients, nurses should introduce themselves as registered nurses who have specific responsibilities to the client. Appropriate identification should clearly identify the nurse and the nurse's position. A positive self-image and personal appearance also promote public perception of professionalism. Furthermore, Kalisch and Kalisch (1984) suggest that nurses develop skills that enable them to answer questions about important nursing and health care issues, write letters to the editor, and participate knowledgeably in public forums.

SUMMARY

Power is an invaluable nursing tool, the effects of which can be positive or negative, depending on the way in which it is used and the ends toward which it is applied. Historically, nurses have not wanted or been prepared to exercise the various power forms available to them. Today's nurse, however, is more willing to exercise the referent, position, physical, expert, economic, and political power available to anyone. Others believe that nurses have the opportunity to develop special powers that they can use in client care.

Nurses must become more knowledgeable and skillful in the exercise of power in their personal lives, in their work environment, and at the state and national levels. Such abilities affect the nurse personally as well as the nursing profession and health care in general. By viewing the exercise of power as a skill that can be learned and effectively practiced, nurses can more successfully advocate for themselves, their clients, and the nursing profession.

APPLICATION EXERCISE

Evaluate your own strengths and weaknesses in the following areas. Of the power sources listed below, identify three you would like to develop further, and describe one short-term action (6 months to 1 year) and one long-term action (5 or more years) that might facilitate your development.

1. Physical Power. Describe your physical strengths and weaknesses. To what degree are you satisfied with your abilities? In what ways would you like to change?

2. Expert Power. Describe your knowledge base and nursing skills. Which areas do you most want to develop?

3. Position Power. What positions do you hold, formally or informally, that give you influence or decision-making authority? How did you achieve these positions?

4. Economic Power. Identify a nursing setting in which you would like to practice after graduation. Evaluate the economic power of nurses working in that institution. Are they members of a collective bargaining group? If not, do they have other sources of economic power that give them input into decisions regarding wages, working conditions, and nursing responsibilities? How might you begin to develop economic power working in this environment?

5. Political Power. Are you active politically in campus, local, or state issues? How might you become more involved at the local or state level in advancing these causes?

6. Referent Power. Describe your present referent power. To what degree are you satisfied with the image you present as a future professional nurse?

REVIEW QUESTIONS

1. What does "advocacy power" mean?

2. How does expert power enhance position power?

3. What are the arguments in favor of nurses using strike power to obtain goals? What are the counterarguments?

4. How is a grievance against an employer conducted under a collective bargaining agreement?

References

Benner, P. *From Novice to Expert: Excellence and Power in Clinical Nursing Practice.* Menlo Park, Calif.: Addison-Wesley Publishing Co., 1984.

Benton, T. "Union Negotiating," *Nursing Management* 23(30):70-72, March 1992.

"CNA Directory 1992," *California Nurse,* June 1992.

Donley, R., and Flaherty, M.J. "Strategies for Changing Nursing's Image," in *Current Issues in Nursing.* Edited by McCloskey, J.C., and Grace, H.K. St. Louis: C.V. Mosby Co., 1990.

Gray, B.B. "Nurses Enter the Fray," *Nurseweek* 5(21):10-12, August 1992.

Kalisch, P.A., and Kalisch, B.J. "Psychiatric Nurses and the Press: A Troubled Relationship," *Perspectives in Psychiatric Care* 22(1):5, 1984.

Larson, E., et al. "An Update on Nursing Research and HIV Infection," *Image* 23(1):4-12, Spring 1991.

Mason, D.J. "Politics, Nursing and You." in *Concepts Fundamental to Nursing.* Edited by Ismeurt, R.L., et al. Springhouse, Pa.: Springhouse Corporation, 1990.

Meyer, C. "Nursing on the Political Front," *American Journal of Nursing* 92(10):56-64, October 1992.

Porter-O'Grady, T. "Of Rabbits and Turtles: A Time of Change for Unions," *Nursing Economics* 10(3):177-182, May-June 1992.

Recommendations for Further Study

Ambrose, Y. "Nursing in 2001: Are You Ready?" *Nursing Management* 21(12):45-48, December 1990.

Beyer, E. "Legislation and You," *California Nursing Review* 44-48, January-February, 1988.

Bushy, A., and Smith, T.O. "Lobbying: The Hows and Wherefores," *Nursing Management* 21(4):39-45, April 1990.

"Denver Nurses Go on Warpath to Get Raise: Mass Walkout Proves Winning Strategy," *American Journal of Nursing* 88:1132, 1139-1140, August 1988.

13

USING RESEARCH FINDINGS

OBJECTIVES

After studying this chapter, the reader should be able to:

1. Distinguish between basic and applied research.

2. Compare and contrast quantitative and qualitative research approaches.

3. Describe descriptive, exploratory, and explanatory research.

4. Compare and contrast the scientific method and the research process.

5. List the steps of the research process.

6. Describe three quantitative and two qualitative research designs.

7. Describe legal and ethical concerns in nursing research.

8. Describe how nurses can appropriately care for research subjects and can avoid threats to the integrity of the study.

9. Describe how nurses can use research findings in practice.

INTRODUCTION

Nursing research can be a valuable tool not only for increasing personal understanding but also for advancing nursing knowledge in general. All nurses can and should be involved in research, whether they conduct research studies, apply findings from published research, or identify everyday clinical practice problems. Professional nurses should be familiar with the research process and with findings from research studies that affect their practice area. They should also incorporate research findings into everyday nursing practice.

This chapter describes the development of nursing research, the different types of research designs, legal and ethical concerns in conducting research, and nursing opportunities for supporting and assisting the research process.

DIVISIONS OF RESEARCH

Nurses should understand that research is conducted in different ways and for various purposes. Research is described as being either basic or applied, depending on whether it focuses on description and theory building or on application and utilization. Research can also be classified as quantitative or qualitative, depending on the approach used. The nurse should understand the distinctions between basic and applied research and between quantitative and qualitative research methodologies.

BASIC RESEARCH

Basic research, as its name suggests, consists of recording basic empirical observations about the subject under study. These basic observations may lead to a theory about how something operates or why something changes; however, the intention of basic research is simply to advance knowledge about the particular subject. For example, researchers who identified the human immunodeficiency virus (HIV) were engaged in basic research; they were attempting to describe the agent causing acquired immune deficiency syndrome (AIDS). Although this research has had significant implications for the care of HIV and AIDS clients, the immediate goal was simply to identify the infection's cause.

APPLIED RESEARCH

Applied research builds on basic research. The researcher takes the empirical observations and any related explanations and theories that have resulted form basic research and applies them to a specific problem. This is usually done as a means of finding a solution to the problem. Unlike basic research, the aim of applied research is to improve a situation. For example, applied research is being conducted to evaluate the effects of different drugs and treatment protocols on AIDS clients. In the course of this process, researchers may discover additional information that further explains the HIV infection and that expands related theory. Nevertheless, the focus of the research remains the practical application of knowledge.

QUANTITATIVE RESEARCH

Quantitative research uses numerical data to describe phenomena and the relations among them, and it uses statistical analysis to determine the significance of findings. Quantitative research is the best known research form, and many terms specific to research come from the language of quantitative research. Characteristics of quantitative research include:

- client groups called treatment or control groups
- random assignment of clients to groups
- active experimentation
- statistical methods to analyze data.

Quantitative research methods might be used to investige the effectiveness of a new drug in treating AIDS clients, half of whom are given the drug and half of whom are given a placebo, by random assignment. A statistical test would measure whether or not the control population responded significantly differently to the new drug.

The researcher using quantitative methods remains as objective as possible. Remaining so can help the researcher to isolate the factor or the interaction being studied and to prevent incidental events from influencing the experiment's outcome.

QUALITATIVE RESEARCH

According to Strauss and Corbin (1990), qualitative research is any kind of study that produces findings not arrived at by statistical procedures or other quantification means. The qualitative researcher uses subjective data to discover under-

---

BASIC AND APPLIED RESEARCH

- *Basic research: seeks to understand and describe*
- *Applied research: seeks to solve problems and apply knowledge*

lying patterns and themes. Rather than isolate the subject from its environment, qualitative researchers try to include as many variables as possible in their description of the subject. The usual statistical tests for significance are not used.

Qualitative research is often used effectively when experimental methods are not feasible or are inappropriate, as is often the case in nursing. For example, randomly assigning clients to control groups or withholding treatment from one group to assess its effectiveness is often not feasible or desirable. A researcher in a laboratory can isolate a particular reaction and measure its effects, but in a client care setting, such isolation of variables is impossible. A noisy roommate or a distressing visit from upset relatives are among the many possible factors that cannot always be controlled.

Qualitative research might be used to describe the experience of terminally ill AIDS clients in both hospital and home environments. Like the quantitative study, the aim would be to compare two client groups. However, rather than randomly assigning clients to groups, the qualitative researcher would select from among clients who have themselves chosen the environments in which they will die. Rather than focusing on the effects of a new drug or experimenting on one group and comparing its response to the control group, the quantitative researcher might try to describe as completely as possible the experience of both client groups.

Quantitative and qualitative research also differ in their methods of data analysis. In the quantitative study, a statistical analysis would determine, for example, a drug's effectiveness. The qualitative study might identify and compare major themes in the experiences of home and hospital clients. Researchers would draw comparisons but in a limited manner because the qualitative study seeks to describe personal experiences, which might not be appropriately subject to generalization. The sections that follow provide additional information on qualitative and quantitative research strategies.

TRIANGULATION RESEARCH

Quantitative and qualitative research can sometimes comple-
ment each other. In a given research situation, some components may best lend themselves to an experiment and quantitative analysis, whereas others may be better described
using quantitative methods. Furthermore, when the findings
of one type of research confirm those of the second, the
overall conclusions are more strongly supported. The combination of both approaches is called triangulation research.

RESEARCH TERMINOLOGY

Because it involves a specialized language, nursing research
has often seemed inaccessible or unrelated to everyday practice. Nevertheless, nurses should understand the concepts
underlying nursing research and the terminology used in
research reports. The following example of nursing research
should help to illustrate the frequently used research vocabulary subsequently defined.

To explore how motivation level and knowledge about
breast-feeding relate to the mother's success or failure, Rentschler (1991) undertook a research study involving 150
women, who were volunteers in childbirth education classes.
The women's knowledge about breast-feeding was measured
by a questionnaire titled "Information on Breastfeeding
Questionnaire." Motivation level was measured by a questionnaire called the "Questionnaire Measure of Individual
Differences in Achieving Tendency" (QMIDAT). Rentschler
used a "Personal Data Inventory" (PDI) to gather information
about the mothers themselves. The PDI data included age,
race, marital status, educational level, occupation and income, information sources on breast-feeding, and length of
intended breast-feeding time. Breast-feeding success was
measured by the "Breastfeeding Experience Questionnaire"
(BEQ). The women answered the PDI at a childbirth class
session and the QMIDAT and IBQ at subsequent sessions. Six
weeks after delivery, the women received the BEQ.

Statistical analysis of the results demonstrated that motivation and knowledge did positively affect breast-feeding. Of

the 150 participants, 107 successfully breast-fed for at least 6 weeks. Based on this finding, Rentschler suggested that nurses working with prenatal clients provide basic breast-feeding information early in the pregnancy to allow the women to make conscious decisions about breast-feeding and to commit themselves to a course of action. Rentschler also advocated providing additional information about breast-feeding and bottle-feeding after the women had decided on a method. In particular, breast-feeding women benefit from instruction about possible problems and their solutions while continuing to breast-feed.

Population. This term refers to the entire group of individuals in which the researcher is interested. Rentschler's population comprised all breast-feeding women. Studying all members of a population is usually not feasible, so a smaller, representative group must be selected.

Sample. A sample is a group representative of the population. Rentschler's sample consisted of 150 women attending childbirth classes who volunteered for the study.

Subject. Each member of the sample is called a subject. To be included in a sample, each subject must meet certain criteria. Rentschler's subjects were women who were pregnant for the first time and who planned to breast-feed. They were also all students in childbirth classes. Although this last characteristic did not specifically interest Rentschler, it may have had an influence on how representative the sample was of the total population. For example, the basic knowledge of and motivation to breast-feed might be higher in women enrolled in prenatal classes than in women who do not enroll in such classes.

Representativeness. This term refers to the degree to which a sample adequately represents a targeted population. If the researcher is drawing conclusions about a population on the basis of a sample response, the sample should include the population's major characteristics. In Rentschler's study, representativeness is somewhat limited by the use of childbirth class volunteers. In such cases, generalizations about the population should be made cautiously.

Randomization. Ideally, when a researcher wants to compare two groups, the groups should comprise the same sorts of subjects. This helps ensure that different responses are not caused by factors other than the independent variable. Randomly assigning subjects to the two groups can help ensure the groups' similarity.

Experimental and control groups. Research studying the effectiveness of a drug or intervention frequently requires that the sample be divided into two groups. An experimental group would receive the treatment, drug, or other intervention being studied. The control group, which resembles as much as possible the experimental group, would not receive the treatment. At the end of the process, the researcher would compare the two groups. Groups that were alike before the intervention but different at the end would suggest that the drug or intervention had produced a change. Because Rentscher did not use experimental and control groups, he could not say for certain that the education and support provided the mothers caused their success; other variables (educational level, supportive environment, socioeconomic level), might have influenced success. When used appropriately, experimental and control groups allow researchers to draw more definite conclusions.

Variable. A variable is something that can change, or vary. The terms "independent variable," "dependent variable," and "extraneous variable" frequently appear in published research. An independent variable is the characteristic or element thought to be responsible for change. Rentschler believed that prenatal education and support contributed to breast-feeding success and as such were the independent variables in his research. A dependent variable is a characteristic that changes as a result of the independent variable. In Rentschler's research, the dependent variable is the women's success or nonsuccess in breast-feeding. Usually, researchers use the terms *independent* and *dependent* variables with research that uses experimental and control groups.

An extraneous or chance variable might also affect the dependent variable and could confuse the relations between the independent and dependent variable. In Rentschler's study, the presence in the successful group of supportive grandmothers or the economic means to hire housekeeping help might have been extraneous variables. The researchers must identify as many extraneous variables as possible and seek to control their effects so as to more accurately measure the effect of the independent variable on the dependent variable.

Validity and Reliability. "Validity" describes the degree to which the thing being measured is the thing being studied. For example, the validity of Rentscher's research would be enhanced to the degree that the questionnaires he used comprehensively measured the subjects' level of knowledge about breast-feeding. "Reliability" refers to the consistency of measured results. Rentscher's questionnaires would demonstrate reliability if they produce similar results when used repeatedly, as long as the subjects' knowledge level had not changed.

Probability and Level of Significance. Researchers use these two terms when discussing the implications of their findings. Probability refers to the likelihood of something happening. It is determined by statistical tests and stated as a mathematical expression, such as P. 05, which means that the probability of a result being the result of chance factors is less than 5%. (Researchers are concerned about the probability of a result being caused by factors other than the independent variable.) If Rentschler had reported the probability of successful breast-feeding as P .018, he would have meant that the probability of success being the result of chance was less than 1.8%; this might have led to the conclusion that the independent variables (knowledge and motivation level) were related to successful breast-feeding.

The term "level of significance" refers to a number chosen by the researcher that identifies the level at which a result is judged to be significant. Frequently seen levels of significance include .05 and .01. Statistical significance may differ from clinical significance, and statistical significance by itself does not mean that a particular finding has clinical significance. For example, in one study, researchers examining the results of rapid bladder decompression noted statistically significant differences in vital signs between groups of clients whose bladders were emptied rapidly and those whose bladders were emptied by stages. The differences had no clinical significance and did not indicate any important change in the clients' physical condition (Bristoll et al., 1989).

PURPOSES OF NURSING RESEARCH

Nursing research has the same purposes as all scientific research: to describe, to explore, to explain, to predict, and to control. A study usually begins with descriptive research and proceeds through other levels as researchers gain more knowledge about the subject.

DESCRIPTIVE RESEARCH

Descriptive research is used to provide a picture of something (a disease, a client response, or a new drug) about which little is known and for which no theory exists. It might be described as "first-level" research because it represents a first attempt at describing what exists and provides a basis for further research, which can explain what occurs and how prediction and control over the events can be achieved.

Descriptive research frequently uses qualitative research methods. An example is the research that has been undertaken to describe the health care practices of new groups of immigrants, such as the Hmong. Rather than trying to isolate variables and to experiment with different ways of providing health care (quantitative research methods), descriptive research uses qualitative research methods to obtain a more complete picture of the new citizens' general health care status and practices.

RESEARCH PURPOSES AND LEVELS

When researchers know little about a phenomenon, research focuses primarily on trying to describe it. Later research will help to explore and to explain the phenomenon. At the final level, researchers can predict and control.

EXPLORATORY RESEARCH

Once the phenomena have been described, exploratory research can proceed. Exploratory research extends descriptive research by defining interrelations and connections among phenomena. An example of exploratory research might be the investigation of what constitutes, from the client's point of view, a caring nurse. Riemen (1986) studied the perceptions of clients and identified specific factors that she suggests are associated with the perception of caring. Such things as the nurse being available and stating concern as well as the client's perception of being accepted and valued by the nurse were all important factors.

EXPLANATORY RESEARCH

Explanatory research uses observations about phenomena and the relations among them to form explanations that can then be tested. Researchers at this stage begin to articulate theory. For example, after describing the relations between nursing actions and clients' perceptions of caring, the researcher could begin to develop a theory explaining how nurses can enhance clients' feelings of being cared for. The researcher might theorize that the interpersonal relations between client and nurse is as important as the client's perception of nursing competence.

PREDICTION AND CONTROL

By understanding the factors responsible for a certain action or outcome, the researcher becomes able first to predict and then to control the action or outcome. Being able to predict and control outcomes allows researchers to generalize about others in similar circumstances. For example, Riemen (1986) described the relationship between specific nursing actions and client perceptions of caring. A theory developed through explanatory research might suggest that nursing actions such as communicating acceptance and concern to clients help clients perceive that they are being cared for. Such a theory may then lead to a study that could predict similar outcomes in other settings with similar clients.

DEVELOPMENT OF NURSING RESEARCH

Early nursing research focused on nurses and nursing students rather than on what nurses did or the impact nursing care had on clients. Today, nursing research not only provides information about the effectiveness of particular nursing interventions but also helps to advance nursing theory about the nature of nursing. It also helps nurses to gain a better understanding of the nurse-client relations, to evaluate the cost-effectiveness of various health care delivery forms, and to assess the impact of technology on nurses and clients.

Nursing research began with the detailed records and observations kept by Florence Nightingale during the Crimean war. She described the conditions under which wounded soldiers were cared for and recorded her efforts to produce a clean, well-lighted, supportive environment conducive to recovery. She observed the changes produced by her interventions and documented these changes. Her documentation helped to identify the environmental impact on healing.

Most subsequent nursing research, conducted by nurses or by others studying nursing, focused on what nurses did, who nurses were, and what type of nursing education was most effective. For example, time and motion studies, popular around the turn of the century, were conducted to determine the most efficient way for nurses to perform specific tasks, such as bathing clients or making beds (see Chapter 3, How organizations are structured).

Between 1900 and 1940, most studies dealt with nursing education and relied heavily on educational research theories, designs, and assessment instruments. During the 1940s, research began to support the movement of nursing education from hospitals to colleges and universities. Social anthropologist E.L. Brown (1948) recommended the move to the academic setting to provide students with the scientific basis they needed for their practice. Brown's recommendation had been preceded by the Goldmark report of 1923, which had pointed out the inadequacies of hospital-based education.

During the 1950s, nursing research accelerated. The number of studies undertaken increased; nurses themselves, rather than educators, physicians, and psychologists, began to conduct more nursing research, and more research dealt with the actual nursing performance and its effect on clients. Several factors were responsible for this development, including the establishment of the American Nurses' Foundation, which promoted nursing research, and the 1952 publication of the first nursing journal devoted to research reports, *Nursing Research.*

As nursing schools moved into academic settings, more students were exposed to research concepts and models; nurses began to undertake research themselves, principally studying the types of people who became nurses, what constituted the best nursing education, and what the public thought of nurses. At the request of the American Nurses' Association (ANA), sociologist Everett C. Hughes (1958) conducted an important study titled "Twenty Thousand Nurses Tell Their Story." Hughes' study described nurses, the nursing practice, and how nurses felt about their profession and identified the contribution that research could make to an understanding of the nursing practice. The study served as a basis for later statements regarding nursing functions, qualifications, and standards. Despite these advancements, the majority of nursing research conducted during this period did not address the practice of nursing itself.

During the 1960s, as nursing's theoretical base expanded, the need for nursing research into the effects of nursing interventions on client care outcomes increased. Nurses undertook collaborative investigations with researchers in other disciplines and in the process gained experience in how to conduct research. The nursing archive at Mugar Library, Boston University, was established. Also during this period, the Western Interstate Council for Higher Education in Nursing studied and recommended graduate nursing education and provided faculty workshops on the application of scientific knowledge.

Nursing curricula began to include research methodologies, and nursing organizations began to sponsor research workshops and conferences at which nursing research was regularly reported. In the 1970s, the nursing research journals *Advances in Nursing Science, Western Journal for Nursing Research*, and *Research in Nursing and Health* began publication. These provided a forum for research being done by various regional groups and individual researchers and helped to disseminate the results of the proliferating nursing research studies.

Important developments during the 1980s included the establishment of a National Commission for the Study of Nursing and Nursing Education through the efforts of the ANA and National League of Nurses (NLN). Emphasizing the importance of nursing research to the development of nursing, the commission recommended that:

- research be done on the impact of nursing practice on the quality, effectiveness, and economy of health care
- research on the nursing curriculum; articulation between curricula at the 2, 3, and 4-year levels and instructional methodologies be carried out to produce the most effectively prepared nurses
- each state develop a master plan to ensure that nursing education become part of the educational mainstream.

A fourth recommendation emphasized the importance of increased support for nursing research and education. The only recommendation not specifically addressing the need for research was the third, in which the focus was on ensuring that nurses obtained the scientific grounding that would prepare them as practitioners *(National Commission for the Study of Nursing and Nursing Education*, 1970)

Also during the 1980s, the development of the National Center for Nursing Research (NCNR) within the National Institutes of Health stimulated research on several levels. The NCNR has continually supported "studies on innovative approaches to the management and delivery of nursing care of [clients] and families, enhancing disease prevention and promoting the speed of recovery, minimizing the effects of acute and chronic illnesses and disability, and maintaining health" *(Reflections*, 1989). This emphasis on broadly based research was typical during the 1980s. NCNR fellowships have allowed many researchers to conduct studies that directly benefit the clinical practitioner and client. Finally, during the 1980s, Sigma Theta Tau, the international nursing honorary society, began raising funds for the Center for Nursing Scholarship, which includes the International Nursing Library. The center, along with the NCNR, should provide a firm foundation for nursing research in the future.

NURSING RESEARCH IN THE 1990s

Several developments reinforce the importance of nursing research in the 1990s. As health care settings and the nurse's role become more diverse, research is needed to document the efficiency and cost-effectiveness of the various modes of health care delivery. Funding for nursing research, particularly research dealing with preventive health care, is expected to increase. As the focus on promoting and maintaining health, rather than treating disease, gains support, additional funds to examine the effectiveness of preventive strategies will be needed. Research in nursing education will also be important in the 1990s, especially as traditional lecture and laboratory instruction is replaced by alternative methodologies using computer-assisted instruction, distance learning, and student-directed learning. Research on the effectiveness of these methods of instruction will be important to ensure that money allocated for nursing education is properly spent. Culture-related research ranging from studies on the different effects of drugs on clients from various racial groups to investigations into the relations between culture and nutrition will be of significance.

Research into ethical dilemmas will become important as families and clients explore options for care termination, refusal of foods and fluids, and euthanasia. Several propositions have already appeared on state ballots that would allow physicians to help terminally ill clients to end their lives. California Proposition 161, which failed in 1992, would have allowed terminally ill, competent adult clients to sign a directive allowing the attending physician to terminate their lives. Qualitative research may provide information on how to better understand the needs of terminally ill clients and to better support them during the final phases of life.

SCIENTIFIC METHOD AND RESEARCH

Scientific methodology and the research process provide a way of observing nature, drawing conclusions from observations, and testing those conclusions to determine their accuracy. Like the nursing process—assessment, planning, diagnosis, intervention, and evaluation—the scientific method and the research process are structured to allow decisions based on empirical observations and rational deductions and to provide a series of steps by which a problem or phenomena can be studied. The scientific method consists of the following steps:

1. Identify the problem.

2. Collect information.

3. Formulate a hypothesis or statement of belief about the problem.

4. Design an experiment to test the belief.

5. Test the hypothesis.

6. Generalize from the test results.

7. Test the generalization.

Steps 1 and 2 resemble the assessment step in the nursing process. Step 3 resembles the diagnosis step. Steps 4 and 5 are similar to the intervention step, the difference being that the nurse engages in a client care activity, whereas the researcher engages in an experiment. The final steps in the scientific method resemble the nursing process evaluation step; in each case, the results of the previous steps are evaluated, and conclusions are drawn.

The research process more comfortably fits the model used by quantitative researchers who rely on experimentation and the collection of quantitative data. Like the scientific method, the research process begins with a problem description and then sets out the steps the researcher will take in performing the study or experiment.

1. State the problem. The researcher clearly defines the problem to be studied. For example, a nurse researcher may be interested in whether a needle-recapping device reduces the incidence of needle sticks when needles need recapping. The problem is to determine whether fewer needle sticks occur when using the new device compared with standard practice.

2. Review the literature. The researcher refers to published studies in nursing, medicine, and other fields to determine what is already known about the problem and what other research has been done. This step can save time and prevent duplication of effort.

3. Develop the theoretical framework. A theoretical framework for research helps to ensure that the research design is appropriate and that findings can be linked with other nursing knowledge. For example, a theory that includes the concept of self-care might provide an appropriate foundation for a study on needle stick prevention.

4. Identify variables. The researcher identifies the variables that will be studied. In the needle stick study, an important variable would be the use or nonuse of the needle-recapping device.

5. Form a hypothesis. The researcher develops a hypothesis related to the problem or phenomena under study. The researcher conducting a needle stick study might hypothesize that using the needle-recapping device will result in fewer needle sticks when compared with other recapping strategies.

6. Select a research design. A researcher can design an experiment in many ways, depending on the things to be observed, the measurement methods, and whether or not an actual treatment is involved. The research design, however, must fit the study because an inappropriate design can lead to inaccurate or inappropriate conclusions. The researcher studying the needle-recapping device might use a design involving experimental and control groups.

7. Collect data. The researcher collects data related to the study or experiment. The researcher of the needle-recapping device study might collect data on the ages, work experience, and education level of the nurses involved in the study and on the results of the experiment. The researcher would also record the number of recappings that occurred in the two groups and the number of needle sticks in each group.

8. Analyze data. The way in which the researcher analyzes data depends on the type of data collected. In the needle-recapping study, the researcher could determine the average age, experience, and education of the nurses involved and whether the outcomes in the two groups were similar or the number of needle sticks was significantly different from one group to the other. This latter analysis would involve a statistical test to see whether the differences were attributable to the needle-recapping device or merely to chance.

9. Present findings. The researcher reports the study results. For example, having completed the study on the needle-recapping device, the researcher may report that the average age of the nurses in the two groups was 36 years. The researcher might also have found that both groups displayed a similar range of experience, from 1 to 20 years, and that 75% of the nurses had associate degrees and 25% had baccalaureate degrees.

10. Interpret findings. The researcher draws conclusions. If the nurses using the needle-recapping device had a much lower incidence of needle sticks, the researcher might recommend its use. The researcher might also have analyzed the relation between nursing experience and the incidence of needle sticks in both groups. Having found that nurses with more experience had fewer incidents of needle sticks, the researcher might conclude that experience is an important factor in preventing needle sticks. Such a conclusion could affect future training and supervision of new nurses.

RESEARCH DESIGNS

To read research reports and apply the findings to clinical practice, nurses must understand the main types of research designs used. This section describes three types of quantitative designs and two qualitative designs. The quantitative designs are experimental, quasi-experimental, and nonex-

RESEARCH PROCESS

- *State the problem*
- *Review the literature*
- *Develop the theoretical framework*
- *Identify variables*
- *Form a hypothesis*
- *Select a research design*
- *Collect data*
- *Analyze data*
- *Present findings*
- *Interpret findings*

perimental. Phenomenology and ethnography are discussed as examples of qualitative research designs.

Of the quantitative designs, the experimental is the most rigorously controlled; the nonexperimental is the least controlled. Control refers to the extent to which the quantitative researcher can direct components of the experiment; the more controlled a research design is, the less likely that chance factors can affect the outcome.

EXPERIMENTAL DESIGNS
Experimental designs have three characteristics:
- Two groups—the control group and the experimental group—are used; the experimental group receives the treatment and the control group does not.
- Subjects are randomly assigned to groups to help ensure comparability between groups.
- The researcher manipulates the independent variable; that is, the experimental group receives the treatment or intervention after which the response of the two groups is compared.

QUASI-EXPERIMENTAL DESIGNS
When it is not possible to use a purely experimental design, a quasi-experimental design might be used. This type of design differs from the experimental design in that one of the three elements listed above is missing. For example, researchers may decide to use volunteers to make up the experimental group. Because this group may differ from the comparison group, the non-experimental group is often referred to as the non-equivalent control group. The weakness of this design is that the two groups may differ substantially in ways that could influence the outcome of the experiment. Although researchers can compare specific variables, such as age, sex, marital status, and other significant factors, they cannot assume that other characteristics will be randomly distributed among the subjects in the two groups.

Another quasi-experimental design uses no control group. The researcher measures some parameter within an experimental group before a treatment and again afterward. This pretest-post-test design gives some indication of the treatment's effect; however, without the use of a control group, the researcher cannot with certainty conclude that the treatment caused the effect observed. For example, a nurse is studying the effects of a presurgery video teaching program on a group of clients without the benefit of a control group. If all the clients report that they were relaxed and well prepared for their surgeries, the researchers might conclude that the video teaching program had produced these effects. In fact, additional attention paid to these clients may have produced their positive feelings. Without a control group to provide comparison, the researcher cannot say for certain what caused the client effects.

Another quasi-experimental design called a time series also lacks a control group but uses the treatment group itself as a sort of control. Researchers take a number of measurements before and after treatment so that they can more accurately evaluate the actual effect of the intervention. For example, a researcher interested in the effects of a teaching program on stress reduction might measure stress levels in participants at regular intervals over a 4-week period before the teaching program. The researcher could then make a similar series of measurements after the teaching program. If the stress level is significantly higher during the preteaching period and significantly lower during a comparable post-teaching period, the researcher may with some certainty, suggest that the teaching program had beneficial effects.

NONEXPERIMENTAL DESIGNS

Nonexperimental research designs provide even less control than the quasi-experimental designs and are used only when the researcher cannot control the variable of interest. For example, a nurse researcher might want to learn what effect the loss of a sibling has on children's anxiety upon admission to the pediatric unit. The nurse cannot manipulate the loss nor randomly assign clients to groups. The nurse can, however, compare the responses of the two naturally occurring groups—those who have experienced loss and those who have not—to determine response differences. This type of nonexperimental design is called "ex post facto," or "after the fact" research. The weakness of this design is that other causes for the difference may go undetected by the researchers.

PHENOMENOLOGY

Unlike quantitative designs, which attempt to control the variables measured and the way in which the experiment proceeds, the qualitative designs maximize the number of variables observed and provide for subjective data interpretation rather than statistical analysis.

One quantitative design, phenomenology, aims "to describe the experience as it is lived by people" (Munhall and Oiler, 1986). Riemen's work is an example of phenomenological research that focuses on subjects' perceptions of others' actions. Riemen (1986) selected 10 clients 18 years or older who were able to communicate their experiences. After gaining their consent, Riemen asked the clients to respond to five items and tape-recorded their answers. Items included:

1. Describe a personal interaction you have had with a registered nurse whom you thought was caring.

2. Try to describe how you felt in that interaction.

3. Describe an interaction you have had with a registered nurse whom you thought was noncaring.

4. Try to describe how you felt during that interaction.

5. Do not stop until you believe that you have discussed your feelings as completely as possible.

Having obtained responses from the 10 subjects, Riemen looked for significant statements and meanings. She identified theme clusters and noted similarities and differences among the respondents. Finally, Riemen attempted to describe as exhaustively as possible the experiences of clients as they received treatment from caring and noncaring registered nurses. By sharing the information with the subjects themselves, Riemen was able to confirm the experiences and conclude that the clients who experienced caring were those who believed that their nurses had genuine regard and interest in them, were available to them, and had listened to their concerns.

The phenomenological approach focuses on the perceptions of subject and validates the findings of the study by having the themes that emerge confirmed by the individuals themselves. Generalizing from such studies may be harder to do than with quantitative studies, but replications of the qualitative study with other groups can provide evidence of its implications for other patients.

ETHNOGRAPHY

Cultural anthropologists who want to describe the characteristics of a particular group of people may use an ethnographic approach. The researcher becomes part of the culture being investigated, as either an observer, a participant-observer, or a fellow participant. Madeline Leininger (1985), using an ethnographic approach that she termed "ethnonursing research," lived 10 months among rural blacks and whites in central Alabama. She wanted to study the health care beliefs and values of these people from their own perspective and to identify how their health care practices differed from urban health care practices. During the 10 months, Leininger observed the customs and living habits of the residents and interviewed 90 subjects. Based on her findings, Leininger was able to determine that the people in this culture conceived of health as "being able to do your work in the home, church, and community" (Leininger, 1985). She also demonstrated the important role religion played in maintaining the spiritual and overall health of these people. Leininger's research has significantly affected the way nurses work with rural clients whose definitions of health and illness may differ from those of urban clients.

In phenomenological and ethnographic research, the researcher is more actively involved in the process than is the researcher using traditional quantitative studies. Additionally, the researcher examines the subject of interest, whether it be client conceptions of caring or definitions of health, within its context rather than in isolation.

LEGAL AND ETHICAL CONCERNS IN RESEARCH

To protect research subjects, educational and health care institutions have established research protocols and procedures. These protocols and controls are based on research codes developed in the aftermath of World War II during the Nuremberg Tribunal. The code was a response to the unethical research conducted by the Nazis on prisoners. The code included the following stipulations:

1. Voluntary consent of the human subject is essential.

2. Experiments should be so designed and based on the results of animal experimentation and knowledge of the natural history of the disease or other problems that the anticipated results will justify the experiment.

3. The degree of subject risk should never exceed the potential humanitarian importance of the problem to be studied.

4. Through all stages of the experiment, those who conduct or engage in it should exhibit the highest degree of skill and care, and only scientifically qualified people should conduct the experiment.

5. At any time during the course of the experiment, the human subject should be at liberty to end participation in the experiment.

6. The scientist in charge must be prepared to terminate the experiment at any stage if the scientist has any probable cause to believe that continuing the experiment is likely to result in injury, disability, or the death of the subject (LoBiondo-Wood and Haber, 1986).

Formal, informed consent is as important in research as it is in client treatment. The researcher should inform the subject about the conditions of participation, including any entailed risks. Usually, a written consent form describes the reasons for undertaking the study, the benefits that will result, the responsibilities of the participating subject and the researcher, and the degree to which anonymity or confidentiality is guaranteed. The consent form also states that participation is voluntary and that the client has the right to withdraw from the study at any time. The institution with which the researcher is affiliated or the one in which the research is conducted usually oversees the consent and approval process. Occasionally, if the institutions are different, both must sanction the approval.

During the 1960s, the World Medical Association in the Helsinki Declaration developed further medical research guidelines. The Helsinki Declaration differentiates between research directly designed to have therapeutic value for clients and that designed to build a basic knowledge base. The Helsinki Declaration states that researchers must clearly communicate the expected self-benefit to subjects before asking for their consent to participate.

The ANA issued *Guidelines for the Investigative Function of Nurses* in 1981 and *Human Rights Guidelines for Nurses in Clinical and Other Research* in 1985. These documents stress the importance of securing informed subject consent that ensures confidentiality or anonymity and provides for voluntary withdrawal without penalty at any point during the study. The documents also protect specific populations, such as young and institutionalized clients as well as those mentally unable to make decisions for themselves, to ensure that their rights are protected.

SCIENTIFIC MISCONDUCT

The National Institutes for Health defines scientific misconduct as fabrication, falsification, plagiarism, or other practices that seriously deviate from those that are commonly accepted within the scientific community for proposing, conducting, or reporting research. It does not include honest error or honest differences in interpretations or judgments (U.S. Department of Health and Human Services, 1989).

Despite safeguards such as the ANA guidelines, instances of scientific misconduct do occur. Hawley and Jeffers (1992) describe multiple examples of data falsification, record alteration, and plagiarism in scientific research. Although nurses have not been involved in any published scientific misconduct incidents, the authors suggest that nurses must be aware of the dangers of such conduct and that nurse researcher socialization should include specific ethical training.

Reasons for scientific misconduct include pressures to publish to receive tenure at educational institutions and pressures to obtain grants and other funding. Hawley and Jeffers (1992) recommend three proactive steps to ensure that nurse researchers are assisted to avoid scientific misconduct:

- careful socialization of new researchers
- adjustment of tenure and promotion guidelines
- increased number of replication studies.

Young researchers should understand that data falsification and plagiarism of another's work are unethical and unprofessional. By creating reasonable expectations concerning publication, educational institutions can create an environment in which meaningful, ethical research can be conducted. Finally, by promoting replication studies, both accidental error and falsification can be detected and corrected.

NURSING RESPONSIBILITIES IN ASSISTING WITH RESEARCH

Not all nurses become researchers, but almost all become involved in some way in nursing research. Nurses identify conditions and problems that suggest the need for research. They also help to evaluate and expand nursing research by applying the findings to other settings.

Other nurses care for clients who are subjects in research studies. In these circumstances, the nurses must have a thorough understanding of the research project and its protocols to avoid invalidating the study. Nurses who are to care for research subjects usually receive instruction related to client safety and the integrity of the research process.

To care for clients who are research subjects and to understand published research, the nurse must understand certain potential threats to the integrity of a research study.

These threats to integrity include measurement errors and the subject variables maturation, testing, history, selection, and mortality (see *Sources of Research Errors*, page 436).

MEASUREMENT ERROR

Measurement error results from the incorrect reading of a parameter under investigation. Vital signs (temperature, blood pressure, pulse, and respiratory rates) are often important research parameters. If certain protocols are not observed when the readings are taken, the nurse may unintentionally allow differences that may affect the validity of the study. Usually, the nurse receives specific guidelines for taking measurements.

Using faulty or outdated equipment and supplies can also lead to measurement error; however, experimental protocols usually require a premeasurement equipment check. Other environmental factors can hamper accurate measurement; for example, temperature and humidity can affect the action of chemical reagent strips.

To avoid measurement errors, nurses caring for research project subjects can identify potential sources of measurement error and vigilantly follow research protocols for taking and recording measurements.

SUBJECT VARIABLES

Subject variables, or characteristics associated with the subjects themselves, can also threaten the integrity of a research study. Subject variables include maturation, testing, history, selection, and mortality.

Maturation refers to an individual's growth and development. It becomes a research problem when an observed effect is the result of normal growth rather than of some independent variable. Researchers working with pediatric clients in long-term studies usually discuss maturation effects in their findings; the researchers must determine whether maturation has affected the variable in question and, if so, describe how the phenomenon was isolated or accounted for.

SOURCES OF RESEARCH ERRORS

Despite the best intentions of careful researchers, errors and extraneous factors can mar a study and make its results questionable. Nurses knowledgeable about sources of error and threats to research integrity can help minimize the likelihood of such errors.

Measurement errors
- *Errors resulting from incorrect instrument readings caused by failure to adhere to research protocols*
- *Errors resulting from faulty equipment*

Subject variables
- *Maturation: variation resulting from natural growth and development*
- *Testing: variation resulting from familiarity with the testing situation*
- *History: variation resulting from extraneous events occurring at the same time the study is under way*
- *Selection: variation resulting from the way in which groups are formed*
- *Mortality: variation resulting from the loss of subjects from one group or another*

Because *testing* itself can produce change, it can threaten the integrity of a research study. For example, a study of stress may require that subjects respond to a questionnaire. If the researcher uses the same question each time, the subject, who has already completed the questionnaire several times, may begin to respond less spontaneously and perhaps less accurately.

History refers to events happening in the subject's environment. These events can affect the subject's responses. For example, if the questionnaire evaluating stress were administered on a day when other events occurred—another client's death in an adjacent bed, a fire drill, a disruptive family visit—the subject's response may reflect stress caused by the immediate event and not long-term stress.

Selection refers to the bias that can unwittingly characterize groups used for comparison purposes. For example, if the researcher wanted to evaluate stress in hospitalized clients and wanted to know if private rooms decreased stress, the researcher might simply compare those who were admitted to private rooms with those who were admitted to semiprivate rooms. By doing so, the researcher might introduce bias into the groups. Those admitted to private rooms may be more affluent and have fewer monetary worries and, consequently, less stress than those admitted to semiprivate wards. On the other hand, the clients selecting semiprivate rooms may be more gregarious and relieve stress by visiting and talking with other clients. The best way to ensure that the groups to be compared are not affected by bias is to assign subjects to groups randomly. If this is not possible, the researcher should carefully evaluate the groups to ensure that they are similar in all important respects, including age, sex, ethnicity, socioeconomic group, and other factors significant to the study.

Mortality refers to the loss of subjects from a study. Subjects may die, no longer meet the qualifications for inclusion, or choose to exercise their right to withdraw. In a study of breast-feeding mothers, subjects could be lost because of fetal demise or because they changed their minds and decided to bottle-feed. If qualified research subjects failed to return a questionnaire, the researcher would have to drop them from the study.

As the number of subjects decreases, the researcher's degree of certainty also decreases. This is especially true in quantitative research methodologies. Researchers usually report the number of subjects lost to a study and describe any related impact on data analysis.

USING NURSING RESEARCH IN PRACTICE

This chapter should help the nurse understand the research process, research terminology, and the various ways in which research can be conducted. Too frequently, however, nursing research has little impact on nursing practice. To combat this unfortunate result and to increase the use of published research, nurses can read nursing journals, participate in research discussion groups, and work to create institutional support for nursing research.

READING NURSING JOURNALS

Some research articles seem unnecessarily complex, and their application to clinical nursing unclear. To help correct this problem, nursing researchers are attempting to demystify research and to present findings in clear, understandable language. Researchers are also more carefully describing the implications of their research results for clinical practice, future research, and theory development.

Many beginning readers of nursing research reports find starting with the abstract, which briefly describes the study and expected outcomes, helpful. They then can read the sections dealing with findings and implications. With an understanding of research terms such as *probability* and *level of significance*, the nurse should be able to understand the outcomes of a study without having an advanced background in statistics.

After reading the abstract and concluding sections of the report, the nurse can review the remainder of the article with a more complete understanding. The nurse should note the conditions under which the research was conducted; an outcome in one clinical setting may not necessarily occur in another, especially if environmental factors are not similar.

PARTICIPATING IN NURSING JOURNAL CLUBS

Forming a journal club within a hospital or health care agency can help nurses wanting to better understand and apply research findings. The group may enlist the aid of a clinical nurse specialist or nursing faculty member who can provide assistance in understanding research strategies or statistical analyses. The journal clubs can meet on a regular basis to discuss research articles of mutual interest; at such meetings, nurses can share information, ask and answer questions, and examine the study's implications for personal nursing practice. Members seek to apply the information to their own client care and report their experiences to the group.

INSTITUTIONAL SUPPORT FOR NURSING RESEARCH

Krouse and Holloran (1992) point out that institutional support for nursing research depends on availability of adequate resources and services. However, they also suggest that nursing research is no longer considered "an elite segment of the discipline, but rather. . . a component integral to everyday practice" (Krouse and Holloran, 1992). The authors suggest that all nurses, from the nurse manager to the bedside practitioner, should understand the contribution research can make.

Institutions can foster support by setting up continuing education programs, including those that focus on research methodology and others that focus on communicating the results of completed research. Institutions can also support staff participation in research conferences as a way to create interest in and appreciation for research and to demonstrate the value of nurses engaging in research.

In health care institutions too small to have a research department or a position devoted to nursing research, Krouse and Holloran (1992) suggest four ways to encourage research:

1. Identify where nurses interested in conducting research can obtain help. Nurses may collaborate with faculty or researchers from a local university or college who can help develop the research design, select data collection instruments, and analyze data.

2. Identify valuable library resources, both within the institution and without. Library resources of other health care institutions, which can often be accessed on a reciprocal basis, can enhance the amount of materials available for use.

3. Identify the availability of computer support for data processing. Institutions may make computers available to nurses on off-peak hours, evenings, or weekends.

4. Identify ways to develop seed money for research. A fund with sufficient money to cover costs of photocopying, travel, postage, and supplies can help to launch a small pilot project, which can then be used as the basis for a larger grant proposal. Collaborating with nursing faculty who have expertise in proposal development and grant writing can also be helpful (Krouse and Holloran, 1992).

SUMMARY

This chapter provided an overview of nursing research, beginning with a description of basic and applied research, and the different approaches embodied by quantitative and qualitative research. The various levels of nursing research include descriptive, exploratory, and explanatory research as well as research aimed at prediction and control. The chapter traced the historical development of nursing research and compared the research method with the scientific method. It then reviewed the legal and ethical requirements for research, including the importance of socializing young researchers to the dangers of scientific misconduct. The chapter concluded with nursing responsibilities in assisting with and using nursing research, along with ways to promote acceptance and use of research in clinical nursing practice.

APPLICATION EXERCISE

With the assistance of your instructor, identify a nursing research article in an area that interests you. Use the following questions to help guide and organize your analysis.

1. What does the research address? Is the problem clearly stated early in the article?

2. What is known about the problem? Do the researchers thoroughly review the literature, including already discovered findings? Does the research build on that of others?

3. How does the problem fit into the whole of nursing knowledge? Do the researchers provide a conceptual framework for the study?

4. If the study is quantitative, do the researchers identify the dependent and independent variables? If the study is qualitative, do the researchers identify topics of investigation?

5. What are the researchers' hypotheses?

6. How is the research structured? Do the researchers identify the research design they are using? Have the researchers overlooked factors that may threaten the integrity of the study? How were research subjects selected? Does the selection method seem appropriate?

7. How was data collected? What things did the researchers measure? Was voluntary subject consent and withdrawal guaranteed?

8. How was the data analyzed?

9. What does the study reveal?

REVIEW QUESTIONS

1. How does basic research differ from applied research?

2. What are the main differences between quantitative and qualitative research designs?

3. Compare the four levels of nursing research.

4. What are the steps in the research process?

5. Contrast the three quantitative research designs (experimental, quasi-experimental, nonexperimental).

6. Compare phenomenology and ethnography.

7. What are the ethical and legal expectations for nurses involved in research?

8. How can nurses use nursing research more effectively in practice?

REFERENCES

American Nurses' Association, Commission on Nursing Research. *Guidelines for the Investigative Function of Nurses.* Kansas City, Mo.: American Nurses' Association, 1981.

American Nurses' Association. *Human Rights Guidelines for Nurses in Clinical and Other Research*. Kansas City, Mo.: American Nurses' Association, 1985.

Bristoll, S.L., et al. "The Mythical Danger of Rapid Urinary Drainage," *American Journal of Nursing* 89(3):344-345, 1989.

Brown, E.L. *Nursing for the Future*. New York: Russell Sage, 1948.

Hughes, E.C. *Twenty Thousand Nurses Tell Their Story*. Philadelphia: J.B. Lippincott Co., 1958.

Krouse, H.J., and Holloran, S.D. "Nurse Managers and Clinical Nursing Research," *Nursing Management* 23(7):62-66, July, 1992.

LoBiondo-Wood, G., and Haber, J. *Nursing Research: Principles and Methods*. Philadelphia: J.B. Lippincott Co., 1986.

Munhall, P. and Oiler, C. *Nursing Research: A Qualitative Perspective*. East Norwalk, Conn.: Appleton-Century-Crofts, 1986.

National Commission for the Study of Nursing and Nursing Education. "Summary Report and Recommendations." American Journal of Nursing 70:279, February 1970.

Riemen, D.J. "The Essential Structure of a Caring Interaction; Doing Phenomenology." In *Nursing Research: A Qualitative Perspective*. Edited by Munhall, P., and Oiler, C. East Norwalk, Conn.: Appleton-Century-Crofts, 1986.

Rentschler, D.D. "Correlates of Successful Breast-feeding," *Image* 23(3):151-154, Fall 1991.

Sharp, N. "$40 Million for Nursing Research: Is It Enough?" *Nursing Management* 22(2):22-23, February 1991.

Strauss, A., and Corbin, J. *Basics of Qualitative Research*. Newbury Park, Calif.: Sage Publications, 1990.

U.S. Department of Health and Human Services. "Responsibilities of Awardee and Applicant Institutions for Dealing with and Reporting Possible Misconduct in Science," *National Institutes of Health Guide* 18, Washington, D.C., Government Printing Office, 1989.

RECOMMENDATIONS FOR FURTHER STUDY

Bull, M.J. "Using Qualitative Methods in Teaching Undergraduate Students Research," Nursing and Health Care 13(7):378-381, September 1992.

Mariano, C. "Qualitative Research," *Nursing and Health Care* 11(7):354-359, 1991.

14

NURSING AS A DEVELOPING PROFESSION

OBJECTIVES

After studying this chapter, the reader should be able to:

1. Define the concept of paradigm shift, and explain why detecting significant social and technological changes can be difficult.

2. Describe changes in nursing's professional paradigm.

3. Describe developments in nursing education.

4. Describe changes in nursing research, particularly in non-acute-care settings.

5. Discuss the five changes that the American Organization of Nurse Executives (AONE) predicts will occur in health care delivery.

6. Describe why cultural awareness will become increasingly important for nurses in the next decade.

7. Discuss the impact of new management techniques such as total quality management (TQM) and continuous quality improvement (CQI) on acute-care and non-acute-care nursing settings.

8. Describe how the political realignment of the 1990s will affect the nurse's role.

9. Identify recent changes in nursing organizations and describe their implications.

10. Describe your personal and professional development, and identify goals you would like to achieve within 5-year and 10-year periods.

INTRODUCTION

Nursing, like health care in general, is in a state of rapid transition. Changes in health care delivery, technology and information systems, and the ways nurses interact with clients, employers, and one another are occurring at an accelerated pace as the end of the century approaches. Nurses are already directing their attention to the 21st century and the ways in which client and practitioner needs can be met.

Earlier chapters described the essential tools and components of professional performance. They discussed communication and interpersonal relations; the theoretical basis of nursing practice and research; nursing's organizational structure; the health care delivery system; cultural, legal, and ethical considerations for nursing practice; and the nurse's role as teacher, leader, decision-maker, change agent, and researcher.

This chapter begins by discussing paradigms, their usefulness and the problems they can cause, and how shifting paradigms can facilitate acceptance of required changes. The chapter then describes the status of the nursing profession and the evolutionary and revolutionary changes occurring within it. The chapter also reviews nursing education and its future. It concludes by identifying the challenges and opportunities that nurses will confront in research, politics, and professional organizations.

PARADIGM SHIFTS

Previous chapters have discussed concepts, models, and theories that nurses can use to help them structure and view reality. Such reality structures, called paradigms, can provide an integrated and comprehensive approach to work and life. However, because these paradigms form a screen through which information must filter, they sometimes make the reception of new information difficult. In other words, individuals using a particular paradigm may have trouble accepting information that does not fit the paradigm in question.

Paradigm shifts in business are numerous. Huey (1991) describes the shift that occurred when Ray Kroc opened the first McDonald's restaurant and changed the way many people around the world eat. Huey also points out that individuals implementing such changes are sometimes viewed as impractical or unrealistic. Fred Smith, who established Federal Express, was told by his Yale professors that his idea for package delivery was "stupid." Ted Turner, when developing Cable News Network, was widely looked on as a crackpot whose vision of a satellite television network that continuously broadcast nothing but news was doomed to failure.

Paradigm shifts in politics can cause drastic changes in how we perceive the world. The political paradigm through which much of the world viewed international relations recently underwent a radical change with the reunification of Germany and the dissolution of the Soviet Union. With these two changes, the cold war paradigm was made obsolete, and a new paradigm began to evolve in its place.

Individuals can usually detect drastic changes, regardless of the paradigm being used. More gradual changes can be much harder to detect, even though they may be equally important. Today, the gradual but persistent change in the way workers accomplish their tasks represents an important paradigm shift. Drucker (1989) describes the development of the "knowledge worker," the professional whose knowledge makes him or her a specialist in a particular discipline and whose relationship with management and other workers has changed from the traditional worker-boss relationship. Drucker predicts that in the future, highly skilled workers will organize their own responsibilities and accomplish work through collaborative effort. These workers will be loyal not to the business or company but to their profession. In nursing, the emergence of shared governance structures represents a paradigm shift from the old, hierarchical way of doing business. Such changes influence the way nurses view one another and their profession.

NURSING AS A PROFESSION

In the traditional nursing paradigm, the nurse is the physician's handmaiden, the loyal subordinate dedicated to working for the clients' benefit under the watchful direction of administrators who make decisions about health care delivery. Drucker (1989) describes a newer, developing paradigm in which the nurse exists as a professional with a unique body of knowledge and independent responsibilities to clients, a nurse whose allegiance is not to an employer but to the nursing profession.

According to Shein and Kommers (1972), a profession has:

- a body of knowledge on which performance is based
- the ability to deliver a unique service to others
- a standardized education based in the collegiate setting
- control over practice standards
- members who are accountable and responsible for their own practice
- the career commitment of its members
- the independent function of its members.

Recent changes in nursing are moving the profession towards this definition. At the same time, the paradigm of "profession" is also undergoing change. Concepts of shared decision making at all levels emphasize the collaborative approach to practice, whether it involves clients, fellow nurses, physicians, or employers. Nurses in the future will retain individual responsibility for their actions but will exercise that responsibility in a much more collaborative way.

NURSING EDUCATION

As the nursing profession is changing, so, too, is nursing education. Although three traditional and separate educational programs—associate degree, diploma, and baccalaureate degree—exist to prepare students for licensure, greater articulation is developing among the programs, along with a clearer delineation of the distinctions and interrelations among them. Students are also becoming more able to move from one level to another.

Larson (1992) describes how the faculty from Augustana College, the University of South Dakota, and nursing leaders at Sioux Valley Hospital have developed a differentiated practice model in which students at the associate and baccalaureate levels care for clients in the clinical setting. Called the "Healing Web" model, this approach to education and health care delivery relies on a curriculum based on the concept of caring and is endorsed by each of the participating institutions and individual members. Within this structure, students at both levels develop a mutual respect and understanding of the differences between the two levels in terms of preparation and role. According to Larson, each nurse's role is differentiated not in terms of importance but in terms of function in overall collaborative care. The associate degree role and baccalaureate role are distinguished as follows:

- *Time frame:* The associate role focuses primarily upon the activities performed during the shift worked, whereas the baccalaureate role focuses on events leading to the illness and the needs remaining at discharge.
- *Interpersonal scope/focus:* The associate role focuses on resolving problems and issues that arise from daily activities of client care and on reporting complex problems. The baccalaureate role is concerned with developing solutions to complex problems, implementing refined skills in confrontation, and negotiating and resolving issues.
- *Structure:* The associate role is conducted in a structured setting with established policies and is supported by a full range of services and providers. The baccalaureate role supports the associate role but may also be conducted in unstructured settings without well-defined policies.
- *Orientation to lifelong learning:* The associate role is oriented to maintaining competencies necessary for the actions and outcomes. The baccalaureate role is additionally oriented to mastering the expanding body of knowledge for use in planning and integrating client care.

Researchers will assess the effects of this integrated educational model, illustrating yet another change in nursing's educational paradigm: the use of well-structured research focused on the effectiveness of educational methodologies. Such research will enable pilot projects, such as the Healing Web, to evaluate effectiveness, while allowing for effective dispersal of methodologies to other educational settings.

The increased articulation between associate degree programs and baccalaureate programs in many states allows nurses to move more easily from one professional level to another. This development represents a paradigm shift from the older education model in which each level was considered separate and nonrelated. Educators now acknowledge that an individual may have multiple career changes during a lifetime and that facilitating change within the nursing profession is both logical and imperative. They also understand that removing unnecessary barriers and artificial distinctions will help attract the diverse practitioners that nursing needs.

The AONE, joining with the American Association of Colleges of Nursing, the American Nurses' Association (ANA), and the National League for Nursing (NLN), has called for reform of the nursing educational system. "Not only must the educational system for tomorrow's students be reformed, but also the degree completion programs for the thousands of currently employed registered nurses working in acute care hospitals" (Lopresti and Whetstone, 1993). Pressing issues include the differentiation of nursing practice roles to match consumers' needs and the providers' competencies, the inclusion in all curricula of primary care processes and skills, the integration of structures and systems information, the inclusion of an economic framework as part of all delivery decisions, the initiation and enhancement of interdisciplinary collaboration, and a curriculum to support multiple non-physician providers in all health care settings.

Other nursing education issues that will continue to be important include specialization versus generalization and the master of science in nursing (MSN) degree as the entry point for professional practice. The degree to which basic nursing education should prepare students for practice in a specialty area varies widely from school to school and from area to area. In rural areas, where associate degree graduates may fill most nursing and management positions in a given health care setting, schools have tended to provide a comprehensive education, including orientation to specialty areas and to leadership and management concepts. In other areas, specialization is seen as the province of the master's-level nurse. Some advocate the MSN degree for entry-level professional practice, arguing that only preparation at that level allows the nurse to function effectively alongside physicians and other health care providers. Increased emphasis on computer use and nursing informatics in general can be expected at all educational levels. The rapidly proliferating body of knowledge, all of which cannot possibly be taught during a normal education, makes the ability to obtain knowledge even more important.

TRANSITION FROM EDUCATION TO PRACTICE

Preparing the nursing student for the realities of the workplace is also becoming more important. Reality shock—finding that nursing school values and goals are not necessarily those found in practice—still concerns educators and employers. The student who has focused on providing the highest-quality client care to a select group of clients may be deeply disconcerted when confronting a routine client care load. Students will find less time to provide care, more clients to care for, and multiple non-nursing responsibilities from which they may have been shielded.

Students may react to reality shock in several ways: They may disavow the values of the academic setting, feeling that such values are unrealistic; they may reject the values of the new environment and become disillusioned with nursing; or they may make a sensible transition to the workplace, recognizing the constraints of normal practice and continuing to strive for their ideals.

A nursing internship can help ease the transition from school to practice. Usually occurring during the student's final semester, the nursing internship places the student in a client care setting under the direct supervision of a registered nurse preceptor. (Preceptors receive special training in supporting student interns and in aiding the transition to the practice.) Although the clinical instructor remains responsible for overall supervision, the student is able to assume responsibilities (supported by the preceptor) that are similar to those of a beginning registered nurse. As students gain experience, they assume more responsibilities until their practice approaches, as nearly as possible, that of the practicing registered nurse.

The work-study program is another strategy for easing the transition from school to practice. Although work-study programs are not new, recent modifications have prove successful in reducing student anxiety about work and in developing skill competency (Borland et al. 1991). Students in work-study programs are employed by a health care agency and paid a wage; at the same time, they are registered in a nursing class, usually on a credit-no credit basis. As with the student internship, a nursing faculty member has overall responsibility for setting up the work-study format and for assisting the student to negotiate goals and expectations, and a specially prepared registered nurse preceptor directly supervises the student. Borland et al. (1991) found that students who participated in work-study programs during the summer before their final year of school displayed more confidence and better clinical skills than did their colleagues. In addition, hospital evaluations of new employees suggest that students participating in work-study programs have less difficulty making the transition from student to practicing nurse and make more rapid progress as new employees.

After finding that new nurses frequently felt frustrated because they couldn't seem to perform at a satisfactory level, the nursing staff at Bryan Memorial Hospital undertook a study of nurse managers' expectations of new graduates (Butts and Witmer, 1992). They developed a list of critical behaviors that managers identified as essential to competent performance and compared this list with the skills and knowledge new nurses were exposed to during their 90-day orientation. In general, the Bryan Memorial Hospital staff discovered that they were covering the topics the nurse managers expected. They also found that personal support was necessary for new nurses' success. Such support could include mentoring by more experienced nurses, support groups for new nurses headed by an experienced leader, and careful cultivation of the nurse's role in the institution. This study suggests that in addition to communicating clear expectations to new graduates, health care agencies should develop a system of personal and professional support for new graduates.

NURSING RESEARCH

Nursing research will continue to concentrate on client care issues but will increasingly focus on settings outside the acute-care area. Albrecht (1992) states that "in the 21st century the home may become the center of care as [clients] are discharged from the hospital 'quicker and sicker.'" Albrecht (1992) identifies these priorities for nursing research related to home settings:

- *Care outcomes:* What is the result of care provided in non-acute settings? How do outcomes compare with those in acute settings? How does quality of life compare?
- *Home care costs:* What is the cost of delivering care in non-acute settings compared with that in acute-care settings?
- *Policy analysis:* What policies should guide health care delivery, particularly to underserved populations? What role does direct reimbursement of nurses play?
- *Client classification systems:* What is the validity of client acuity systems and case load measures? How reliable are they?
- *Nature of information to be collected regarding client care:* What is the minimum client information that should be collected to assist in nursing research?
- *Predictors of care and managed care:* What are the best predictors of care need in certain settings? What role does

nursing diagnosis and client classification play in predicting needs?

- *Coordination of care and managed care:* How can continuity of care be better provided for through managed care, case management, and other care systems? What has been the impact of diagnosis-related groups on care?
- *Productivity:* What is the best way of ensuring maximum productivity? What roles do case mix, management styles, and interdisciplinary methods play?
- *Documentation forms:* What has been the impact of computer-assisted record-keeping? of computer information systems?
- *Use of health care services:* Who are the users of the health care system? Is this effective use? What are unmet needs?

Similar research needs could be compiled for the other health care delivery settings, including outpatient clinics and wellness centers.

NURSING PRACTICE

Nursing practice will continue to implement more collaborative working relationships and shared governance management structures. It will grow in areas outside the acute-care hospital, including nurse-run health care centers, outpatient clinics, and home care settings.

The AONE has identified five important health care delivery changes that it expects will occur in the near future (Lopresti and Whetstone, 1993):

1. Health care delivery will become consumer driven with "tremendous responsibilities placed upon individuals for their own health care behaviors." Emphasis will shift to disease prevention and health promotion.

2. The system will become community-based. The acute-care health facility, no longer the focus of health care, will be part of a broader-based system involving a range of settings and providers.

3. Cultural diversity and technological complexity will increase, and worker expectations will change.

4. Registered nurses and other non-physician providers will be better able to serve as basic health care providers for populations that have traditionally been underserved.

5. The relation between cost and care outcome will be more carefully evaluated.

Nursing care being delivered in the acute-care setting will also change as new techniques and technologies are developed. Nurses will constantly need to evaluate their knowledge level and to seek out opportunities for expanding their knowledge base. Such developments will affect acute-care nursing practice.

For example, Kupper-Grubbs (1992) describes how as organ transplant becomes more common, so do the chances that affected clients will be part of a nurse's routine assignment in the general acute-care setting.

She describes the arrival in the emergency department of a stab wound client. Stab wounds are certainly not infrequent in most large-city emergency departments, but this particular client had an additional complication: He had the year before received kidney and pancreas transplants. Nurses caring for such a client needed to know not only how to care for a stab wound but also how to care for a client who had previously undergone transplant surgery. When faced with such a situation, the nurses had to identify their knowledge needs and quickly ascertain information resources. In this case, immediate resources included the client and the client's family and the transplant center where the surgery had been performed.

In dealing with clients whose care involves new technologies, new procedures, new drugs, or other innovations, nurses must evaluate their knowledge base and promptly request assistance from others, including clinical specialists, clients, and medical centers specializing in the treatment of such clients. As care becomes more complex, knowing how to get an answer becomes more important than having all the answers.

CULTURAL AWARENESS

As the United States becomes culturally and ethnically more diverse, nurses will need to become more aware of the impact such diversity has on health and illness. Pharmacoanthropology, a developing field, has already begun investigating variations in response to drugs based on racial differences (Kudzma, 1992). This is an important development, especially in light of the fact that most clinical trials of drugs are still done in the Western world, primarily on white male subjects. As a result, drugs may be given to clients who exhibit physiologic responses quite different from those of the test subjects. For example, several studies indicate that African American clients may require higher doses of antihypertensive drugs, whereas Asian clients may require lower doses. Other drugs, including psycotrophic drugs, such as alprazolam (Xanax) and haloperidol (Haldol), and antimalarial drugs, such as chloroquine, also appear to have different effects, depending on the client's ethnicity.

Different responses to drugs may be caused by nutrition or genetic variations in the way drugs are processed and eliminated from the body. Both factors may be culturally influenced. Because of these differences and because of the fact that nonwhite groups are not adequately represented in drug trial samples, nurses must become aware of the potentially different responses to commonly given medications.

Women, also, have been historically underrepresented in clinical drug trials and in research studies in general. The Food and Drug Administration and the National Institutes of Health are now more actively reviewing subject selection. New studies focusing on the effects of aspirin, beta-carotene, and vitamin E on heart disease in women are now under way. Nurses must become aware of this type of new research.

In addition to becoming aware of the impact of culture on health care in our own country, nurses should understand its impact on a worldwide basis. The United States and the European Economic Community will be called on to assist other nations in meeting social and political needs. With the dissolution of the Soviet state, the United States remains one of the few countries able to mount large-scale humanitarian efforts such as that begun in 1992 in Somalia to combat starvation and disease.

Researchers in the United States will also be studying health care models in other countries as they develop the health care delivery system necessary for the 21st century. Canada, which has had a national health care system since 1968, may represent an example of how the U.S. structure might evolve. The Canadian system, nonetheless, has definite shortcomings, including long waits for some surgeries and physician domination of basic health care provider roles. Laschinger and McWilliam (1992) point out that the Canadian system, which is positioned between the free enterprise U.S. system and the socialized medicine system of Britain, is moving closer to the American model in some respects; they maintain that Canadian nurse activists are seeking many of the same reforms being called for by U.S. nurses. The advantages of Canada's public insurance model, which provides for health care to all citizens, is undeniable; the cost of the Canadian system, at 8.6% of the gross national product, compares favorably with the more than 12% spent in the United States. Many problems, however, remain to be addressed before any such system can be implemented in this country.

In 1987, the World Health Organization (WHO) targeted the year 2000 as the point at which all peoples of the world should have attained "a level of health that permits them to live socially and economically productive lives" (Little, 1992). Although this is unlikely to be fully achieved by the turn of the century, Dr. Erick Goon of WHO points out that all member states have made some progress toward better health promotion, disease prevention, and health care resources provision. The economic downturn of the late 1980s and early 1990s hindered greater advances.

ETHICAL AND LEGAL DEVELOPMENTS

Nurses can no longer depend on direction from physicians or hospital administrators to determine their responsibilities

BECOMING INVOLVED IN WHO

Margaret Truax, a nurse scientist for WHO, emphasizes that nurses can become involved in WHO initiatives in various ways. Interested nurses can contact 20 collaborating centers around the world (4 are located in the United States) for further information.

to clients, employers, or themselves (see Chapter 6, Legal implications for nursing practice, and Chapter 7, Ethical implications for nursing practice). They must be aware of their clients' legal and ethical rights and develop an individual plan for confronting dilemmas as they arise. Grant (1992) describes such a dilemma involving a nursing student, a Jehovah's Witness who died as the result of refusing a transfusion 3 weeks before her expected graduation from nursing school. Although the caregivers fully supported the client's right to self-determination, they needed assistance in dealing with their own feelings about being ineffectual and with their own sadness at this "preventable" death.

As questions about the right to die and the right to terminate treatments, including foods and fluids, are more frequently encountered, nurses must learn to deal with bioethical dilemmas. Working with hospital or professional committees that address these concerns and developing a personal and professional commitment to honor the rights of others as they make decisions about health care will help prepare the nurse for the eventual confrontation with difficult choices.

NURSES AS LEADERS AND MANAGERS

The function of leaders and managers in all settings is changing rapidly with the development of the professional "knowledge worker," using the term used by Drucker (1989). New planning and decision-making methods are replacing the old bureaucratic ones. Management strategies that build on new collaborative relations are known as total quality management (TQM), continuous quality improvement (CQI), and quality assessment and improvement (QAI). All stress the importance of involving employees in problem identification and decision making. Perhaps the best known of the strategies is TQM.

Developed from the work of Edward Deming (1982) and first applied in the business sector, TQM differs from the usual quality assurance (QA) approach in several fundamental ways. First, unlike QA, TQM takes a more positive approach to problems; rather than focusing on the difficulty of not meeting the identified standard or the shortcomings of the personnel involved, the TQM approach focuses on the system and changes that need to be made to improve it. According to Deming, the system rather than individuals are responsible for 94% of all errors. Also, within the TQM environment, everyone has responsibility for improving the system, not just specifically designated QA managers or evaluators.

Under the TQM approach, employees focus on serving the needs of the individual or group identified as the "customer." In health care, both external customers, such as clients, and internal customers, such as professionals in other areas, exist. For example, a nurse waiting for laboratory results is an internal customer of the laboratory. TQM provides a structured way of allowing individuals most affected by problems within the system to identify potential solutions and to form task groups to accomplish the solutions. TQM also emphasizes the importance of appropriate data collection as a means of understanding the problem and identifying workable solutions.

Deming has identified 14 principles that underlie the TQM approach. Lopresti and Whetstone (1993) have applied these principles to the health care setting:

1. *Create constancy of purpose for product and service improvement.* This principle identifies the importance of all workers at all levels to see their jobs as part of a continuous search for ways to improve functioning.

2. *Adopt the new philosophy.* This principle emphasizes the shift from focusing on performance standards to continuous striving for system improvement.

3. *Cease dependence on inspection to achieve quality.* This principle replaces inspection with process improvement.

4. *End the practice of awarding business on price alone.* This principle allows decisions to be made on long-term costs and product appropriateness; it allows managers to make decisions on more realistic bases.

5. *Constantly improve every planning, production, and service process.* This empowers workers by inviting and expecting them to contribute to the improvement process.

6. *Institute on-the-job training and retraining.* This principle emphasizes the need for employees to be encouraged, rather than forced or driven to comply; such encouragement requires intensive training and support so that employees can alter their own style from that of compliance with standards to the continuous search for improvement.

7. *Assure qualified leadership for system improvement.* This emphasizes the importance of leaders working collaboratively using the new decision-making and problem-solving approaches.

8. *Drive out fear.* Deming points out that employees must be encouraged to make suggestions regarding system functioning. Support for such behaviors must be constant and visible because in the past, employees were frequently expected to adhere to established standards rather than propose changes in the underlying system.

9. *Break down barriers among staff areas.* Each area should become aware of the needs and responsibilities of other areas. The concept of the internal customer is important here. Employees should see their responsibilities not only to clients but also to others involved in serving the client.

10. *Eliminate slogans, exhortations, and targets for the work force.* Deming emphasizes that employees react less positively to externally established standards and expectations than they do to mutually developed improvement strategies. In this regard, management must inform employees about any steps being taken to make their job performance easier.

11. *Eliminate numerical quotas both for the work force and for management.* Again, this principle focuses on establishing a continuous striving for improvement rather than on achieving specific goals that may not address underlying systemic problems. Lopresti and Whetstone emphasize "quality first, quantity will follow."

12. *Remove barriers to professional pride.* Employees should be recognized for collaborative as well as individual efforts.

13. *Institute a vigorous educational and self-improvement program for everyone.* Personal development, even in areas not job-related, results in long-term benefits for the organization. **14.** *Put everyone to work on the transformation.* Without the total involvement of all individuals, the transformation from a traditional standards-based management style to one of continuous improvement will not succeed.

One of the major breakthroughs that TQM exemplifies is the shift from competition to collaboration. An individual's contribution should not be based on position or title but on the person's contribution. To be effective, institutions must promote self-esteem, equality, and self-renewal in all workers (see *Quality Management Techniques,* page 460). Such a management system will require considerable changes in the way many health care institutions are run today.

POLITICAL CHANGES

Sharp (1993) points out that nurses need to work actively for a voice in reshaping the health care delivery system. She points out that when Medicare legislation was enacted in the 1960s, nurses had no role or voice in determining how this significant legislation developed. She suggests several ways in which nurses can actively work to make Congress aware of nursing's health care agenda. These include writing directly to the White House to communicate concerns, personally visiting legislators' offices at home or in Washington, writing position papers and statements regarding proposed legislation, and testifying before governmental bodies. Nurses can work to set up Health Advisory Committees for Congress and can offer to review pending legislation dealing with health care. Another effective way of eliciting greater understanding and political support is to invite a legislator to "walk a day in a nurse's shoes." Although spending an entire day in a health care setting may not be feasible for a legislator, visiting specific problem areas and talking with clients and health care providers may be.

QUALITY MANAGEMENT TECHNIQUES

TQM and associated management techniques such as CQI exist in many versions. Generally, they have the following common concepts:
- *Improve the system. Rather than focusing on the individual, quality management techniques stress improving the overall system in which the individual works.*
- *Abandon generalized standards. Rather than focusing on abstract performance standards, quality management seeks constantly to improve individual performance.*
- *Involve all workers. Rather than dictating to workers how their jobs should be done, quality management techniques stress that workers have the best information with which to solve problems at their level.*
- *Obtain data before acting. Rather than patching up a problem without gaining sufficient information, analyze the situation completely with input from all affected.*
- *Use ongoing training and in-service to ensure that workers and managers all see their jobs as continuously improving the system.*
- *Recognize group accomplishment. Emphasize the collaborative nature of work and achievement, rather than individual "stars."*
- *Extend quality improvement to each individual. By assisting each member of the team to develop personally, the contribution to the system as a whole can be improved.*

PROFESSIONAL NURSING ASSOCIATIONS

Current trends in professional nursing association membership suggest that an increasing number of nurses will ally themselves with specialty organizations, perhaps at the expense of belonging to the older, more generally organized associations. Two multipurpose nursing organizations, the ANA and the National League for Nursing (NLN), remain. Their roles are broad and, to some degree, overlap.

The ANA is the oldest American nursing association, dating back through several transformations and mergers to 1893. It works to:
- improve health standards and the availability of health care services for all people
- foster high standards of nursing

- stimulate and promote the professional development of nurses, and advance their economic and general welfare.

The ANA is the only U.S. nursing association with membership in the International Council of Nurses. It has been influential in advancing the purposes of nursing but recently has experienced a membership decline from a peak of 24.1% in 1970 to 12.1% (Hegyvary, 1990).

The NLN was established in 1952 after the need for a second multipurpose organization was identified at the 1950 ANA convention. Although ANA membership is limited to registered nurses, NLN membership includes both institutional and individual membership of nurses and nonnurses. The NLN seeks to strengthen and support nursing services, promote research for the knowledge base of nursing education and practice, maintain responsiveness to the nursing membership, promote public understanding and support for nursing, and explore new avenues for nursing practice in alternate health care settings. Like the ANA, the NLN's membership has declined during the past decades.

By contrast, specialty organizations such as the American Association of Critical Care Nurses have shown considerable membership growth. Other specialty groups exhibited considerable growth in the 1970s and 1980s. In 1984, an umbrella group, the National Federation of Specialty Nursing Organizations, was formed to represent the interests of nursing specialty organizations.

Other nursing groups expected to show strong member support include the American Association of Colleges of Nursing (AACN) and the AONE. The AACN exists to advance the quality of baccalaureate- and graduate-level education and has actively promoted nursing interests in the academic setting. As changes occur in nursing education, the AACN will exert important influence over how educational structures evolve. The AONE, once a component group of the American Hospital Association, has developed rapidly into an effective, independent voice for nursing administration. The organization's primary purpose is to promote safe and effective client care. The AONE also seeks to participate

NURSES WITH CONNECTIONS

Nurses can network with nurses already in health policy positions. About 400 nurses are already in such positions, and they are listed in The Nurses' Directory of Capitol Connections. The first nurse to enter the U.S. Congress, Eddie Bernice Johnson, was elected in 1992.

in the formulation of public policy dealing with health care and nursing at local, state, and national levels.

Nursing organizations are also tending to develop alliances with one another. The Tri-Council, which includes the ANA, NLN, AACN, and AONE, was formed to deal with issues that affect all nursing groups and to serve as a vehicle for voicing nursing concerns on a national level. As the nursing knowledge base continues to expand and as client care in all settings becomes increasingly complex, membership in multipurpose national and state organizations and in specialty organizations can help nurses remain current and contribute to the changes in health care delivery.

SUMMARY

As the nursing profession continues to evolve, nurses must adapt to changes. This may require a shift in the paradigm with which nurses approaches their jobs and lives. Any new professional paradigm must, however, take into account the new systems of shared governance and the emergence of the "knowledge worker," the worker who is loyal not so much to an employer as to the profession. Accompanying the professional changes are changes in nursing education and the nurse's role. Primary among the educational changes is the increased cooperation among the different levels of preparation.

Nursing research must also change to adapt to the times and must include a greater focus on health care practices and outcomes, particularly in the nonacute setting. Nurses must furthermore incorporate new knowledge and technologies into their practice. Doing so requires that nurses remain current within their field and know how to access information. Nurses must also become more aware of cultural ramifications as they relate to nursing and medicine and develop a means of dealing with ethical and legal dilemmas that will more frequently be encountered. One way to ensure that all these changes are instituted is for nurses to become politically involved on local, state, and national levels in seeing that nursing's agenda is considered by government.

Nurses can take particular care to foster innovative thinking, to support pilot projects that challenge the established way of doing things, and to use their own ingenuity to best advantage in helping to solve the health care problems of the emerging century.

APPLICATION EXERCISE

Consider your current situation and aspirations as a beginning professional nurse. Anticipate where you would like to be, professionally and personally, in the next 5 years and then in the next 10 years. To do this, you may need to think in new ways about work, education, family, and community. Rather than focusing on impediments and the status quo, try to begin from the goal itself and consider what changes you would need to make to accomplish the goals you have envisioned.

Goals in 5 years

Education. In 5 years, I would like to have achieved the following educational goals:

Profession. In 5 years, I would like to have achieved the following professional goals, related to organization membership and activity in health care promotion or civic groups:

Practice. In 5 years, I would like to have achieved the following practice goals, related to clinical skills development and achievement of work-related position:

Personal. In 5 years, I would like to have achieved the following goals related to my family, community, and culture:

Goals in 10 years

Education. In 10 years, I would like to have achieved the following educational goals:

Profession. In 10 years, I would like to have achieved the following professional goals, related to organization membership and activity in health care promotion or civic groups:

Practice. In 10 years, I would like to have achieved the following practice goals, related to clinical skills development and achievement of work-related position:

Personal. In 10 years, I would like to have achieved the following goals related to my family, community, and culture:

Beginning to explore your personal goals, however unspecific and undefined they may be, will allow you to begin to think more concretely about the future as you would have it evolve.

REVIEW QUESTIONS

1. How is nursing evolving as a profession, and in what ways does the new professional paradigm differ from the classical definition of a profession?

2. Why is cultural awareness important for nurses in all areas of practice?

3. What is TQM and how does it differ from the traditional QA approach?

4. How can nurses become more effective politically in advancing nursing's agenda for health care?

REFERENCES

Albrecht, M. "Research Priorities for Home Health Nursing," *Nursing and Health Care* 12(10):538-540, December 1992.

Borland, K., et al. "Collaborating to Develop a Student Intern Program," *Nursing Management* 22(10):56-59, October 1991.

Butts, B.J., and Witmer, D.M. "New Graduates: What Does My Manager Expect?" *Nursing Management* 23(8):46-48, August 1992.

Deming, E.W. *Out of the Crisis.* Cambridge, Mass.: MIT Press, 1982.

Drucker, P.F. "How Schools Must Change," *Psychology Today* 18-20, May 1989.

Hegyvary, S.T. "A Guide to Nursing Organizations," in *Current Issues in Nursing.* Edited by McCloskey, J.E., and Grace, H.K. St. Louis: C.V. Mosby Co., 1990.

Huey, J. "Nothing Is Impossible," *Fortune*, 135-139, September 23, 1991.

Kudzma, E.C. "Drug Response: All Bodies Are Not Created Equal," *American Journal of Nursing* 92(12):48-50, December 1992.

Kupper-Grubbs, E. "When a Transplant Complicates Your Care," *RN* 55(12):24-32, December 1992.

Larson, J. "The Healing Web," *Nursing and Health Care* 13(5):246-252, May 1992.

Laschinger, S.K.H., and McWilliam, C.L. "Health Care in Canada," *Nursing and Health Care* 134:204-207, April 1992.

Little, C. "Health for All by the Year 2000," *Nursing and Health Care*, 13(4):198-203, April 1992.

Lopresti, J., and Whetstone, W.R. "Total Quality Management: Doing Things Right," *Nursing Management* 24(1):34-36, January 1993.

McCloskey, J.E., and Grace, J.K. *Current Issues in Nursing.* St. Louis: C.V. Mosby Co., 1990.

Sharp, N. "Getting Ready for the New Tomorrow," *Nursing Management* 24(1):28-32, January 1993.

Shein, E.H., and Kommers, D.W. *Professional Education.* New York: McGraw-Hill Book Co., 1972.

RECOMMENDATIONS FOR FURTHER STUDY

Barker, A.M. *Transformational Nursing Leadership: A Vision for the Future.* New York: National League for Nursing Press, Pub. No. 15-2473, 1992.

Dixon, I.L. "Continuous Quality Improvement in Shared Leadership," *Nursing Management* 24(1):40-45, January 1993.

Erickson, M.E. "General and Liberal Education: Competing Paradigms," *Community College Review* 19:15-20, 1992.

Levine-Ariff, J., and Groh, D.H. *Creating an Ethical Environment.* Nurse Managers' Bookshelf; Vol. 2, No.1 Baltimore: Williams & Wilkins, 1990.

Ventura, M.R., et al. "Quality Indicators: Control Maintains—Propriety Improves," *Nursing Management* 24(1):46-49, January 1993.

INDEX

A

Abdellah, Faye, 53
Abortion, 218
Accreditation, 198-199
Acquired immunodeficiency syndrome (AIDS), 129-134, 250-253
Adaptation model (Roy), 62-64
Adkins, Janet, 245
Adult ego state, 7-8
Advance directives, 215-216, 248-249
Agir, Terry, 401
Alcohol abuse, 128-129
American Nurses Association, 460
    Code for Nurses, 226-227
    Standards of Clinical Practice, 261
Angelo, Richard, 247
Apache culture, 156
Arbitration, binding, 396
Assault, 206-207
Autocratic management, 300-301
Autonomy, 233
Autopsy, 218-219

B

Barnard, Chester, 88
Battery, 206-207
Behavioral learning theory, 263-264
Behavioral objectives, 275
Beneficence, 232
Bentham, Jeremy, 234
Berne, Eric, 6-8
Bertalanffy, Ludwig von, 94
Betts, Virginia Trotter, 402
Biological variation, 178-179
Body motions, 22-23
Brainstorming, 338-339
Bureaucracy, 81-86
Burns, 202-203

C

Carnegie approach (organizational structure), 88-89
Certification, 197-198

Change
    agent of, 366-370
    clients and, 372-375
    employees and, 370-372
    natural disasters and, 375-377
    stress and, 351-352
    theories of, 352-366
    types of, 349-351
Charismatic theory, 295
Child ego state, 8-10
Chinese medicine, 177
Chiropractic, 176
Client rights, 192-195
Clinton, William, 141-142, 218, 401
Cognitive learning, 264-265
Collective bargaining, 389-399
Collins, Virginia, 403
Communication
    assertive, 33-38
    definition of, 2
    difficult, 31-38
    hindrances to, 16-19
    models of, 3-10
    nonverbal, 3, 22-28
    therapeutic, 29-31
    verbal, 3, 10-19
    written, 20-21
Community health education, 287
Concepts, 45-48
Conceptual models, 48-49
Confidentiality, 208, 250-253
Confrontation, communication and, 33-35
Contingency approach (organizational structure), 92-94
Contingency theory, 296-298
Contracts, 199-201, 394-399
Credentialing, 195-201
Critical path methodology, 341-342
Critical path plans, 21
Cruzan, Nancy, 214-215
Cultural assessment, 179-181
Cultural barriers, 157-159
Cultural orientation, 162-173

Culture
    client diversity in, 159-162, 237
    demographic changes and, 151-152
    health and, 153-157, 454-455

D

Death certification, 218-219
Decertification (collective bargaining), 399
Decision making, 322-347, 400-401
Delegation, 312-314
Delphi technique, 339-340
Democratic management, 301-302
Deontological theory, 235
Depositions, 211
Dewey, John, 229
Diagnosis-related groups (DRGs), 120
Discrimination, 159
DNR orders, 216
Drug abuse, 128-129
Duty, ethics and, 232

E

Education, nursing, 446-451
Ego states, 7-10
Elderly clients, 127-128
Elopement, 206
Empirical-rational model, 358-360
Entropy, 95
Environment
    communication and, 25-26
    concept of, 47-48
Equipment defects, 205
Ethics
    acquired immunodeficiency and, 250-253
    advance directives and, 248-249
    confidentiality and, 250-253
    euthanasia and, 244-247
    health care policy and, 238-240
    morality and, 228-230
    pain and, 243-244
    principles and, 232-234
    rights and, 227-228
    substance abuse and, 249-250
    technology and, 236-237
    theories of, 234-236
    values and, 231
    withholding nutrition and, 240-242

Ethnocentrism, 158
Ethnography, 431-432
Euthanasia, 214, 244-247

F

Facial expressions, communication and, 23
Fact finding, 396
Faith healing, 177-178
Falls, 203
Families
    teaching plan for, 286
    types of, 165-168
Fayol, Henri, 80-81
Feedback, 95
Fidelity, 233-234
Fiedler, Fred, 296
Follett, Mary Parker, 87
Follower, types of, 306-309
Foreign objects, 203
Fraud, 207

G

Gantt, Henry, 80
Gaze, communication and, 24
Gilbreth, Frank, 80
Goldwater, Marilyn, 402
Graduates as followers, 311
Great man theories, 294-295
Groups
    developmental stages of, 103-104
    formal and informal, 101-102
    formation of, 99-101
    nominal, 340-341
    open and closed, 102
    primary and reference, 98-99
    religious, 168-173
    teaching, 284-286

H

Hahnemann, Samuel, 174
Hawthorne effect, 87
Health
    concept of, 47
    culture and, 153-157

Health care
    costs of, 134-137
    problems associated with, 126-134
    providers of, 124-125
    reform of, 137-143, 238-240
    restructure of, 108-110
    settings of, 125-126
    types of, 116-124
Health maintenance organizations (HMOs), 121
Helicy, 61
Henderson, Virginia, 53
Hierarchy of needs communication model, 4-6
Home care, nursing liability and, 221
Homeopathy, 174-175
Human caring model (Watson), 64-67
Humanistic learning, 265
Human relations (organizational structure), 86-88

I

Informed consent, 217
Integrality, 61
Interaction theories, 54-55

J

Jarvis, Judy, 403
Johnson, Dorothy, 55
Johnson, Eddie Bernice, 403
Judicial process, 209-210
Justice, 233

K

Kevorkian, Jack, 245
Kinesics, 22-23
King, Imogene, 54-55
Knapp, Cheryl Davis, 403
Knowledge, patterns of, 329

L

Laissez-faire management, 302
Law, types of, 189-192
Leadership
    evolution of, 316-318
    theories of, 294-299

Learning
    barriers, 267
    domains, 262
    styles, 326-331
Leininger, Madeline, 431
Levine, Myra, 56
Lewin, Kurt, 264, 352
Liability, 209, 219-221
Libel, 207-208
Licensure, 196-197
Living wills, 213-215
Lust, Benedict, 176

M

Magnet hospitals, 104-105
Malpractice, 201-202, 221-222
Management
    Fayol's rules of, 81
    styles of, 299-305
March, James, 88
Maslow, Abraham, 4-6
McGregor, Douglas, 90
Mediation, 396
Medicare and Medicaid, 122-123
Medication errors, 204
Military services, 123-124
Mill, John Stuart, 234
Misconduct, scientific, 433-434
Mistaken identity, 204
Modern systems approach (organizational structure), 94-98
Moral development, 229-230
Multicratic management, 303

N

National Labor Relations Act, 389
National League for Nursing, 460
Naturopathy, 176
Needs, human, 4-6
Negligence, 201-202
Nightingale, Florence, 48, 51-52, 291, 402, 421
Nominal groups, 340-341
Nonmaleficence, 232-233
Normative-reeducative model (Lewin), 352-358
Nurse practice acts, 191, 196-197
Nursing centers, 106
Nursing outcomes, 55-56

Nursing process, 43-44
Nursing rights, 192-195
Nursing theory
  contemporary, 56-67
  evaluation of, 67-68
  evolution of, 51
  interaction and, 54-55
  levels of, 50-51
  needs and, 53-54
  nursing outcomes and, 55-56
  research and, 68-69
  types of, 49-50

O

Open system, 47-48, 94
Operant conditioning, 263
Orem, Dorothea, 56-60
Organ donation, 218-219
Organizations
  Carnegie approach to, 88-89
  centralization of, 76-77
  classical theory and, 79-86
  contingency approach to, 92-94
  complexity of, 76
  formalization of, 77-79
  groups and, 98-104
  human relations and, 86-88
  modern systems approach to, 94-98
  Theory Y approach to, 90-92
Orlando, Ida Jean, 54
Osteopathy, 175

P

Pain relief, 243-244
Palmer, David Daniel, 176
Paradigm shifts, 444-446
Paradoxical model, 360-362
Paralinguistics, 26-27
Parent ego state, 7
Path-goal theory, 298
Patient Self-Determination Act, 215
Pavlov, Ivan, 263
Peer review organizations (PROs), 120
Peplau, Hildegard, 52-53
Phenomenology, 430-431
Philosophy, nursing and, 44
Piaget, Jean, 229, 264

Pluralism, 235
Politics, nursing and, 401-406
Power
  economic, 388-401
  expert, 387
  nursing practice and, 384-386
  physical, 386-387
  political, 401-406
  position, 387-388
  referent, 406-408
Power-coercive model, 362-366
Prejudice, 159
Privacy, invasion of, 208
Probability, 418
Problem solving, 331-337
Property loss or damage (client's), 205
Proxemics, 24

Q

Quality assurance, 220
Quinlan, Karen Ann, 214

R

Randomization, 417
Reddin's 3D theory of leadership, 304
Registration, 196-197
Religion, health care and, 168-173
Research
  designs used in, 427-432
  development of, 421-425
  divisions of, 412-415
  errors in, 436
  ethical and legal issues in, 432-434
  home care and, 451
  nursing responsibilities in, 434-440
  purposes of, 419-420
  scientific method and, 425-427
  terminology of, 415-419
Resonancy, 61
Rights, 192-195, 227-228
Risk management, 220
Rogers, Carl, 29, 31
Rogers, Martha, 60-62
Roy, Sister Callista, 62-64

S

Scanlon, Joseph, 90-91
Self-care model (Orem), 56-60
Sender-receiver communication model, 3-4
Shared governance, 315, 400-401
Simon, Herbert, 88
Situational theory, 296
Skinner, B.F., 263
Slander, 207-208
Steady state, 95
Stereotyping, 158
Still, Andrew, 175
Substance abuse, 249-250
Synectics, 340-341
Systems theory, 94

T

Taft-Hartley Act, 390
Taylor, Frederick, 80
Teaching plan, 275-282
Technology, nursing and, 93, 107-108, 135, 236-237
Teleological theory, 234
Theory Y approach (organizational structure), 90-92
Therapeutic relationships, 29-31
Thinking, critical, 324-326
Total quality management, 456-457
Touching, communication and, 27-28
Trait theories, 295-296
Transactional analysis communication model, 6-10

U

Uniform Anatomical Gift Act, 218
Unitary man model (Rogers), 60-62

V

Values, ethics and, 231
Validity, 418
Variable, 417, 435-437

W-Z

Wagner Act, 389
Watson, Jean, 64-67
Watson, John B., 263
Weber, Max, 81
Withholding nutrition, 240-242
Witness (material and expert), 211-213
Woodward, Joan, 92-93
Work stoppage, 396-397
World Health Organization, 455